HIV and AIDS: Selected Topics

HIV and AIDS: Selected Topics

Edited by **Roger Mostafa**

hayle medical

New York

Published by Hayle Medical,
30 West, 37th Street, Suite 612,
New York, NY 10018, USA
www.haylemedical.com

HIV and AIDS: Selected Topics
Edited by Roger Mostafa

International Standard Book Number: 978-1-63241-253-9 (Hardback)

Printed in the United States of America.

Contents

Preface

This book brings forth some important selected topics in HIV and AIDS. The ongoing AIDS pandemic reminds us that in spite of the ceaseless quest for knowledge and information since the early 1980s, we have a lot to learn and comprehend about AIDS and HIV. This syndrome represents one of the biggest challenges for humanity, science and medicine. The aim of this book is to provide a source of encouragement for researchers and serve as an efficient guide for graduate students in their ongoing search for a cure of HIV, and aid clinicians. Therefore, this book provides both basic as well as advanced clinical knowledge regarding HIV/AIDS transmission, diagnosis and treatment.

This book has been the outcome of endless efforts put in by authors and researchers on various issues and topics within the field. The book is a comprehensive collection of significant researches that are addressed in a variety of chapters. It will surely enhance the knowledge of the field among readers across the globe.

It is indeed an immense pleasure to thank our researchers and authors for their efforts to submit their piece of writing before the deadlines. Finally in the end, I would like to thank my family and colleagues who have been a great source of inspiration and support.

Editor

Part 1

From the Clinic to the Patients: HIV and Clinical Manifestations

Pathology of HIV/AIDS:
Lessons from Autopsy Series

Andrey Bychkov[1,2], Shunichi Yamashita[1] and Alexander Dorosevich[2]
[1]Nagasaki University Graduate School of Biomedical Sciences
[2]Smolensk Regional Institute of Pathology
[1]Japan
[2]Russia

1. Introduction

HIV infection is a global disease and despite considerable efforts of the international community it is a main cause of human mortality (UNAIDS, 2009). Morphological insights into HIV/AIDS are based on the study of clinical cases by means of biopsy and autopsy. Morphological changes during development of HIV infection and, especially, through AIDS progression are variable and specified mainly by characteristics of widespread secondary infections and tumors. Opportunistic infections account for approximately 80% of deaths in patients with AIDS and their spectrum is constantly changing, as a result of improvements in treatment options and prophylaxis along with the increasing life span of HIV-infected individuals. Postmortem examinations provide important diagnostic and epidemiological data and represent a most reliable source for estimation of the full spectrum of diseases in individual patients and the general population.

2. Pathomorphology of HIV/AIDS

Morphology of HIV/AIDS is manifested by wide range of indicative (secondary) diseases while specific changes caused by HIV are mainly detected in immune system at the early stages of infection and in central nervous system.

Lymphadenopathy is the marked feature of acute HIV infection defined as generalized enlargement of lymph nodes. Histologically, this process passes through a series of changes: hyperplasia, involution, depletion, and sclerosis (Baroni & Uccini, 1993). In the stage of hyperplasia, the lymph nodes are characterized by disorderly grouped multiple follicles with 'starry sky' pattern due to arrangement of macrophages. Formation of multinuclear cells resembling symplasts is result of merging of lymphocytes infected by virus. With the progression of disease, lymphoid depletion becomes extensive and a fibrovascular carcass appears more evident along with increasing vascularity (angiomatosis). Finally, lymph nodes harbor 'burnt-out' appearance. Although profound depletion of lymphoid tissues is driven by cytotoxic effect of HIV but there is no histologic picture diagnostic of this condition (O'Murchadha et al., 1987).

Large proportion of patients at different stages of disease has morphological proofs of HIV-induced brain damage (Kibayashi et al., 1996). HIV neuropathology is comprised of following patterns (in order of appearance): lymphocyte infiltration of the leptomeninges, microglial nodules formation and HIV encephalitis. The latter lesion consists of numerous foci with mononuclear cells typical of small macrophages, microglia, and multinucleated giant cells. The giant cells are the hallmark of HIV infection since viral antigens can be detected in their cytoplasm (Gyorkey et al., 1987).

Development of indicative diseases which include opportunistic infections and secondary neoplasms which reflects severe deficiency of immune system and in most of cases determines progression of the disease to full-blown AIDS. Morphological descriptions given below represent our common findings of infectious and neoplastic diseases in AIDS.

2.1 Morphology of mycobacterial Infections in HIV patients

Tuberculosis in HIV-patients is characterized by a prevalence of its generalized form with extensive dissemination and acute progression of specific processes. Notable histological features are loss of granuloma formation and abundance of necrotic changes. Generally, all the forms of tuberculosis seen in the terminal stages are actively progressive. The main forms of tuberculosis are generalized, pulmonary (often disseminated) and extrapulmonary. Thus, various organs are affected, most often the lungs, lymph nodes, liver, kidneys, spleen, intestine, and central nervous system (Smith et al., 2000). Tissue reaction in the terminal stage shows typical tuberculous granulomas with giant and epithelioid cells in only 20% of lesions, whereas the remaining 80% demonstrates numerous foci of nonreactive caseous necrosis abundant of acid-fast bacilli (Parkhomenko et al., 2003).

Pulmonary tuberculosis is manifested as a bilateral disseminated type or polycavernous variant. In disseminated tuberculosis, foci of specific lesions (granulomas) comprise large central zones of caseous necrosis surrounded by a few inflammatory cells. Giant cells are uncommon. Ziehl-Neelsen staining shows numerous acid-fast bacteria in the foci of caseous necrosis. All these histological signs characterize tuberculosis as progressive and highly active. Macroscopic study of the lungs often reveals miliary disseminated tuberculosis, while macrofocal dissemination and caseous pneumonia are rare. The pattern of dissemination is bilateral, with a predominance of micronodular, miliary and submiliary types. Tubercles evenly spread to the whole organ or localized to one of the lobes. In a large proportion of cases, macroscopic detection of tuberculous changes in lungs is difficult, but histological examination reveals miliary and submiliary necrotic foci (Berdnikov et al., 2011). The characteristic microscopic picture is a predominance of alterative and exudative changes with the lack of a productive component of inflammation or its minimal manifestation (Fig. 1a). The latter is marked by the absence of signs of encapsulation and organization of inflammatory foci. Classic granulomas are infrequent and only few of them contain giant cells of Langhans (Fig. 1b). Initially, there is formation of colonies of *Mycobacteria* in the pulmonary parenchyma, which is accompanied by cellular infiltration with a significant predominance of polymorphonuclear leucocytes. The cells phagocytose the bacteria and this step is marked by karyorrhexis. Later, this process is associated with massive breakdown of leucocytes resulting in necrosis and microabscesses. Tissue sections stained by Ziehl–Neelsen showed numerous acid-fast bacteria in the foci of caseous necrosis. An exudative reaction in the form of serous-fibrinous pneumonia or fibrinous-purulent pneumonia with predominance of neutrophilic leucocytes is detected at the periphery of caseous foci. Such exudation may extent from lobular up to sub-lobar area. Some alveoli contain accumulations of foamy macrophages that are characteristic for typical tuberculous inflammation. There is an increase in the thickness of the pleura caused by extensive hyperemia and edema. The intrathoracic lymph nodes are also affected, enlarged (3–4 cm in diameter), and aggregated. Partial or total caseous lymphadenitis is detected with the spread of inflammatory processes to the surrounding soft tissues. Evident reduction of follicular structures and lymphoid depletion is a characteristic feature of these lymph nodes.

Extrapulmonary tuberculosis is detected as a component of a generalized type of tuberculosis. Monomorphic miliary foci of caseous necrosis are found in various internal organs, more often in the spleen, kidneys, liver, and rarely in the meninges, peritoneum, exo- and endocrine glands (pancreas, adrenals, prostate, thyroid, ovaries). As a whole, in cases of generalized tuberculosis, *Mycobacteria* cause alterative and exudative reactions simultaneously in several organs with the mean number of organs involved is 5.4 (own data). Most of the foci are suspected to be spread via hematogenous dissemination from lungs. Histopathology of the parenchymatous organs reveals monomorphic miliary nodules of caseous necrosis with rare giant cells, as in the lungs. In many cases, tubercles are not visible by visual inspection. In the spleen, the foci of caseous necrosis have a tendency to fuse and may cover up to 50% of the cut surface.

Tuberculous meningitis is characterized grossly by typical basilar localization with poorly detected gray-white exudates and tubercles in the subarachnoid space. Microscopic examination of the meninges reveals evident hyperemia and edema accompanied by alterative reactions. The latter is manifested as areas of caseous necrosis extensively infiltrated by polymorphs, lymphocytes, and macrophages. Various types of vasculitis such as endovasculitis, panvasculitis, thrombovasculitis, and perivasculitis are evident. Perivasculitis is more often present with edema and excessive mononuclear, neutrophilic, eosinophilic, and plasma cell infiltration in all layers of the vessel wall (Fig. 1c). Destructive process may extent into brain tissue with formation of localized abscesses.

Mycobacterium avium-intracellulare (MAI) infection leads to massive necrotic destruction of lymph nodes with minor involvement of the lungs. Mostly granulomas are difficult to detect throughout the inner organs by naked eye. The only exception is spleen which is filled with miliary granulomas in roughly half of cases. Different groups of visceral lymph nodes are enlarged and show characteristic yellow tone of cut surface. Microscopically, proliferation of large round to elliptical striated pale blue macrophages is noted. Cytoplasm of these cells is packed with huge number of acid-fast bacilli. Well-formed granulomas with fibrosis, necrosis, and epithelioid histiocytes are present in less than one third of cases (Klatt et al., 1987).

2.2 Morphology of bacterial infections

Bacterial Pneumonia

There is a broad spectrum of causative agents of pneumonia revealed by microbiology. Besides typical microflora, bacterial pneumonia can be caused by opportunistic agents, which are activated under immunodeficiency. The most common causative agents of pneumonia are *Staphylococcus aureus*, *Pseudomonas aeruginosa*, *Klebsiella pneumoniae*, *Streptococcus pneumoniae*, *Haemophilus influenzae* and *Escherichia coli* (Afessa et al., 1998).

Hematoxylin and eosin together with Gram staining of sections of lungs helps in revealing nonspecific microflora. At autopsy, staining of smears of lung sections using Romanovskii–Giemsa and Gram stains is also useful in establishing the nonspecific character of microflora in cases of bacterial pneumonia. Bacteriological culture of lung tissue helps in revealing the nature of the causative agents of pneumonia most accurately. Grossly, patchy areas of red or grey consolidation involve more often the lower zones of the lungs. On cut surface, these patchy consolidated lesions are dry, granular, firm, red or grey in color, slightly elevated over the surface and are often located around a bronchiole. Histologically, suppurative exudate, consisting of neutrophils with admixture of fibrin, fills alveoli and alveolar septa are dilated by congested capillaries and leucocytic infiltration. Often, the course of pneumonia in HIV-infected patients has a tendency to form microabscesses, and in such cases, the microscopic changes resembles to microfocal dissemination in pulmonary tuberculosis. In microabscesses, purulent necrotic foci are found with expressed perifocal exudative reaction, which strengthened their resemblance to pulmonary tuberculosis in HIV-infected patients.

Sepsis

Pneumonia and primary bloodstream infections are the main sites of infections for almost all patients with sepsis, followed by angiogenic-related bacteremia originated from thrombophlebitis in intravenous drug users or from venous catheter in bedridden patients and urinary tract infections. Nosocomial infections compose the major part of etiology of severe sepsis. Microbiology of infections is comprised of different species, mostly *Pseudomonas aeruginosa*, *Klebsiella pneumoniae* and *Staphylococcus spp.*, while *Streptococcus spp.*, *Escherichia coli* and *Salmonella spp.* are detected with lower frequency (Japiassú et al., 2010). Microorganisms impact small vessels in the primary site and cause local injury both by obstructing the vessels and by releasing toxins. Subsequently a combination of necrosis, hemorrhage and suppuration occurs, with further formation of pyemic abscesses in the various organs and their distribution depends on the site of the original septic thrombosis. Microscopically, pyemic abscesses are typically surrounded by a zone of hemorrhage and an early lesion may show a central zone of necrosis often containing huge numbers of bacteria. This is surrounded by a zone of suppuration and an outermost zone of acutely inflamed and often hemorrhagic tissue. In septic thrombosis of major veins, larger fragments may be released into the circulation, and by impacting in arteries give rise to correspondingly larger foci of necrosis and suppuration (septic infarcts). In case if it involves heart, pyogenic bacteria may produce endocarditis and severely damage cardiac valves. The vegetations on valve are tend to break down and the valve cusps are largely covered by crumbling masses, which consist of layers of fibrin containing clumps of bacteria enclosed by a zone of leukocytes, macrophages and granulation tissue. The substance of the cusps may be extensively destroyed by suppuration.

2.3 Invasive fungal infections

Pneumocystis jirovecii (former *Pneumocystis carinii*) typically produces pneumonia that is widespread throughout the lungs with a chronic course of disease and rapid progression. Pulmonary pneumocystosis is a disease caused by intense multiplication of relatively pathogenic single-celled saprophyte *Pneumocystis jirovecii* in the human respiratory tract.

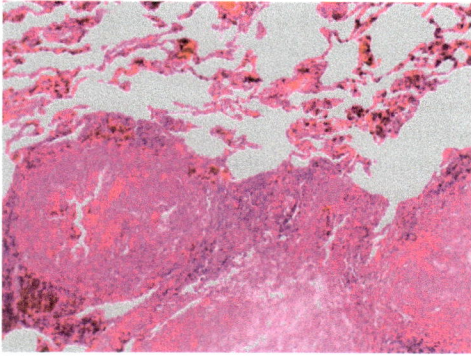

(a) Pulmonary tuberculosis,
foci of caseous necrosis. H&E, × 100

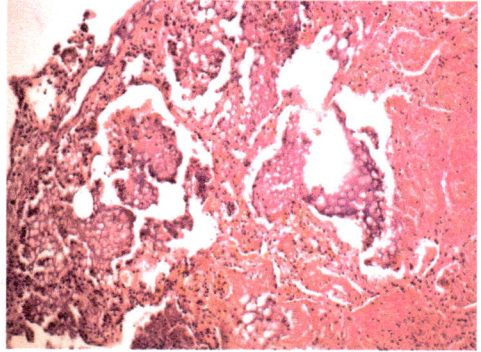

(d) Pneumocystic pneumonia,
foamy exudate. H&E, × 100

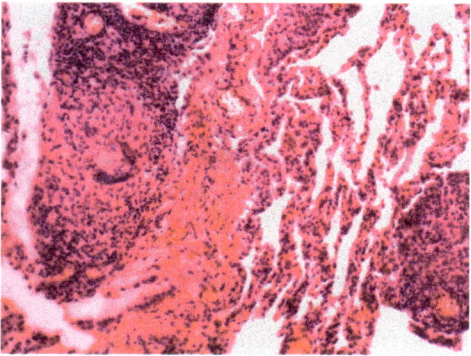

(b) Pulmonary tuberculosis,
granuloma with giant cell. H&E, × 140

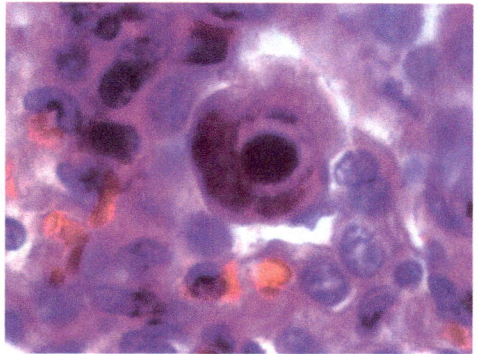

(e) Cytomegalovirus infection of lung,
cell with 'owl-eye' appearance. H&E, × 1200

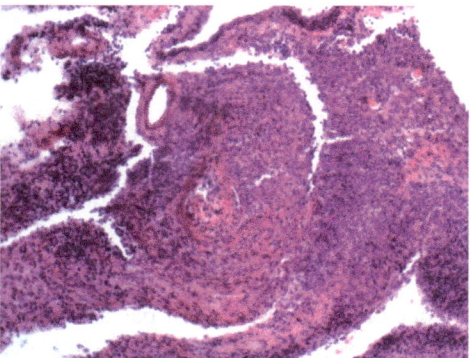

(c) Tuberculous meningitis,
panvasculitis with alteration. H&E, × 140

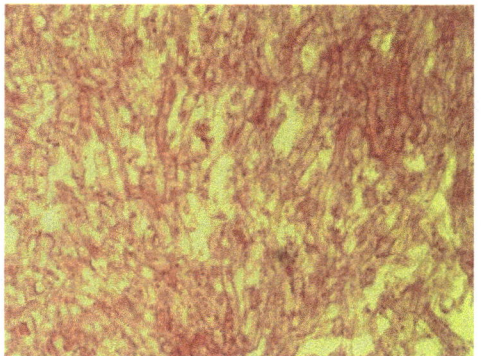

(f) Pulmonary aspergillosis,
branching hyphae of fungus. PAS, × 600

Fig. 1. Microscopic patterns of opportunistic infections in AIDS

The terminal period of pneumocystosis is pneumonia, manifested in the later stages of HIV infection, which often leads to death. The gross appearance resembles to pneumonic consolidation. The cut surface of the lung is pale pink with scattered areas of congestion and rarely hemorrhages. Microscopically, in the edematous stage, characteristic homogenous, foamy protein-containing eosinophilic exudate is found in the alveolar lumen (Fig. 1d). This is a pathognomonic sign of pneumocystic pneumonia. Neutrophils, macrophages and plasma cells are detected around the collections of *Pneumocystis jirovecii*.

Cryptococcus neoformans in immunocompromised hosts may spread from lungs, which is the site of primary infection, to distant organs anh most frequently affecting the central nervous system and causes meningitis. Pulmonary manifestations exhibit pneumonitis, pulmonary nodules or less commonly pleural effusions. Sometimes variably sized pale soft granulomas are grossly visible in the lungs. If fungi with capsules are numerous, a grossly apparent mucoid exudate may be seen in the cerebral ventricles or on the meninges. Microscopically, the yeast cells appear pale blue and ovoid while the capsule is round and clear. Inflammatory reaction is weak and represented by a few scattered lymphocytes or macrophages with phagocytized organisms. PAS stain is effective for detection of the capsule and nucleus of the organisms.

Candida albicans infection is one of the most prevalent in patients with AIDS, ranging from localized skin and mucosa lesions to widely disseminated disease. Characteristic gross findings of candidiasis are prominent in the pharynx, larynx, and trachea with invasion into principle bronchi, which includes a pseudomembranous form with white, elevated mucosal plaques. Bronchopulmonary aspergillosis and candidiasis are characterized by the collection of fungal mycelia in the lumen of small bronchi and invasion of fungus into the acini. *Candida* microabscesses are common and they had a typical polymorphonuclear leucocytes infiltration. Histologically, *Candida* organisms could be identified by their size, budding property, and pseudohyphae. The pseudohyphae could be distinguished from *Aspergillus* hyphae by the lack of branching, the smaller size, and frequent absence of true septations in the former. Histological diagnosis may be confirmed using the Romanovskii staining technique, which is helpful in differentiation between *Candida* and *Aspergillus*. Bronchopulmonary aspergillosis is characterized by the collection of branching mycelia of *Aspergillus* in the bronchial lumen with involvement of the bronchial wall and further invasion of the fungus into the acini (Fig. 1f).

2.4 Viral and parasitic infections

Cytomegalovirus (CMV) *infection* is one the most prevalent secondary diseases in AIDS. It is featured by multiple organs involvement, including lungs, digestive system, brain and eyes. CMV infection proceeds diversely from latent infection to severe acute generalization in the later stages of HIV infection. Microscopically, CMV lesions appear as characteristic metamorphosis of alveolar and bronchial epithelium (Fig. 1e). The persistence of viruses in the epithelial cells leads to cytomegalic giant cell formation. Alveolar cells increase in size up to 25–40 μm. About 1–2 nuclear inclusions are detected containing viral particles in the chromatin in each cell and there is a thin perinuclear clear halo. The nucleus of each affected cell is usually eccentrically positioned and the cell border is not prominent. Additionally, the cytoplasm of affected cells may contain coarse dark basophilic bodies. Characteristic infiltrative changes and CMV transformations are numerous. Moderate cytomegalic transformation of alveolar and bronchial epithelial cells (2–3 typical cells in the form of an 'owl-eye' in the field of view) is accompanied with focal accumulations of serous fluid and protein masses in the alveolar cavities along with admixtures of macrophages and weak infiltration of interstitial tissue. If the lung changes consist of diffuse persisting alveolitis with CMV transformation (up to 20 cells per field of view), then this process is accompanied by extensive fibrosis, but uncommonly leads to the formation of a 'honeycomb-like' appearance of the lungs. The outcome of CMV infection of the lungs is peribronchial and widespread interstitial fibrosis with thickening and vast deformation of the interalveolar septa. Thus, heterogeneous patterns of CMV infection of the lung represent continuous progression of disease and include the following events as virus-induced transformation of the cells, pneumonias with cavity formation, productive granulomatous alveolitis and eventually pulmonary fibrosis (Parkhomenko et al., 2004).

Toxoplasma gondii is a protozoan parasite which is highly prevalent among humans and animals throughout the world. Immunocompromised patients are especially prone to develop disseminated toxoplasmosis, either from acute exposure to the organisms or from reactivation of latent infection. Multiple organ systems are often involved, including the CNS, heart, lungs and skeletal muscle. Damage to the CNS by *Toxoplasma gondii* is characterized by numerous foci of enlarging necrosis and microglia nodules. The former are often resolved with cyst formation or calcification. Presence of many brain abscesses with almost universal involvement of the cerebral hemispheres is the most characteristic feature of toxoplasmic encephalitis in AIDS patients. The diagnosis of toxoplasmosis is readily made from histologic analysis of tissue specimens by observing any of the three infectious stages of *T. gondii*: tachyzoites in groups, bradyzoites (parasitic tissue cysts) or sporozoites within oocysts. Tachyzoites and cysts are seen in and adjacent to necrotic foci near or in glial nodules, perivascular regions, and even in uninvolved cerebral tissue. Reactive inflammatory reaction is comprised of mixed infiltrate distributed in patchy pattern.

2.5 HIV-associated neoplasia

Kaposi's sarcoma is a low-grade mesenchymal tumor which arises initially as an angioproliferative disorder caused by *Kaposi's sarcoma-associated herpes virus* (Du et al., 2007). Skin involvement is common and manifested by the presence of red to red-purple lesions ranging from flat patches to slightly raised plaques and nodules. Visceral involvement frequently includes the lung, lymph nodes, and gastrointestinal tract. Microscopically, Kaposi's sarcoma features clusters of tiny apparent capillaries budding off normal blood vessels. It grows as massed bundles of spindle cells, with red blood cells in slits between them. Hemosiderin pigmentation and hyaline globules usually accompany the spindle cell proliferation. Tumor has an ability to infiltrate around large vascular structures, near epithelial or mesothelial surfaces, or near the capsules of organs.

Non-Hodgkin lymphomas (NHL) risk in AIDS patients is increased more than 70 times comparing with general population (Frisch et al., 2001). Malignant non-Hodgkin's lymphomas (mostly intermediate- to high-grade tumors) exhibit two major patterns which include systemic and CNS lymphomas. These lymphomas often show evidence of *Epstein-Barr virus* as etiologic agent (Fassone et al., 2002). AIDS-related lymphomas consistently determine a B-cell phenotype and are histogenetically related to germinal center or postgerminal center B-cells in the vast majority of cases. About 80% of NHL's in AIDS arise systemically, either nodally or extranodally, while 20% arise in the central nervous system. Almost any extranodal site can be involved with predominance of bone marrow, gastrointestinal tract and liver. NHLs appear as small infiltrates, focal nodular lesions, or larger tumor masses with accompanying necrosis and hemorrhage. Microscopically, tumors generally referred to diffuse large B-cell lymphomas or high-grade B-cell (small non-cleaved) Burkitt-like lymphomas, according to REAL classification. Immunohistochemistry is a routine diagnostic tool in typing of these lesions.

3. Autopsy series

AIDS was recognized in 1981 for the first time, resulting in the deaths of more than 25 million people. Since the late 1990s approximately 2 million HIV-infected persons are reported to have died annually (UNAIDS, 2009). Distribution of the regions with the highest death tolls is determined by the prevalence of HIV infection. Countries of Sub-Saharan Africa are the worst-affected, followed by South and South-East Asia. Most countries with high rates of AIDS prevalence have published reports on autopsy series to date (Fig. 2). Currently, there is a global decline of autopsy rates as a consequence of improved patient management, introduction of etiologic therapy and preventive measures. However such advances are available only in developed countries, where postmortem examination has lost the status of routine diagnostic procedure. Concurrently only few recent reports from Sub-Saharan Africa are available while the pace of HIV epidemics is still very high. Moreover, some countries with high AIDS burden (more than 500,000 infected) including Thailand, China and Ukraine are yet to present large autopsy series.

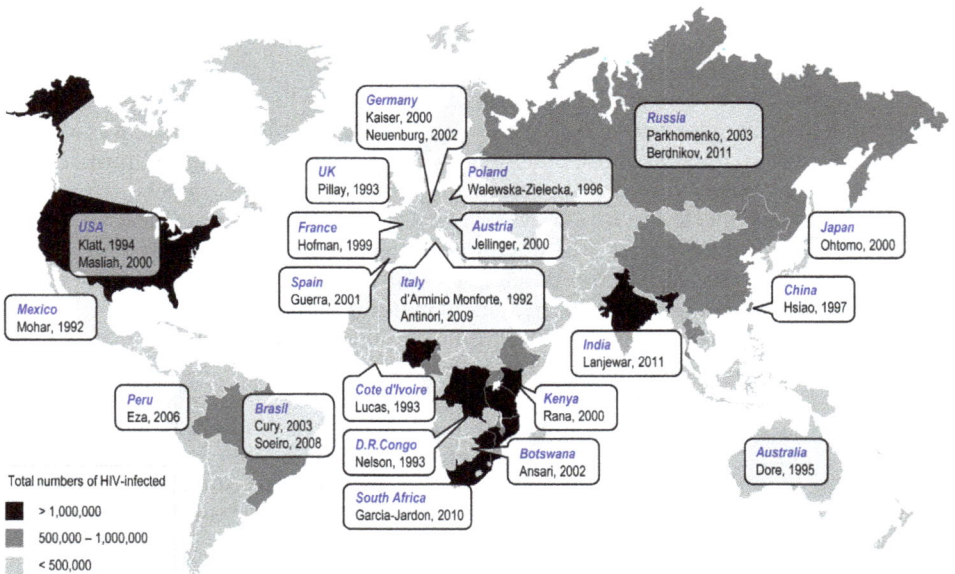

Fig. 2. Worldwide representative autopsy series

3.1 Value of autopsy

Since the first years of HIV/AIDS pathology has contributed significantly to study of new disease. Before mid-1990s various changes of organs and systems studied with different pathological techniques were described in numerous publications. The data taken from the study of autopsy series have shown that postmortem examination is extremely valuable for determining wide range of AIDS-related diseases. Diagnostic role of the autopsy is enhanced considerably by employment of histological examination of the organs. Such specimens can be further proceeded to staining with special techniques useful in detection of microorganisms or immunohistochemistry and even to molecular biological techniques. Thus, complete postmortem study allows determining the cause of death and contributed pathologies, it may identify diseases and etiological agents that were clinically unsuspected or undiagnosed. By providing these types of data, the autopsy serves as an important measure in monitoring the quality of care, basically comparing antemortem with postmortem findings. Autopsy remains established tool for obtaining epidemiological information about diseases and producing vital statistics, since systematic postmortem examination provides representative data on the main pathologies in distinct communities and permits evaluation of changes that may occur over time (Lanjewar, 2011; Lyon et al., 1996). Postmortem surveillance is vital for monitoring the course of HIV-infection and promotes clinicians awareness (Sehonanda et al., 1996).

However, over the past decades, autopsy rates have markedly declined all over the world due to various reasons (Table 1). Advances in laboratory and radiological diagnostics contribute in recognizing different AIDS-related diseases and diminish diagnostic value of autopsy.

Benefits	Limitations
Diagnostic value: - gross findings, - histological analysis, - correlations with antemortem diagnosis *Epidemiological needs:* - death records, - trends over time periods *Educational goals:* - for students, - for professionals (clinical conferences) *Scientific potential:* - case reports, - series reports, - sample collection/further reevaluation	*Difficulties in obtaining consent* *High efficiency of clinical diagnostic tools:* - laboratory diagnostics, - diagnostic radiology, - endoscopy *Risk of infection for staff* *Choice of 'alternative autopsy' techniques:* - needle autopsy, - virtual autopsy, - verbal autopsy *High costs*

Table 1. The AIDS autopsies today: *Pros & Cons*

Health care systems of developed countries offer high-quality diagnostic opportunities for HIV patients, while in developing countries such options have limited availability. Another one concern is that most relatives of died patients are not willing to provide consent for an autopsy because of cultural, traditional and other beliefs (Garcia-Jardon et al., 2010). It is important for clinicians to approach families for autopsy consent. From the other hand, some pathologists and technicians avoid to carry out autopsies on HIV infected cases, because of risk to be infected (Lanjewar, 2011). A major challenge in applying autopsy for AIDS cases is the rising trend of so-called 'alternative autopsy' techniques. Whereas incomplete autopsies such as examination of selected organs or needle autopsy may be accepted partially as being equivalent to a full autopsy, non-invasive procedures like virtual autopsy and echopsy cannot substitute for conventional necropsy techniques (Burton & Underwood, 2007). Verbal autopsy which appears to be gaining acceptance in developing countries (Bhattacharya & Neogi, 2008) is in no way an objective diagnostic technique. Postmortem examination should include collection of organs specimens for histological study; any exception to this rule will markedly decrease the value of autopsy.

3.2 Results

We have analyzed the largest autopsy series from different continents that covered the time period from 1982 to 2011 (Table 2). The main focus was on the prevalence of AIDS-indicative diseases and their distribution according to time periods and geography. Opportunistic infections were the most common autopsy findings, followed by less frequent secondary neoplasms.

Mycobacterial infections were detected in all the series with the lowest frequency around 20% (Afessa et al., 1998; Guerra et al., 2001; Soeiro et al., 2008). In developed countries such as Italy, Germany and Japan, the prevalence of tuberculosis in autopsies of patients with HIV/AIDS is 5-7%, whereas these rates were found to be 38-59% mostly in developing countries (Ansari et al., 2002; d'Arminio Monforte et al., 1992; Hsiao et al., 1997; Kaiser et al., 2000; Lucas et al., 1993; Ohtomo et al., 2000). Pulmonary lesions tend to hematogenous spread, thus the disseminated variant was described in 60-90% cases (Ansari et al., 2002; Cury et al., 2003; Parkhomenko et al., 2003; Rana et al., 2000; Soeiro et al., 2008). Extremely high rates of tuberculosis were reported in recent studies from Russia and India, 82% and 68%, respectively (Berdnikov et al., 2011; Lanjewar, 2011). Emergence of tuberculosis became obvious only in the last decade, when dramatic increase of this infection was implicated as a prime cause of death in AIDS patients. The main reason for such burden in Russia is the overlapping of prior independent epidemics of HIV and tuberculosis with subsequent merging and fast spread through neglected population groups like intravenous drug users, prisoners, alcoholics, homeless persons. Modern HIV-associated tuberculosis is a highly aggressive destructive process in the lungs caused by multidrug resistant strains of *Mycobacteria* and characterized by widespread dissemination and extrapulmonary involvement (Berdnikov et al., 2011).

Currently MAI infections are not of major significance, but they featured notably in the early series from USA and Europe (Guerra et al., 2001; Jellinger et al., 2000; Klatt et al., 1994; Masliah et al., 2000).

	USA	USA	USA	USA	USA	Austria	Spain	Botswana	Brasil	Russia	Brasil	SouthAfrica	Russia	India	Russia
Source	Klatt, 1994	Lyon, 1993	Sehonanda, 1996	Afessa, 1998	Masliah, 2000	Jellinger, 2000	Guerra, 2001	Ansari, 2002	Cury 2003	Parkhomenko, 2003	Sceiro, 2008	Garcia-Jardon, 2010	Berdnikov, 2011	Lanjewar, 2011	own data (unpublished)
Period	1982-1993	1984-1993	1982-1993	1985-1996	1982-1998	1953-1999	1987-1997	1997-1998	1993-2000	1991-2001	1990-2000	2000-2008	2003-2010	1988-2007	2000-2011
Cases	565	279	168	233	390	260	150	104	92	321	250	86	264	223	155
MycoBact															
TB	76 13%	64 23%	45 27%	13 5%	85 21%	15 6%	12 8%	42 40%	25 27%	99 31%	36 14%	25 32%	216 82%	152 68%	72 46%
MAI	104 18%	81 29%	26 15%	31 13%		36 14%	17 11%	2 2%			15 6%		7 3%		1 1%
Bacterial															
Pneum	52 9%			98 42%	149 41%	138 53%	14 9%	24 23%	13 14%	48 15%	91 36%	17 22%	26 10%	48 21%	40 26%
Sepsis	32 6%						1 1%	4 4%	5 5%	23 8%	36 14%	4 5%	10 4%		6 4%
Meningitis								2 2%		5 2%	4 2%	8 10%			1 1%
Viral															
CMV	286 51%	128 46%	36 21%	40 17%	196 50%	127 49%	19 13%	16 15%	16 17%	59 19%	33 13%		3 1%	35 16%	10 7%
HSV	92 16%	20 7%				11 4%	1 1%								1 1%
Fungal															
PCP	308 55%	80 29%	55 33%	56 24%	100 26%	30 12%	21 14%	11 11%	15 16%	6 2%	68 27%	7 9%	6 2%	11 5%	17 11%
Asperg	6 1%	3 1%	9 5%	2 1%		12 5%	3 2%		4 4%		1 1%		1 1%		1 1%
Cryptoc	78 14%	25 9%	9 5%	23 10%		25 10%	3 2%	7 7%	6 6%	3 1%	9 3%	6 7%	9 3%	18 8%	5 3%
Cand	240 42%	30 11%	23 14%	6 2%	119 30%	46 18%	1 1%		5 5%	3 1%			44 17%	6 3%	9 6%
Histoplasm	13 2%	29 10%	3 2%	2 1%		2 1%					3 1%	1 1%	3 1%		
Parasitic															
Toxo	51 9%	9 3%	5 3%		11 3%	18 7%	1 1%	1 1%	9 10%	22 7%	18 7%	1 1%		15 6%	
Cryptosp	5 1%	7 3%		3 1%							5 2%	1 1%		6 3%	
Helminthes												1 1%		3 1%	
					Secondary Neoplasms										
KS	138 24%			19 8%	41 10%	41 16%	1 1%	11 11%	2 2%	33 10%	11 4%	1 1%	2 1%	2 1%	
NHL	81 14%			3 1%	20 5%	17 7%	13 9%	3 3%		3 1%	5 2%		6 2%	8 3%	2 2%
Frequency hierarchy	CMV / PCP-Bact	PCP-CMV / TB-CMV	PCP / TB-CMV	Pneum / PCP-CMV	CMV-Bact / PCP	Bact-CMV	PCP-CMV	TB / Pneum-CMV	TB / Bact-CMV	TB / CMV-Pneum	Pneum-PCP	TB / Pneum	TB / Pneum-CMV	TB / Pneum	TB / Pneum

Table 2. Autopsy findings from the largest autopsy series.

Abbreviations: MycoBact, mycobacterial infections; TB, tuberculosis; MAI, *Mycobacterium avium-intracellulare* infection; Pneum, pneumonia; CMV, *Cytomegalovirus* infection; HSV, *Herpes Simplex Virus* infection; PCP, pneumocystis pneumonia; Asperg, aspergillosis; Cryptoc, cryptococcosis; Cand, candidiasis; Histoplasm, histoplasmosis; Toxo, toxoplasmosis; Cryptosp, cryptosporidiosis; KS, Kaposi's sarcoma; NHL, non-Hodgkin's lymphoma; Bact, bacterial infections

Similarly, bacterial infections in the same way as tuberculosis showed a marked rise in the last decades and represent an important cause of mortality in AIDS patients. Bacterial pneumonias were identified in 21-36% of cases from low- and middle-income countries (Ansari et al., 2002; Garcia-Jardon et al., 2010; Lanjewar, 2011; Soeiro et al., 2008). Early American sets often not mentioned pneumonias apart from pyogenic infections like sepsis, because they were included in the list of AIDS criteria subsequently. HIV patients are prone to nosocomial pneumonias caused by bacterial associations which demonstrate relapsing course with complications such as abscess formation and pleural effusion (Parkhomenko et al., 2003).

The prevalence of *Cytomegalovirus* infection ranges from 13-19% in African, Indian and Brasilian series to 46-69% cases from USA and Europe (Jellinger et al., 2000; Klatt et al., 1994; Lyon et al., 1996; Masliah et al., 2000; Pillay et al. 1993; Walewska-Zielecka et al., 1996). The highest rates of 74-76% were described in Japan and Australia (Dore et al., 1995; Ohtomo et al., 2000). Among invasive fungal infections pneumocystosis exhibits most significant decline due to effective prophylaxis and introduction of highly active anti-retroviral therapy (HAART). Early reports described high prevalence of pneumocystic pneumonias in more than half of all patients (Klatt et al., 1994), however recent studies could reveal *Pneumocystis jirovecii* pneumonia in less than 10% cases (Parkhomenko et al., 2003). Low levels of pneumocystosis are also specific for African countries regardless time period (Garcia-Jardon et al., 2010; Lucas et al., 1993; Nelson et al., 1993). A large retrospective study of an Italian cohort showed that the prevalence of opportunistic mycoses decreased over time, owing mainly to a significant decrease in pneumocystosis and cryptococcosis, whereas the prevalence of aspergillosis and histoplasmosis remained relatively stable while that of candidiasis tended to increase in the last years (Antinori et al., 2009). Rates of toxoplasmosis showed no significant variation for decades and comprise 1-10% of cases (Cury et al., 2003; Guerra et al., 2001; Sehonanda et al., 1996). The levels of HIV-related neoplasms seem to be decreasing over time, which was demonstrated for both non-Hodgkin's lymphomas and Kaposi's sarcomas in reviewed series (Jones et al., 1999; Launay & Guillevin, 2003).

The main patterns of organ/system involvement in AIDS are pulmonary, generalized or system isolated (CNS, digestive system). In most autopsy series of HIV-infected patients, pulmonary pattern was the most common with an incidence of 60–88%, followed by the CNS (60–80%), and the gastrointestinal tract (Concepcion et al., 1996; Cox et al., 2010; Hofman et al., 1999; Jellinger et al., 2000; Mohar et al., 1992; Sehonanda et al., 1996). Opportunistic monoinfection was observed on the highest level only in 40% cases, while most postmortem studies detected several microbial agents (Rana et al., 2000; Soeiro et al., 2008).

Cases with advanced CNS alterations have a high frequency of opportunistic infections and neoplasms (Masliah et al., 2000). A generalized pattern may be caused by virtually all opportunistic agents, but the most disseminating microorganism today is *Mycobacterium tuberculosis* (Parkhomenko et al., 2003).

Not all deaths of AIDS patients are related to HIV. The percentage of deaths from AIDS-related diseases has decreased, especially in those countries where highly active antiretroviral therapy is widely available. Non-AIDS causes in high-income countries account for at least a third of deaths, and include non-natural causes such as drug overdose, suicide, and violence along with various somatic diseases (Kohli et al., 2005; Krentz et al., 2005). Important non-HIV-related complications contributing to mortality of AIDS patients are chronic liver diseases, cardiovascular pathology and malignancies (d'Arminio Monforte, 2009; Friis-Møller et al., 2010; Lucas et al., 2008; Sackoff et al., 2006). Cases of hepatic involvement are extremely common in HIV-infected cohort of intravenous drug users with HCV co-infection which may die from liver cirrhosis or necrotizing liver failure (Guerra et al., 2001).

One of the important utilities of autopsy is the correlation between antemortem and postmortem diagnosis. A recent review from the UK spanning 23 years showed that the autopsy findings altered the primary diagnosis in 70% of cases, and that 36% of opportunistic infections were not diagnosed prior to death (Beadsworth et al., 2009). An Indian series showed discordance between antemortem and postmortem diagnosis in 42% cases (Lanjewar, 2011). Russian authors reported that in 7% of cases HIV infection (!) was detected only postmortem (Berdnikov et al., 2011). Both false positive as well as false negative antemortem diagnoses are described (Martinson et al., 2007). Infections such tuberculosis, *Cytomegalovirus* and invasive mycoses are missed with the highest rate (Antinori et al., 2009; Beadsworth et al., 2009; Eza et al., 2006; Tang et al., 2006; Wilkes et al., 1988).

3.3 Current trends

The most notable changes described in reviewed series are the rise of tuberculosis infection and bacterial pneumonias for last 10 years (Fig. 3). Tuberculosis is often represented by generalized and disseminated forms. Bacterial infections still occur more frequently than other opportunistic infections in patients with HIV. Multiple infections with involvement of several organs are common.

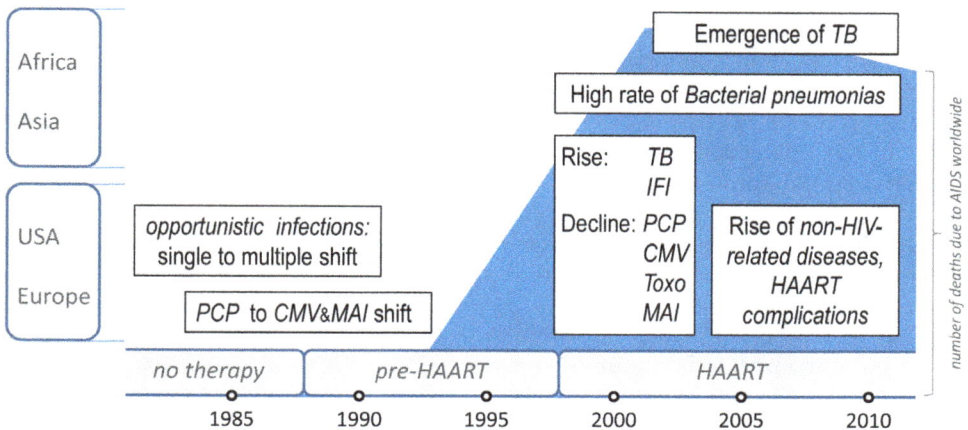

Abbreviations: PCP, pneumocystic pneumonia; CMV, *Cytomegalovirus* infection; MAI, *Mycobacterium avium-intracellulare* infection; TB, tuberculosis; IFI, invasive fungal infections; Toxo, toxoplasmosis

Fig. 3. Major changing patterns of AIDS reported in retrospective studies.

Lungs and central nervous system are the most common targets for pathological processes. The incidence of pneumocystic pneumonia has declined significantly as a result of antiretroviral therapy and chemoprophylaxis. Rates of CMV infection also had been decreased, but not so markedly as pneumocystosis.

The possible concern of described results is that early autopsy series from our set represent high-income developed countries and the most recent series are from low- and middle-income countries. Therefore, it is more correct to report about emergence of HIV-related tuberculosis in developing countries than all over the world. Actually, in Western world (high-income model) tuberculosis spreads through HIV-infected cohort, while in Russia and India social conditions drives tuberculosis in neglected population (alcoholics, imprisons, homeless), that is superimposed by HIV. Contribution of non-HIV-related pathology in AIDS mortality depends on availability of HAART and, consequently, economical development of the country.

Finally, we may suppose that current trends in AIDS mortality for low- and high-income countries are different. Emergence of tuberculosis and high prevalence of bacterial infections are typical for Sub-Saharan Africa, South-East Asia and Eastern Europe. Growth of non-AIDS-related diseases is observed in USA and Western Europe.

4. Conclusion

Through the whole timeline of HIV epidemics significant differences in epidemiology contributed to evolution of disease. Thus, changing patterns of geographic distribution, modes of infection, spectrum of secondary diseases were widely described and explained. Since the first reports on AIDS autopsy has playing an important role in study of HIV infection. Autopsy series and case reports provided abundance of data on various aspects of AIDS. Soon after introduction of HAART large retrospective autopsy studies covering several thousand cases were published (Jellinger et al., 2000; Morgello et al., 2002; Neuenburg et al., 2002; Vago et al., 2002). Results of comprehensive post-mortem examinations were in concordance with data from numerous clinical studies declaring efficacy of therapy and marked reduction of mortality from AIDS (de Martino et al., 2000; Mocroft et al., 1998; Palella et al., 1998). HAART contributed the most important shift in the history of HIV epidemics. However, currently only 10% (roughly) of HIV patients globally are receiving ART (Brown et al., 2010). Moreover, rates of non-adherence to antiretroviral therapy has been shown to range from 33% to 88% (Mills et al., 2006). Access to antiretroviral therapy in developing high-burden countries is restricted and number of AIDS-related deaths in only Sub-Saharan Africa for the last 10 years has exceeded 10 million (UNAIDS, 2009).

The total number of HIV autopsies declined worldwide after the advent of combination therapy. It is thought, that recruiting of such sophisticated studies like autopsy series to analysis of morbidity and mortality trends is not reasonable. Instead of that new methods are established to assess mortality statistics in developing countries (Bhattacharaya & Neogi, 2008). Currently, the popularity of studies evaluating AIDS-related mortality by means of verbal autopsy is increasing (Bundhamcharoen et al., 2011; Lopman et al., 2010; Negin et al., 2010).

We believe that autopsy series represent most reliable sources in estimation of mortality trends. While in the early years of HIV epidemics autopsy function was largely scientific (e.g. recognizing and describing), nowadays the epidemiological data are of main value. Systematic retrospective study of autopsy series worldwide is a valuable tool that should contribute to the study of AIDS epidemics evolution.

5. Acknowledgment

Authors would like to thank Dr. Jimson W. D'Souza (Smolensk State Medical Academy), Dr. Florence Orim (Nagasaki University Graduate School of Biomedical Sciences), Dr. Jitender Singh (Sir Ganga Ram Hospital, New Delhi) and Dr. Larisa Skrobut (Smolensk Regional Institute of Pathology) for their help in preparation of manuscript.

This work was supported by Grant-in-Aid for Scientific Research by Ministry of Health, Labor and Welfare of Japan #H22-AIDS-nominated type-G009, "Patients' participated clinical research on long term therapy of HIV/HCV co-infected hemophiliacs".

6. References

Afessa, B., Green, W., Chiao, J. & Frederick, W. (1998). Pulmonary Complications of HIV Infection: Autopsy Findings. *Chest*, Vol. 113, No. 5, pp. 1225-1229.

AIDS Epidemic Update: November 2009, UNAIDS, ISBN 978 92 9173 832 8, Geneva.

Ansari, N., Kombe, A., Kenyon, T., Hone, N., Tappero, J., Nyirenda, S., Binkin, N. & Lucas, S. (2002). Pathology and Causes of Death in a Group of 128 Predominantly HIV-Positive Patients in Botswana, 1997-1998. *The International Journal of Tuberculosis and Lung Disease*, Vol. 6, No. 1, pp. 55-63.

Antinori, S., Nebuloni, M., Magni, C., Fasan, M., Adorni, F., Viola, A., Corbellino, M., Galli, M., Vago, G., Parravicini, C. & Ridolfo, A. (2009). Trends in the Postmortem Diagnosis of Opportunistic Invasive Fungal Infections in Patients with AIDS: a Retrospective Study of 1,630 Autopsies Performed Between 1984 and 2002. *American Journal of Clinical Pathology*, Vol. 132, No. 2, pp. 221-227.

Baroni, C. & Uccini, S. (1993). The Lymphadenopathy of HIV Infection. *American Journal of Clinical Pathology*, Vol. 99, No. 4, pp. 397-401.

Beadsworth, M., Cohen, D., Ratcliffe, L., Jenkins, N., Taylor, W., Campbell, F., Beeching, N. & Azadeh, B. (2009). Autopsies in HIV: Still Identifying Missed Diagnoses. *International Journal of STD & AIDS*, Vol. 20, No. 2, pp. 84-86.

Berdnikov, R., Grinberg, L., Sorokina, N., Zhidkova, O. & Nevolin, A. (2011). HIV and Tuberculosis by Data Gained from Pathologic Anatomy Autopsy. *Ural'skiĭ Meditsinskiĭ Zhurnal*, Vol. 79, No. 1, pp. 67-71.

Bhattacharya, M. & Neogi, S. (2008). Estimation of Mortality Due to AIDS – A Review. *Indian Journal of Public Health*, Vol. 52, No. 1, pp. 21-27.

Brown, T., Bao, L., Raftery, A., Salomon J., Baggaley, R., Stover, J. & Gerland P. (2010). Modelling HIV Epidemics in the Antiretroviral Era: the UNAIDS Estimation and Projection Package 2009. *Sexually Transmitted Infections*, Vol. 86, ii3-ii10.

Bundhamcharoen, K., Odton, P., Phulkerd, S. & Tangcharoensathien, V. (2011). Burden of Disease in Thailand: Changes in Health Gap between 1999 and 2004. *BMC Public Health*, Vol.11:53.

Burton, J. & Underwood, J. (2007). Clinical, educational, and epidemiological value of autopsy. *Lancet*, Vol. 369, No. 9571, pp. 1471-1480.

Concepcion, L., Markowitz, G., Borczuk, A. & Factor, S. (1996). Comparison of Changing Autopsy Trends in the Bronx Population with Acquired Immunodeficiency Syndrome. *Modern Pathology*, Vol. 9, No. 10, pp. 1001-1006.

Cox, J., Lukande, R., Lucas, S., Nelson, A., Van Marck, E. & Colebunders, R. (2010). Autopsy Causes of Death in HIV-Positive Individuals in sub-Saharan Africa and Correlation with Clinical Diagnoses. *AIDS Reviews*, Vol. 12, No. 4, pp. 183-194.

Cury, P., Pulido, C., Furtado, V. & da Palma, F. (2003). Autopsy Findings in AIDS Patients from a Reference Hospital in Brazil: Analysis of 92 Cases. *Pathology, Research & Practice*, Vol. 199, No. 12, pp. 811-814.

d'Arminio Monforte, A., Vago, L., Lazzarin, A., Boldorini, R., Bini, T., Guzzetti, S., Antinori, S., Moroni, M. & Costanzi, G. (1992). AIDS-Defining Diseases in 250 HIV-Infected Patients; a Comparative Study of Clinical and Autopsy Diagnoses. *AIDS*, Vol. 6, No. 10, pp. 1159-1164.

d'Arminio Monforte, A. (2009). Malignancy-Related Deaths Among HIV-infected Patients. *Clinical Infectious Diseases*, Vol. 48, No. 5, pp. 640-641.

de Martino, M., Tovo, P., Balducci, M., Galli, L., Gabiano, C., Rezza, G. & Pezzotti, P. (2000). Reduction in Mortality with Availability of Antiretroviral Therapy for Children with Perinatal HIV-1 Infection. Italian Register for HIV Infection in Children and the Italian National AIDS Registry. *Journal of American Medical Association*, Vol. 284, No. 2, pp. 190-197.

Dore, G., Marriott, D. & Duflou, J. (1995). Clinico-Pathological Study of Cytomegalovirus (CMV) in AIDS Autopsies: Under-Recognition of CMV Pneumonitis and CMV Adrenalitis. *Australian and New Zealand Journal of Medicine*, Vol. 25, No. 5, pp. 503-506.

Du, M., Bacon, C. & Isaacson, P. (2007). Kaposi Sarcoma-Associated Herpesvirus/Human Herpesvirus 8 and Lymphoproliferative Disorders. *Journal of Clinical Pathology*, Vol. 60, No. 12, pp. 1350-1357.

Eza, D., Cerrillo, G., Moore, D., Castro, C., Ticona, E., Morales, D., Cabanillas, J., Barrantes, F., Alfaro, A., Benavides, A., Rafael, A., Valladares, G., Arevalo, F., Evans, C. & Gilman, R. (2006). Postmortem Findings and Opportunistic Infections in HIV-Positive Patients from a Public Hospital in Peru. *Pathology, Research & Practice*, Vol. 202, No. 11, pp. 767-775.

Fassone, L., Cingolani, A., Martini, M., Migliaretti, G., Oreste, P., Capello, D., Gloghini, A., Vivenza, D., Dolcetti, R., Carbone, A., Antinori, A., Gaidano, G. & Larocca L. (2002). Characterization of Epstein-Barr Virus Genotype in AIDS-Related Non-Hodgkin's Lymphoma. *AIDS Research and Human Retroviruses*, Vol. 18, No. 1, pp. 19-26.

Friis-Møller, N., Thiébaut, R., Reiss, P., Weber, R., Monforte, A., De Wit, S., El-Sadr, W., Fontas, E., Worm, S., Kirk, O., Phillips, A., Sabin, C., Lundgren, J. & Law, M. (2010). Predicting the Risk of Cardiovascular Disease in HIV-Infected Patients: the Data Collection on Adverse Effects of Anti-HIV Drugs Study. *European Journal of Cardiovascular Prevention and Rehabilitation*, Vol. 17, No. 5, pp. 491-501.

Frisch, M., Biggar, R., Engels, E. & Goedert J. (2001). Association of Cancer with AIDS-related Immunosuppression in Adults. *Journal of American Medical Association*, Vol. 285, No. 13, pp. 1736-1745.

Garcia-Jardon, M., Bhat, V., Blanco-Blanco, E. & Stepian, A. (2010). Postmortem Findings in HIV/AIDS Patients in a Tertiary Care Hospital in Rural South Africa. *Tropical Doctor*, Vol. 40, No. 2, pp. 81-84.

Guerra, I., Ortiz, E., Portu, J., Atarés, B., Aldamiz-Etxebarría, M. & De Pablos, M. (2001). Value of Limited Necropsy in HIV-Positive Patients. *Pathology, Research & Practice*, Vol. 197, No. 3, pp. 165-168.

Gyorkey, F., Melnick, J. & Gyorkey, P. (1987). Human Immunodeficiency Virus in Brain Biopsies of Patients with AIDS and Progressive Encephalopathy. *Journal of Infectious Diseases*, Vol. 155, No. 5, pp. 870-876.

Hofman, P., Saint-Paul, M., Battaglione, V., Michiels, J. & Loubière, R. (1999). Autopsy Findings in the Acquired Immunodeficiency Syndrome (AIDS). A Report of 395 Cases from the South of France. *Pathology, Research & Practice*, Vol. 195, No. 4, pp. 209-217.

Hsiao, C., Huang, S., Huang, S., Song, C., Su, I., Chuang, C., Yao, Y., Lin, C. & Hsu, H. (1997). Autopsy Findings on Patients with AIDS in Taiwan. *Zhonghua Min Guo Wei Sheng Wu Ji Mian Yi Xue Za Zhi*, Vol. 30, No. 3, pp. 145-159.

Japiassú, A., Amâncio, R., Mesquita, E., Medeiros, D., Bernal, H., Nunes, E., Luz, P., Grinsztejn, B. & Bozza, F. (2010). Sepsis is a Major Determinant of Outcome in Critically Ill HIV/AIDS Patients. *Critical Care*, Vol. 14, No. 4, R152, 8 pages.

Jellinger, K., Setinek, U., Drlicek, M., Böhm, G., Steurer, A. & Lintner, F. (2000). Neuropathology and General Autopsy Findings in AIDS During the Last 15 Years. *Acta Neuropathologica*, Vol. 100, No. 2, pp. 213-220.

Jones, J., Hanson, D., Dworkin, M., Ward, J. & Jaffe, H. (1999). Effect of Antiretroviral Therapy on Recent Trends in Selected Cancers among HIV-Infected Persons. Adult/Adolescent Spectrum of HIV Disease Project Group. *Journal of Acquired Immune Deficiency Syndromes*, Vol. 1, No. 21, Suppl. 1, pp. S11-S17.

Kaiser, A., Weng, L., Brockhaus, W. & Wünsch, P. (2000). Opportunistic Infections and HIV-Associated Malignancies. An Evaluation of 58 autopsy Cases Within 10 Years. *Medizinische Klinik*, Vol. 95, No. 9, pp. 482-486.

Kibayashi, K., Mastri, A. & Hirsch C. (1996). Neuropathology of Human Immunodeficiency Virus Infection at Different Disease Stages. *Human Pathology*, Vol. 27, No. 7, pp. 637-642.

Klatt, E., Jensen, D. & Meyer, P. (1987). Pathology of Mycobacterium Avium-Intracellulare Infection in Acquired Immunodeficiency Syndrome. *Human Pathology*, Vol. 18, No. 7, pp. 709-714.

Klatt, E., Nichols, L. & Noguchi, T. (1994). Evolving Trends Revealed by Autopsies of Patients with the Acquired Immunodeficiency Syndrome. 565 Autopsies in Adults with the Acquired Immunodeficiency Syndrome, Los Angeles, California, 1982-1993. *Archives of Pathology & Laboratory Medicine*, Vol. 118, No. 9, pp. 884-890.

Kohli, R., Lo, Y., Howard, A., Buono, D., Floris-Moore, M., Klein, R. & Schoenbaum, E. (2005). Mortality in an Urban Cohort of HIV-Infected and at-Risk Drug Users in the Era of Highly Active Antiretroviral Therapy. *Clinical Infectious Diseases*, Vol. 41, No. 6, pp. 864-872.

Krentz, H., Kliewer, G. & Gill, M. (2005). Changing Mortality Rates and Causes of Death for HIV-Infected Individuals Living in Southern Alberta, Canada from 1984 to 2003. *HIV Medicine*, Vol. 6, No. 2, pp. 99-106.

Lanjewar, D. (2011). The Spectrum of Clinical and Pathological Manifestations of AIDS in a Consecutive Series of 236 Autopsied Cases in Mumbai, India. *Pathology Research International*, Vol. 2011, Article ID 547618, 12 pages

Launay, O. & Guillevin, L. (2003). Epidemiology of HIV-Associated Malignancies. *Bulletin du Cancer*, Vol. 90, No. 5, pp. 387-392.

Lopman, B., Cook, A., Smith, J., Chawira, G., Urassa, M., Kumogola, Y., Isingo, R., Ihekweazu, C., Ruwende, J., Ndege, M., Gregson, S., Zaba, B. & Boerma, T. (2010). Verbal Autopsy Can Consistently Measure AIDS Mortality: a Validation Study in Tanzania and Zimbabwe. *Journal of Epidemiology and Community Health*, Vol. 64, No. 4, pp. 330-334.

Lucas, S., Hounnou, A., Peacock, C., Beaumel, A., Djomand, G., N'Gbichi, J., Yeboue, K., Hondé, M., Diomande, M., Giordano, C., Doorly, R., Brattegaard, K., Kestens, L., Smithwick, R., Kadio, A., Ezani, N., Yapi, A. & De Cock, K. (1993). The Mortality and Pathology of HIV Infection in a West African City. *AIDS*, Vol. 7, No. 12, pp. 1569-1579.

Lucas, S., Curtis, H. & Johnson, M. (2008). National Review of Deaths Among HIV-Infected Adults. *Clinical Medicine*, Vol. 8, No. 3, pp. 250-252.

Lyon, R., Haque, A., Asmuth, D. & Woods, G. (1996). Changing Patterns of Infections in Patients with AIDS: a Study of 279 Autopsies of Prison Inmates and Nonincarcerated Patients at a University Hospital in Eastern Texas, 1984-1993. *Clinical Infectious Diseases*, Vol. 23, No. 2, pp. 241-247.

Martinson, N., Karstaedt, A., Venter, W., Omar, T., King, P., Mbengo, T. Marais, E., McIntyre, J, Chaisson, R. & Hale, M. (2007). Causes of Death in Hospitalized Adults with a Premortem Diagnosis of Tuberculosis: an Autopsy Study. *AIDS*, Vol. 21, No. 15, pp. 2043-2050.

Masliah, E., DeTeresa, R., Mallory, M. & Hansen, L. (2000). Changes in Pathological Findings at Autopsy in AIDS Cases for the Last 15 Years. *AIDS*, Vol. 14, No. 1, pp. 69-74.

Mills, E., Nachega, J., Bangsberg, D., Singh, S., Rachlis, B., Wu, P., Wilson, K., Buchan, I., Gill, C. & Cooper, C. (2006). Adherence to HAART: a Systematic Review of Developed and Developing Nation Patient-Reported Barriers and Facilitators. *PLoS Medicine*, Vol. 3, No. 11, e438.

Mocroft, A., Vella, S., Benfield, T., Chiesi, A., Miller, V., Gargalianos, P., d'Arminio Monforte, A., Yust, I., Bruun, J., Phillips, A. & Lundgren, J. (1998). Changing Patterns of Mortality Across Europe in Patients Infected with HIV-1. EuroSIDA Study Group. *Lancet*, Vol. 352, No. 9142, pp. 1725-1730.

Mohar, A., Romo, J., Salido, F., Jessurun, J., Ponce de León, S., Reyes, E., Volkow, P., Larraza, O., Peredo, M., Cano, C., Gomez, G., Sepulveda, J. & Mueller, N. (1992). The Spectrum of Clinical and Pathological Manifestations of AIDS in a Consecutive Series of Autopsied Patients in Mexico. *AIDS*, Vol. 6, No. 5, pp. 467-473.

Morgello, S., Mahboob, R., Yakoushina, T., Khan, S. & Hague, K. (2002). Autopsy Findings in a Human Immunodeficiency Virus-Infected Population Over 2 Decades: Influences of Gender, Ethnicity, Risk Factors, and Time. *Archives of Pathology & Laboratory Medicine*, Vol. 126, No. 2, pp. 182-190.

Negin, J., Wariero, J., Cumming, R., Mutuo, P. & Pronyk, P. (2010). High Rates of AIDS-Related Mortality among Older Adults in Rural Kenya. *Journal of Acquired Immune Deficiency Syndromes*, Vol. 55, No. 2, pp. 239-244.

Nelson, A., Perriëns, J., Kapita, B., Okonda, L., Lusamuno, N., Kalengayi, M., Angritt, P., Quinn, T. & Mullick, F. (1993). A Clinical and Pathological Comparison of the

WHO and CDC Case Definitions for AIDS in Kinshasa, Zaïre: is Passive Surveillance Valid? *AIDS*, Vol. 7, No. 9, pp. 1241-1245.

Neuenburg, J., Brodt, H., Herndier, B., Bickel, M., Bacchetti, P., Price, R., Grant, R. & Schlote, W. (2002). HIV-Related Neuropathology, 1985 to 1999: Rising Prevalence of HIV Encephalopathy in the Era of Highly Active Antiretroviral Therapy. *Journal of Acquired Immune Deficiency Syndromes*, Vol. 31, No. 2, pp. 171-177.

Ohtomo, K., Wang, S., Masunaga, A., Iwamoto, A. & Sugawara I. (2000). Secondary Infections of AIDS Autopsy Cases in Japan with Special Emphasis on Mycobacterium Avium-Intracellulare Complex Infection. *The Tohoku Journal of Experimental Medicine*, Vol. 192, No. 2, pp. 99-109.

O'Murchadha, M., Wolf, B. & Neiman, R. (1987). The Histologic Features of Hyperplastic Lymphadenopathy in AIDS-Related Complex are Nonspecific. *American Journal of Surgical Pathology*, Vol. 11, No. 2, pp. 94-99.

Palella, F., Delaney, K., Moorman, A., Loveless, M., Fuhrer, J., Satten, G., Aschman, D. & Holmberg, S. (1998). Declining Morbidity and Mortality among Patients with Advanced Human Immunodeficiency Virus Infection. HIV Outpatient Study Investigators. *New England Journal of Medicine.*, Vol. 338, No. 13, pp. 853-860.

Parkhomenko, I., Tishkevich, O., Shagil'dian, V., Solnyshkova, T. & Nikonova, E. (2004). Pathomorphogenesis of Cytomegalovirus Lungs Lesions in HIV Infection. *Arkhiv Patologii*, Vol. 66, No. 4, pp. 20-23.

Parkhomenko, I., Tishkevich, O. & Shakhgil'dian, V. (2003). Analysis of Autopsies in HIV Infection. *Arkhiv Patologii*, Vol. 65, No. 3, pp. 24-29.

Pillay, D., Lipman, M., Lee, C., Johnson, M., Griffiths, P. & McLaughlin, J. (1993). A Clinico-Pathological Audit of Opportunistic Viral Infections in HIV-Infected Patients. *AIDS*, Vol. 7, No. 7, pp. 969-974.

Rana, F., Hawken, M., Mwachari, C., Bhatt, S., Abdullah, F., Ng'ang'a, L., Power, C., Githui W., Porter, J. & Lucas, S. (2000). Autopsy Study of HIV-1-Positive and HIV-1-Negative Adult Medical Patients in Nairobi, Kenya. *Journal of Acquired Immune Deficiency Syndromes*, Vol. 24, No. 1, pp. 23-29.

Sackoff, J., Hanna, D., Pfeiffer, M. & Torian, L. (2006). Causes of Death among Persons with AIDS in the Era of Highly Active Antiretroviral Therapy: New York City. *Annals of Internal Medicine*, Vol. 145, No. 6, pp. 397-406.

Sehonanda, A., Choi, Y. & Blum, S. (1996). Changing Patterns of Autopsy Findings Among Persons with Acquired Immunodeficiency Syndrome in an Inner-City Population. A 12-Year Retrospective Study. *Archives of Pathology & Laboratory Medicine*, Vol. 120, No. 5, pp. 459-464.

Smith, M., Boyars, M., Veasey, S. & Woods, G. (2000). Generalized Tuberculosis in the Acquired Immune Deficiency Syndrome. *Archives of Pathology & Laboratory Medicine*, Vol. 124, No. 9, pp. 1267-1274.

Soeiro, A., Hovnanian, A., Parra, E., Canzian, M. & Capelozzi, V. (2008). Post-mortem Histological Pulmonary Analysis in Patients with HIV/AIDS. *Clinics*, Vol. 63, No. 4, pp. 497-502.

Tang, H., Liu, Y., Yen, M., Chen, Y., Wann, S., Lin, H., Lee, S., Lin, W., Huang, C., Su, B., Chang, P., Li, C. & Tseng, H. (2006). Opportunistic Infections in Adults with Acquired Immunodeficiency Syndrome: a Comparison of Clinical and Autopsy Findings. *Journal of Microbiology, Immunology, and Infection*, Vol. 39, No. 4, pp. 310-315.

Vago, L., Bonetto, S., Nebuloni, M., Duca, P., Carsana, L., Zerbi, P. & D'Arminio-Monforte, A. (2002). Pathological Findings in the Central Nervous System of AIDS Patients on Assumed Antiretroviral Therapeutic Regimens: Retrospective Study of 1597 Autopsies. *AIDS*, Vol. 16, No. 14, pp. 1925-1928.

Walewska-Zielecka, B., Kamiński, Z. & Nowosławski, A. (1996). AIDS Pathology: Infections and Neoplasms in 55 Fatal AIDS Cases. A Postmortem Study. *Polish Journal of Pathology*, Vol. 47, No. 4, pp. 163-170.

2

AIDS and Trauma

Erik Vakil, Caroline Zabiegaj-Zwick and AB (Sebastian) van As
University of Cape Town
South Africa

1. Introduction

Trauma is a significant cause of mortality (10%) worldwide and is responsible for 15% of all disability-adjusted life years (DALYs) (Murray & Lopez, 1997). Seven of the top 30 contributors to the global burden of disease are due to injury, including motor vehicle accidents, falls, war injuries, self-inflicted injuries, violence, drowning and burns. All of these injuries are seen in the trauma setting and places trauma workers at risk of exposure to blood and other body fluids. The relevance of HIV and trauma is increasing as the global prevalence of HIV continues to rise. Sixty million have been infected with HIV since the beginning of the epidemic and 25 million have died of HIV-related causes (UNAIDS, 2009). Of those newly infected, 40% were young people - the group most likely to be involved in trauma.

2. Universal precaution

In general, the risk of transmission of any infectious disease may be minimised in the trauma setting by implementing universal precautions. The World Health Organization (WHO) has developed universal precaution guidelines which are summarised below (WHO, 2007).

- Hand wash after any direct contact with patients
- Safe collection and disposal of sharps
- Gloves for contact with body fluids, non intact skin and mucous membranes
- Wearing a mask, eye protection and a gown if blood or other body fluids might splash
- Covering cuts and abrasions
- Cleaning of spills of blood and other bodily fluids
- Safe system for hospital waste management and disposal

In addition, the WHO advocates Hepatitis B virus (HBV) vaccination of healthcare workers, development of post exposure protocols for those at risk of contact with infected body fluids, adequate provision of personal protective equipment (PPE) with appropriate means of disposal, and monitoring of staff training and use of PPE.

Historically, trauma workers have generally had poor compliance with universal precaution guidelines. In a Jamaican study, where health care workers were interviewed to determine the reason for not adhering to universal precautions, numerous reason were provided including: (1) increase in workload made adherence difficult, (2) a perceived reduction in dexterity when wearing gloves, (3) insufficient supply of PPE and (4) lack of penalties for not adhering to universal precautions (Vaz et al., 2010). Other studies in the United States have reached similar conclusions and also highlighted that trauma workers have a poor knowledge of infection risk (Kelen et al. 1990; Kim et al., 1999)

3. Post-exposure prophylaxis

Post-exposure prophylaxis (PEP) is the collection of measures taken after exposure to a pathogen in order to prevent or reduce the risk of transmission. In the case of HIV, such measures should include, but are not limited to, first-aid, appropriate HIV testing, counselling, anti-retroviral (ARV) chemotherapy, and follow-up. The risk of occupational exposure to healthcare workers in the trauma setting depends on the relative prevalence of HIV in the trauma population and the level of exposure. The use of PEP in patients attending the trauma service should also be considered in cases of sexual assault and other forms of acute non-occupational exposure. It is strongly recommended that all trauma services have well established PEP protocols, sufficient resources and necessary training for effective implementation.

The only direct evidence supporting the prophylactic use of ARV chemotherapy (zidovudine) for healthcare associated HIV exposure comes from a single case-control study involving patients from the United States, United Kingdom, France and Italy (Cardo et al., 1997). Healthcare workers were 81% less likely to seroconvert if they received zidovudine after a needlestick injury and the risk of seroconversion was linked to the volume of blood transmitted and the HIV blood titre level. Indirect evidence supporting the prophylactic use of ARVs include reduced rates of vertical transmission in HIV positive mothers who received zidovudine and the success of ARVs in raising $CD4^+$ counts, reducing viral titres, and decreasing morbidity and mortality in HIV positive patients (Connor et al., 1996).

3.1 Occupational exposure

The risk of HIV transmission through needlestick injury is 0.3%. The risk of transmission from contact of contaminated fluids with mucous membranes or damaged skin is approximately 0.09%. However, the risk of occupational exposure in trauma may be higher than in other hospital settings. This is because the HIV status of patients is usually unknown, the prevalence of HIV in the trauma population is generally greater than the community, the mechanism of injury is often violent and may increase the level of exposure, and the emergent nature of trauma increases the situational stress and may lead to riskier practice.

PEP is only indicated in cases where there is a risk of transmission (Table 1) and contra-indicated in cases where there is no appreciable benefit (Table 2). For occupational exposure, this includes contact between body fluids at risk of HIV contamination and non-intact skin or mucous membranes. Indirect evidence from animal studies suggest that initiation of PEP after 72 hours following exposure is not effective at reducing rates of seroconversion. PEP should therefore not be offered in such cases and strategies should exist to offer PEP as soon as possible after exposure (Martin et al., 1993). Starter packs are well-suited to the emergency department as they offer quick access to ARVs, may result in less wasted medication if PEP is not continued, requires the patient to attend follow-up to obtain additional ARVs ensuring appropriate testing and counselling, and can easily be placed in small or under-serviced departments. Theoretical risk of HIV resistance may develop if starter packs are inappropriately used or ARV courses are not routinely completed.

Exposure between body fluids suspected of, or confirmed to be, HIV positive and:
• Non-intact skin (needlestick, sharp injury, skin abrasion)
• Mucous membranes (oral cavity, nasal cavity, eyes)
• Sexual contact in cases where a condom was not used, broke or fell off during intercourse
• Oral sex with ejaculation[1]

Table 1. Indications for PEP[2]

• Patient is already HIV positive from previous exposure
• Exposure has been chronic[3]
• Exposure through intact skin
• Sexual contact with condom use that remains intact
• Exposure to non-infectious body fluids such as saliva, faeces, urine, and sweat
• Exposure to HIV negative body fluids
• Greater than 72 hours have elapsed since exposure

Table 2. Contraindications to PEP[2]

3.2 Exposure as a result of sexual assault

The risk of non-occupational exposure depends on the nature of contact with contaminated fluids. In cases of sexual assault, the method of assault, the condition of genital or oral mucosa, the circumcision status, and the level of HIV virulence all play a role. Risk is increased in cases of rape, where there is decreased lubrication and may be associate with violent penetration. Children, especially small children, are also at an increased risk for anatomical reasons. Generalised risk from a single sexual contact depends on the method of exposure. Published estimates of HIV transmission for receptive anal intercourse are 1-30%, insertive anal intercourse 0.1-10%, receptive vaginal intercourse 0.1-10%, and insertive vaginal intercourse 0.1-1% (Boily et al., 2009). Case studies have also reported transmission from oral sex with ejaculation (Lifson et al., 1990; Rozenbaum et al., 1988).

PEP should be offered to all victims of sexual assault attending the trauma service where the act occurred within 72 hours. In many cases, particularly with children, the assault may be on a background of chronic abuse, in which case PEP is not indicated. However, special care should be taken to distinguish between cases of chronic abuse and cases of acute-on-chronic abuse where a different perpetrator is responsible for the most recent assault. In such cases, PEP should be offered.

---

[1] The risk for oral transmission is considered very low but PEP may be offered in cases where the exposure is in association with significat oral disease such as ulceration or dysplasia

[2] Adapted from: WHO. Post-exposure prophylaxis to prevent HIV infection: Joint WHO/ILO guidelines on post-exposure prophylaxis (PEP) to prevent HIV infection. *HIV/AIDS Programme: Strengthening health services to fight HIV/AIDS.* 2007

[3] Chronic exposure should be distinguished from episodic exposure where PEP may still be effective. This distinction may be challenging.

3.3 Other types of exposure

Routine PEP after community-acquired needlestick injury is controversial and administration should be based on risk assessment. At risk populations include children, security workers and cleaners (Celenza et al., 2011). Children from communities with low prevalence of HIV may not warrant PEP (Makwana & Riordan, 2005). Care should also be taken to ensure exposure was within 72 hours as presentation to the emergency department may be delayed (Johnston & O'Conor, 2005).

The risk associated with needle-sharing is approximately 0.67%. PEP for needle-sharing may also be offered if presented within 72 hours and where exposure is likely to be acute rather than chronic.

3.4 PEP regimens

When indicated, the ARV regimen used depends on various factors including national policy, institutional policy, level of resources, toxicity and side-effects, daily pill burden, drug contra-indications and compliance. Although a single drug regimen using zidovudine has shown to be effective, multi-drug regimens are now more commonly used in order to cover drug-resistant HIV clones. The use of two drugs must be weighed against cost, toxicity and availability. A third drug may be considered in cases where the background prevalence of ARV resistance is greater than 15%.

Two drug regimens include fixed-dose dual nucleoside reverse transcriptase inhibitor (NRTI) therapy with combination zidovudine-lamivudine or combination tenofovir-emtricitabine. A protease inhibitor (PI), usually in combination with ritonavir, which increases PI plasma levels, are usually added if a third drug is necessary. Combination ritonavir-lopinavir, -atazanavir, -darunavir have all been used. All PEP regimens are given for 28 days post exposure.

3.5 Testing, follow-up and counselling

Testing of the source patient, in cases where HIV status is unknown, should include rapid-ELISA testing for HIV as well as testing for HBV (surface antigen - HBsAg) and Hepatitis C virus (HCV). In cases where HIV or HCV infection has occurred within the last 2-4 weeks, HIV or HCV RNA PCR may be indicated.

Testing of the exposed patient should be carried out as soon as possible to establish a baseline for follow-up testing. Tests should include a rapid-ELISA for HIV, HBV immunity status (anti-HB antibodies), HBsAg and HCV antibodies. Baseline full blood count, liver enzymes and creatinine should also be obtained to monitor for PEP side-effects and sequelae from hepatitis infection. Screening for other sexually transmitted infections may be warranted in cases of sexual assault or in patients with high risk behaviour.

At the minimum, follow-up testing at 6 months should be performed to document HIV negative status. Seroconversion after 6 months in those receiving PEP has been reported but is extremely rare (Ippolito et al., 1999). More intensive follow-up can include HIV and HCV antibody testing at 4-6 weeks, 3 months, and 6 months. Relevant additional testing should be offered in patients who become symptomatic or experience drug toxicity.

Post-exposure counselling should form an integral part of the PEP protocol. Services should be available to address HIV testing, follow-up testing, ARV treatment, legal issues and compensation claims should they arise. In the event that HIV is contracted, services should be available to address relevant needs. Counselling to address special needs of certain population sub-groups such as children and victims of sexual assault should also be made available.

4. Management and outcome of HIV positive patients in trauma

The function of a trauma unit is to stabilise and treat life threatening injuries. It has been shown that HIV alone is not responsible for mortality in trauma but rather the patient's ability to mount an immune response (Allard & Meintjies, 2005). It is also unethical to not treat life-threatening conditions based on a patient's HIV status (Smit 2010). In fact, a number of studies have suggested that HIV positive patients have the same mortality rate as non-infected patients, especially if they are in the early stages of the disease (Smit, 2010).

With regard to surgical outcomes, early views were often pessimistic. It was felt that HIV positive patients were prone to poor wound healing, high post-operative complication rates, a prolonged post-operative period and higher mortality rates. This helped trigger a number of studies investigating the morbidity and complication rates among HIV positive patients both in general and orthopaedic surgery.

Many such studies have produced conflicting results. Duane et al conducted a retrospective study comparing outcomes of HIV positive and HIV negative patients over a 5-year period in the trauma unit. They found no difference in infection rates or overall complications based on CD4+ count alone (Duane et al., 2008). Conversely, Karpelowsky et al showed that in children who were HIV positive or exposed to HIV had increased rates of poor wound healing and breakdown of reconstruction sites (Karpelowsky et al., 2009). Other post-operative complications cited in the study were likely due to non-HIV related factors. For example, a large proportion of the children studied underwent emergency surgery, which is known to have higher rates of post-operative complications since the children tend to be sicker at presentation. This is true for both HIV positive and HIV negative patients. It was also found that up to 79% of children included in the study were undernourished and 36% had other co-morbid diseases including major respiratory and nutritional problems prior to undergoing surgery.

Stawicki et al found that HIV positive patients had both longer length of hospital stay as well as longer length of stay in ICU (Stawicki et al., 2005). They noted however, that HIV positive patients had more pulmonary, infectious and renal complications than the control group and suggested that the mortality of HIV positive patients was likely linked to these co-morbid processes. They also found that HIV positive patients needed greater numbers of surgical procedures but failed to state what the indication for these procedures were. Studies by Morrison et al and Horberg et al found similar findings to Stawicki et al, stating that HIV positive patients had higher post-operative complication rates, especially respiratory complications (Horberg et al., 2006; Morrison et al., 2010).

Studies comparing complication rates in orthopaedic surgeries have been small and only tentative conclusions can be drawn. It has been shown that HIV positive patients with an open fracture (depending on the contamination of the wound) have a higher rate of infection, especially deep infection. There is also a higher rate of late sepsis with procedures that need internal instrumentation, but sepsis may have been avoided with improved medical management including prophylactic antibiotic use before invasive procedures as well as early evaluation and treatment of possible infections (Luck Jr, 1994; Van Aardt, 2010).

The overwhelming conclusion in all these studies however, has been that there is not enough evidence to properly evaluate the relationship between HIV and outcomes after trauma. There is a significant deficiency in research in this particular area and often available data is extrapolated from studies determining the effect of HIV on patients undergoing surgical procedures, either emergency or elective. Unfortunately, researchers face an ethical challenge when testing for HIV in the trauma setting and it is unlikely that sufficiently powered studies with adequate controls are possible in the current medical climate.

5. Drug interference between ARVs and commonly used trauma drugs

Currently available ARVs inhibit the reverse transcriptase and protease enzymes of the human immunodeficiency virus. These drugs are associated with many side-effects and close monitoring is mandatory. It is also important in the trauma setting to recognise a patient's HIV status and the possible concurrent use of ARVs since administration of drugs with potential for interaction may to lead to adverse outcomes.

First-line treatment of HIV involves the use of 2 NRTIs and a non-nucleoside transcriptase inhibitor (NNRTI). Protease inhibitors are used as second line therapies (Town, 2003). Common side effects of NRTIs include lactic acidosis, hypersensitivity reactions, pancreatitis, peripheral neuropathy and hepatic dysfunction (as most are metabolised in the liver). NNRTIs are known inducers or inhibitors of other drugs due to their effect on the hepatic cytochrome systems, and hypersensitivity reactions are common. Protease inhibitors undergo hepatic cytochrome P450 (CYP450) metabolism and many in this class are potent hepatic inhibitors.

Table 3 outlines the drug interactions between NNRTIs or protease inhibitors and other drugs that are dependent on CYP450 metabolism. Many potential interactions of other commonly used drugs remain unknown and have not been included. It is important to take a drug history to ensure that potential side effects can be avoided or closely monitored. In cases where drugs must be administratered, dose adjustment may limit side-effects.

	Drugs	ARV interaction	Clinical Effects	Management
A	Aminophylline	Protease inhibitors	Decreased theophylline effects	Monitor and adjust theophylline levels as indicated
	Amiodarone	NNRTI Protease inhibitors	Increased amiodarone effects (hypotension, bradycardia, cardiac arrhythmias	Monitor and adjust amiodarone as indicated, with reduction of amiodarone dose as needed Should not be co-administered with PIs

	Drugs	ARV interaction	Clinical Effects	Management
B	Bactrim	Lamivudine	Increased Lamivudine levels?	Unknown at present but no dose adjustment necessary for either drug
	Beta- Blockers	Protease inhibitors	Increased effects of Beta-blockers	Use with caution
D	Diazepam	Zidovudine, Protease inhibitors, Efavirenz	Increased diazepam levels (increased sedation, respiratory depression)	Do not co-administer Alternative agents: Lorazepam, oxazepam, temazepam
	Digoxin	Protease inhibitor	Increased digoxin levels	Monitor digoxin levels closely
	Dilitiazem	Efavirenz	Decreased dilitiazem effects	Titrate dilitiazem to clinical effect
F	Fentanyl	NNRTI Protease inhibitors	Increased effects of Fentanyl	Close monitoring necessary
	Flagyl	Protease Inhibitors	Disulfiram-like reaction	Do not co-administer
	Furosemide	NNRTI Protease inhibitors Lamivudine	Increased effects of ARVS?	Use with caution
H	Haloperidol	NNRTIs PIs	Increased haloperidol effects	Monitor and adjust dosage as indicated
I	Ipecac	All	Decreased effects of ARVs if recently ingested due to induced vomiting	Avoid concurrent use
K	Ketamine	NNRTIs	Reduced effects of ketamine	Monitor and adjust dose as necessary
L	Lidocaine	Protease Inhibitors	Increased lidocaine levels	Monitor and adjust lidocaine dose
M	Methyl-prednisone	NNRTIs Protease Inhibitors	Possibly increased methylprednisone effects	Monitor while using
	Midazolam	NNRTI Protease inhibitors	Increased midazolam effects (increased sedation, confusion, respiratory depression)	Single dose IV midazolam may be used; chronic midazolam administration should be avoided

	Drugs	ARV interaction	Clinical Effects	Management
	Morphine	Protease inhibitors	Increased morphine levels (increased sedation and respir-atory depression)	Monitor closely when using together
N	Nitroglycerine	Protease inhibitors	Possible increase in effects of nitro-glycerine	Not known- but monitor for hypotension
P	Phenergan	NNRTIs Protease inhibitors	Unknown	Monitor closely in used concurrently for side effects
	Phenobarbitol	NNRTIs, Protease inhibitors	Decreased NNRTI and PI levels	Avoid combination if possible
	Phenytoin	NNRTIs Protease inhibitors	Decreased NNRTI and PI levels	Avoid combination if possible
	Prednisone	NNRTIs Protease Inhibitors	Possibly increased prednisone effects	Close monitoring
S	Succinylcholine	NNRTI Protease inhibitors	Possible prolongation of effects of succinylcholine	Use with caution

Table 3. Commonly used drugs in the trauma unit and possible complications (McNicholl 2011; University of Cape Town 2003; University of Liverpool 2010)

6. Conclusion

It is likely that trauma units will see an increasing number of HIV positive patients in the years to come. In an area still lacking adequate research, trauma workers need to be diligent to approach the HIV positive patient in the context of their presentation. They must also stay vigilant to protect themselves against transmission. It is hoped that as HIV prevention and treatment improve, HIV patients will no longer represent a unique cohort and their management, and most importantly, their outcomes, will be as good as those without HIV.

7. References

Allard, D. & Meintjies, G. (2005). HIV and Trauma, In: *Handbook of Trauma for Southern Africa*, A. Nicol, (Ed.), pp. 374-380, Oxford University Press, ISBN 978-019-5780-80-2, Cape Town, South Africa

Boily, M.; Baggaley R. F.; Wang L.; Masse, B.; White, R. G.; Hayes, R. J. & Alary M. (2009). Heterosexual Risk of HIV-1 Infection Per Sexual Act: Systematic Review and Meta-Analysis of Observational Studies. *The Lancet Infectious Diseases*, Vol.9, No.2, (February 2009), pp. 118-129, ISSN 1473-3099

Cardo, D. M.; Culver, D. H.; Ciesielski, C. A.; Srivastava, P. U.; Marcus, R.; Abiteboul, D.; Heptonstall, J.; Ippolito, G.; Lot, F.; McKibben, P. S. & Bell, D. M. (1997). A Case–

Control Study of HIV Seroconversion in Health Care Workers after Percutaneous Exposure. *New England Journal of Medicine*, Vol.337, No.21, (November 1997), pp. 1485-1490, ISSN 0028-4793

Celenza, A.; D'Orsogna, L. J.; Tosif, S. H.; Bateman, S. M.; O'Brien, D.; French, M. A. & Martinez O. P. (2011). Audit of Emergency Department Assessment and Management of Patients Presenting with Community-Acquired Needle Stick Injuries. *Australian Health Review*, Vol.35. No.1, (February 2011), pp. 57-62, ISSN 0156-5788

Connor, E. M.; Sperling, R. S.; Gelber, R.; Kiselev, P.; Scott, G.; O'Sullivan, M. J.; VanDyke, R.; Bey, M.; Shearer, W.; Jacobson, R. L.; Jimenez, E.; O'Neill, E.; Bazin, B.; Delfraissy, J. F.; Culnane, M.; Coombs, R.; Elkins, M.; Moye, J.; Stratton, P. & Balsley, J. (1994). Reduction of Maternal-Infant Transmission of Human Immunodeficiency Virus Type 1 with Zidovudine Treatment. *New England Journal of Medicine*, Vol.331, No.18, (November 1994), pp. 1173-1180, ISSN 0028-4793

Duane, T. M.; Sekel, S.; Wolfe, L. G.; Malhotra, A. K.; Aboutanos, M. B. & Ivatury, R. R. (2008). Does HIV Infection Influence Outcomes After Trauma. *The Journal of Trauma*, Vol.65, No.1 (July 2008), pp. 63-65, ISSN 1529-8809

Horberg, M. A.; Hurley, L. B.; Klein, D. B.; Follansbee, S. E.; Quesenberry, C.; Flamm, J. A.; Green, G. M. & Luu, T. (2006). Surgical Outcomes in Human Immunodeficiency Virus-Infected Patients in the Era of Highly Active Antiretroviral Therapy. *Archives of Surgery*, Vol.141, No.12. (December 2006), pp. 1238-1245, ISSN 0004-0010

Ippolito, G.; Puro, V.; Heptonstall, J.; Jagger, J.; De Carli, G. & Petrosillo, N. (1999). Occupational Human Immunodeficiency Virus Infection in Health Care Workers: Worldwide Cases Through September 1997. *Clinical Infectious Diseases*, Vol.28, No.2, (February 1999), pp. 365-383, ISSN 1058-4838

Johnston, J.J. & O'Conor, E. (2005). Neddlestick Injuries, Management and Education: A Role for Emergency Medicine?. *European Journal of Emergency Medicine*, Vol. 12, No.1, (February 2005), pp. 10-12, ISSN 0969-9546

Karpelowsky, J. S.; Leva, S. E.; Kelley, B.; Numanoglu, A.; Rode, H. & Millar, A. J. W. (2009). Outcomes of Human Immunodeficiency Virus–Infected and –Exposed Children Undergoing Surgery – A Prospective Study. *Journal of pediatric surgery*, Vol.44, No.4, (April 2009), pp. 681-687, ISSN 1531-5037

Kelen, G.D.; DiGiovanna, T.A.; Celentano, D.D.; Kalainov, D.; Bisson, L.; Junkins, E.; Stein, A.; Lofy, L.; Scott, C. R. J.; Sivertson, K.T. & Quinn, T. C. (1990). Adherence to Universal (Barrier) Precautions During Interventions on Critically Ill and Injured Emergency Department Patients. *Journal of Acquired Immune Deficiency Syndromes*, Vol.3, No.10, (October 1990), pp. 987-994, ISSN 0894-9255

Kim, L. E.; Evanoff, B. A.; Parks, R. L.; Jeffe, D. B.; Mutha, S.; Haase, C. & Fraser, V. J. (1999). Compliance with Universal Precautions Among Emergency Department Personnel: Implications for Prevention Programs. *American Journal of Infection Control*, Vol.27, No.5, (October 1999), pp. 453-455, ISSN 0196-6553

Lifson, A. R.; O'Malley, P. M.; Hessol, N.A.; Buchbinder, S.P.; Cannon, L. & Rutherford, G. W. (1990). HIV Seroconversion in Two Homosexual Men After Receptive Oral Intercourse with Ejaculation: Implications for Counseling Concerning Safe Sexual Practices. *American Journal of Public Health*, Vol.80, No.12, (December 1990), pp. 1509-1511, ISSN 0090-0036

Luck Jr., J.V. (1994). Orthopaedic Surgery on the HIV-Positive Patient: Complications and Outcomes. *Instructional Course Lectures*, Vol.43, pp. 543-549, ISSN 0065-6895

Makwana, N. & Riordan, F. A. (2005). Prospective Study of Community Needlestick Injuries. *Archives of Disease in* Childhood, Vol.90, No.5, (May 2005), pp. 523-524, ISSN 1468-2044

Martin, L. N.; Murphy-Corb, M.; Soike, K. F.; Davison-Fairburn, B. & Baskin, G. B. (1993). Effects of Initiation of 3'-Azido,3'-Deoxythymidine (Zidovudine) Treatment at Different Times after Infection of Rhesus Monkeys with Simian Immunodeficiency Virus. *Journal of Infectious Diseases*, Vol.168, No.4, (October 1993), pp. 825-835, ISSN 0022-1899

McNicholl, I. R. (Ed.) (2011). Database of Antiretroviral Drug Interaction, In: *HIV InSite, University of California San Francisco*, 06.05.2011, Available from http://hivinsite.ucsf.edu/insite?page=ar-00-02

Morrison, C. A.; Wyatt, M. M. & Carrick, M. M. (2010). Effects of Human Immunodeficiency Virus Status on Trauma Outcomes: A Review of the National Trauma Database. *Surgical Infections*, Vol.11, No.1, (February 2010) pp. 41-47, ISSN 1557-8674

Murray, C. J. L. & Lopez, A. D. (1997). Global Mortality, Disability, and the Contribution of Risk Factors: Global Burden of Disease Study. *The Lancet*, Vol.349, No.9063 (May 1997), pp. 1436-1442, ISSN 0140-6736

Rozenbaum, W.; Gharakhanian, S.; Duval, C. E. & Coulard, J. P. (1988). HIV Transmission By Oral Sex. *The Lancet*, Vol.331, No.8599, (June 1988), pp. 1395-1395, ISSN 0140-6736

Smit, S. (2010). Guidelines For Surgery in the HIV Patient. *CME*, Vol.28, No.8, (August 2010) pp. 356-358

Sperling, R. S.; Shapiro, D.; Coombs, R. W.; Todd, J. A.; Herman, S. A.; McSherry, G. D.; O'Sullivan, M. J.; VanDyke, R. B.; Jimenez, E.; Rouzioux, C.; Flynn, P. M.; Sullivan, J. L.; Spector, S. A.; Diaz, C.; Rooney, J.; Balsley, J.; Gelber, R. D. & Connor, E. M. (1996). Maternal Viral Load, Zidovudine Treatment, and the Risk of Transmission of Human Immunodeficiency Virus Type 1 from Mother to Infant. *New England Journal of Medicine*, Vol.335, No.22, (November 1996), pp. 1621-1629, ISSN 0028-4793

Stawicki, S. P.; Hoff, W. S.; Hoey, B. A.; Grossman, M. D.; Scoll, B. & Reed 3rd, J. F. (2005). Human Immunodeficiency Virus Infection in Trauma Patients: Where Do We Stand?" *The Journal of Trauma*, Vol.58, No.1, (January 2005), pp. 88-93, ISSN 0022-5282

University of Cape Town. (2003). *South African Medical Formulary*, South African Medical Association: Health and Medical Publishing Group, ISBN 1-875098-39-9 , Cape Town, South Africa.

UNAIDS. (2009). Global Facts and Figures, In: *Data and Analysis*, 06.05.2011, Available from http://data.unaids.org/pub/GlobalReport/2006/200605-fs_globalfactsfigures_en.pdf.

University of Liverpool. (July 2010). HIV Drug Interactions, In: *HIV Drug Interactions*, 06.05.2011, Available from http://www.hiv-druginteractions.org/PrintableCharts.aspx

Van Aardt, P. (2010). The Impact of HIV/AIDS on Orthopedic Surgery. *CME* Vol.28, (August 2010), pp. 384

Vaz, K.; McGrowder, D.; Alexander-Lindo, R.; Gordon, L.; Brown, P. & Irving, R. (2010). Knowledge, Awareness and Compliance with Universal Precautions Among Health Care Workers at the University Hospital of the West Indies, Jamaica. *The International Journal of Occupational and Environmental Medicine*, Vol.1, No.1, (October 2010), pp. 171-181, ISSN 2008-6814

WHO. (2007). Standard Precautions in Healthcare, In: *Global Alert and Response*. 06.05.2011, Available from http://www.who.int/csr/resources/publications/standardprecautions/en/index.html

3

HIV and Lung Cancer

Yusuke Okuma, Naoki Yanagisawa, Yukio Hosomi,
Atsushi Ajisawa and Masahiko Shibuya
Tokyo Metropolitan Cancer and Infectious diseases Center, Komagome Hospital
Japan

1. Introduction

Lung cancer patients with HIV infection are expected to become an emerging issue with respect to morbidity and mortality, as the number of such patients is rapidly increasing. However, few reports or textbooks dealing with this issue have documented the details of these cases. Thus, in clinical settings, infectious disease physicians or medical oncologists occasionally hesitate to treat HIV-infected patients with lung cancer. Since 1996, the outcome of HIV-infected patients has improved, because CD4 cell counts and viral load are generally well controlled with the advent of highly active antiretroviral therapy (HAART), which strongly inhibits HIV viral proliferation and restores the patient's immunological status. Furthermore, the prognosis in the HIV population has improved significantly due to the prevention and treatment of opportunistic infections (OIs). As a result, HIV infection is chronically manageable. In the pre-HAART era, the median survival time in the HIV population was 10 years, while, at present, 85% of patients survive more than 10 years.(Sepkowitz, 2001)

In the pre-HAART era, most HIV-infected patients died of acquired immunodeficiency syndrome (AIDS). Recently, however, one-third of all such patients die of malignant tumor,(Bonnet *et al.*, 2009) and deaths due to AIDS-defining cancers (ADCs), such as Kaposi's sarcoma (KS), primary central nervous system lymphoma (PCNSL) and non-Hodgkin's lymphoma (NHL), and invasive cervical carcinoma, which were defined by the Centers for Disease Control and Prevention (CDC), are decreasing. On the other hand, the number of deaths due to non-AIDS-defining cancers (NADCs) is increasing.(Engels *et al.*, 2008, Silverberg *et al.*, 2009) At present, in the population with HIV infection, lung cancer accounts for 5% of all deaths and 15% of all deaths by malignant tumors.(Bonnet *et al.*, 2009) Of all of the NADCs, lung cancer is the most common,(Engels *et al.*, 2006, Lavole *et al.*, 2006, Patel *et al.*, 2008) followed by breast cancer, soft tissue sarcoma, Hodgkin's lymphoma (HL), penile cancer, lip cancer, and testicular seminoma.(Frisch *et al.*, 2001) In 1984, Irwin *et al.* reported the first case with simultaneous HIV infection and lung cancer,(Irwin *et al.*, 1984) and several dozen patients have since been reported in the United States and Europe. (Table. 1) The clinical demographics of lung cancer with HIV infection differ slightly from the general population and are characterized by younger age, advanced stage at diagnosis, and aggressive tumor extension. Thus, the prognosis of lung cancer in the HIV population is poorer than that of lung cancer in the general population.(Lavole *et al.*, 2006) Moreover, patient fragility to treatment needs to be considered.

In the general population, lung cancer is the most common cause of cancer death worldwide. Furthermore, in the last decade, there has been progress in lung cancer treatment modalities. The development of novel antitumor agents and molecular targeted drugs has increased the lines of chemotherapy, and new treatment strategies, such as maintenance therapy and biomarker-based therapy (personalized therapy), provide diverse options. At present, in front-line chemotherapy for lung cancer patients, platinum-doublet chemotherapy with the third-generation antitumor agent has been shown to prolong survival and contribute to symptom palliation. Before the 1990s, the median survival time with the best supportive care was 4-5 months, and the 1-year survival rate was 10% in Stage IV non-small cell lung cancer (NSCLC). In 1995, the benefits of chemotherapy for Stage IV NSCLC were confirmed, and the median survival time was prolonged to 8 months.(Non-small Cell Lung Cancer Collaborative Group, 1995) At present, median survival time is 12 months, and the 1-year survival rate has improved to 50-60% from 30-35% in 2002.(Azzoli *et al.*, 2009) Thus, the reported data dealing with lung cancer in HIV patients are not comparable. In addition, drug interactions between antiviralagents and antitumor agents

Author	Nº of patients	Years	Median age (y)	Male (%)	Smoking (%)	Median pack-years	IVDU (%)	Homosexual (%)	NSCLC (%)	Adenocarcinoma	Squamous cell carcinoma	SCLC (%)	Median CD4 (cells/μL)	CD4 < 200 cells/μL	Latency (y)	PS > 2 (%)	Stage III/IV	Median Survival (mo)
Sridhar et al.	19	86-91	47	100	94	60	21	32	95	42	31	5	121	53	-	37	79	3
Trielli et al.	36	86-98	38	89	94	40	69	17	86	36	33	14	150	44	-	43	84	5
Brock et al.	92	86-04	46	67	99	30	58	-	91	48	17	9	305	-	5.5	-	87	6.3
Vyzula et al.	16	88-95	45	94	100	30	63	38	88	50	19	12	184	54	-	69	81	5.4
Alshafie et al.	11	90-94	50	82	90	-	81	0	100	46	36	0	329	30	-	-	90	3
Spano et al.	22	93-02	45	86	95	40	23	45	95	36	50	5	364	30	-	-	90	3
Pakkala et al.	80	95-08	52	80	100	37	25	33	91	41	32	9	304	-	-	-	-	-
Lavole et al.	49	96-07	46	67	99	33	17	18	100	67	17	0	350	-	8.6	71	84	8.1
D'Jaen et al.	75	96-08	50	83	99	41	30	47	81	46	35	19	340	-	11	-	77	9
Bertolaccini et al.	26	03-07	39	85	85	30	58	23	81	-	-	19	143	-	-	-	76	23

IVDU: intravenous drug user; NSCLC: non-small cell lung cancer; SCLC: small cell lung cancer; PS: performance status

Table 1. Documented clinical demographics of lung cancer patients with HIV.

must be considered, as they may increase or decrease efficacy by inhibiting cytochrome P450 (CYP450) induction, and the actual efficacy of and tolerance to therapy in such patients are uncertain.

In this chapter, we discuss the epidemiology, frequency, risk factors, clinical management, and treatment of HIV-infected lung cancer patients.

2. Incidence

Between 2001 and 2006, 71% of deaths were due to malignant tumors, as compared to only 20% in the pre-HAART era.(Crum-Cianflone *et al.*, 2009) It is evident that the HIV-infected population has a higher risk for lung cancer. In many studies comparing the incidence of lung cancer in patients with HIV to that in the general population, the standardized incidence ratio (SIR), adjusted for age and sex, has been calculated. SIR is an estimate of the ratio of the incidence of cancer in a given patient subset compared with the projected cancer incidence in the population at large. For instance, an SIR > 1 would indicate that lung cancer occurs more frequently in HIV-infected patients than in the general population; in fact, the SIR was 1.4-4.5. In the period before the advent of HAART, the SIR was 6.5 (95% confidential interval (CI) 4.5-8.9),(Frisch & Hjalgrim, 1999, Parker *et al.*, 1998) from 1978-1996, the SIR was 4.5 with 808 patients,(Frisch *et al.*, 2001) and in most European studies, the SIR did not exceed 1.13.(Bower *et al.*, 2003, Herida *et al.*, 2003, Powles *et al.*, 2009) In the HAART era, the SIR was 2.27-3.3.(Powles *et al.*, 2009, Patel *et al.*, 2008) In a meta-analysis with seven observational studies of NADCs (n=1016), the SIR was 2.72 (95% CI 1.91-3.87).(Grulich *et al.*, 2007) In many studies, the number of lung cancer patients with HIV infection has been shown to increase from the HAART era to the post-HAART era. The incidence, however, has not changed. On the other hand, there are few data from Asian countries. The TAHOD study, a retrospective study of 617 patients between 2000 and 2008 in 10 Asian countries, reported that the number of patients with simultaneous HIV infection and NADCs is increasing, even in developing countries. Infection-unrelated NADCs (NADC-IURs), including lung cancer, account for 22%, with lung cancer being the most common (1.9%, 12 patients). In this study, the authors concluded that the Asian patient demographic differs from the Western demographic.(Petoumenos *et al.*, 2010)

3. Pathogenesis & risk factors

The risk factors for lung cancer in the HIV population are strongly associated with immunity and cigarette smoking. The higher risk for carcinogenesis in immune-compromised patients and the increased risk for lung cancer occurrence are particularly well known; kidney transplant patients have a significantly higher incidence of lung cancer than hemodialysis patients.(Vajdic *et al.*, 2006) Carcinogenesis in lung cancer is not directly associated with viral load and CD4 cell counts, and the mechanism of the increased risk for lung cancer is not fully understood. The reasons for the increased incidence of lung cancer in HIV-infected patients therefore remain uncertain.

3.1 Smoking exposure & other traditional risk factors

Cigarette smoking in the HIV population is a major contributing factor for carcinogenesis, as in the general population. The American Lung Association has reported that 87% of all lung cancer is caused by smoking, and smoking cessation decreases the annual risk.(Samet *et al.*, 1988) The rate of smoking in the HIV population is 57%, higher than in the general population (33%),(Saves *et al.*, 2003) and a smoking history of 30-40 pack-years is seen in the HIV population.(Benard *et al.*, 2007, Friis-Moller *et al.*, 2003) In particular, in the Women's Interagency HIV Study (WIHS) cohort study in the HIV population in the United States, female lung cancer patients with HIV infection were significantly more common than in the general population, showing the increased risk for lung cancer.(Levine *et al.*, 2010) Thus, smoking cessation programs need to be directed to the HIV population when infection is diagnosed. On the other hand, smoking is reported to be an independent risk factor for carcinogenesis in lung cancer.(Kirk *et al.*, 2007)

Recently, the National Cancer Institute reported that an annual low-dose computed tomography (CT) scan in the general population decreased lung cancer death by 80% by detecting the early stages of lung cancer.(Aberle *et al.*, 2010) In a study at Johns Hopkins University and associated hospitals, most of the 92 lung cancer patients with HIV infection died of lung cancer. Overall, 60% of the 32 patients who underwent chest radiography were not diagnosed as having lung cancer within a year. With regard to CT, 1 out of 28 patients was not diagnosed.(James, 2006) Smoking cessation and low-dose CT scans to detect the early stages of lung cancer would therefore be beneficial for HIV population.

Among other behavioral risk factors, intravenous drug users had been considered as a higher risk for developing lung cancer. However, the higher rate of smoking among intravenous drug users may be a confounding factor in some studies.

3.2 Immunosuppression as a risk factor

Immunodeficiency is a significant risk factor for carcinogenesis in some types of cancer. However, there is no evidence that decreased CD4 cell counts are associated with carcinogenesis in NADCs.(Clifford & Franceschi, 2007) In many case-control studies, the incidence of NADCs was not associated with the CDC classification (Table 2).

CD4 Cell Categories	Clinical Categories		
	A Asymptomatic, Acute HIV, or PGL	B Symptomatic Conditions, not A or C	C AIDS-Indicator Conditions
>500/µL	A1	B1	C1
200-500/µL	A2	B2	C2
< 200/µL	A3	B3	C3

CDC = U.S. Centers for Disease Control and Prevention; PGL = persistent generalized lymphadenopathy.

Table 2. CDC Classification System for HIV-Infected Adults and Adolescents

However, the incidence in HL, anal cancer, or hepatocellular carcinoma is affected by decreased CD4 cell counts. CD4 cell counts less than 200 cells/µL were associated with the incidence of NADCs (hazard ratio (HR), 1.67).(Powles *et al.*, 2009) CD4 cell counts increased by 100 cells/µL with the introduction of HAART, and the risk for NADCs decreased by 19%.(Bruyand *et al.*, 2009) However, carcinogenesis in lung cancer is not considered to be associated with immunological status (CD4 cell counts and viral load).(Kirk *et al.*, 2007, Spano *et al.*, 2004)

3.3 HIV as a risk factor

Many cases of carcinogenesis in HIV-related carcinomas are related to viruses such as Epstein Barr virus or Human Herpes virus-8. The International Agency for Research on Cancer (IARC), an agency of the World Health Organization (WHO), is examining the relationship between viruses and carcinogenesis, including: Epstein Barr virus for HL, NHL, nasopharyngeal carcinoma, and Burkitt's lymphoma; human herpes virus-8 for KS and primary effusion lymphoma; human papilloma virus for cervical, vulvar, and vaginal carcinoma, penile carcinoma, anal carcinoma, oral cavity carcinoma, and oropharyngeal and tonsillar carcinoma; hepatitis C virus for hepatocellular carcinoma and NHL; hepatitis B virus for hepatocellular carcinoma; and HIV for cervical and conjunctival squamous cell carcinoma, NHL, PCNSL, KS, and HL (particularly mixed cellularity and lymphocyte depleted subtypes). Of these, HIV is not organ-specific and is unique in that carcinogenesis occurs indirectly through immune suppression. Considering immunological status and infection, carcinomas accompanying HIV infection are classified into three categories: first, KS, NHL, and head and neck cancer, including AIDS-defining disease; second, NADC-IRs (infection-related), related to infection, hepatocellular carcinoma, HL, leiomyosarcoma, anal cancer, bladder cancer, laryngeal cancer, oral cavity cancer, penile cancer, gastric cancer, tongue cancer, and tonsillar cancer; and lastly, NADC-IURs (infection-unrelated), not related to infection, such as lung cancer and breast cancer.

Currently, carcinogenesis in lung cancer is considered not to be associated with HIV infection itself. On the other hand, microsatellite alternation resulting in genetic instability is seen in lung cancer patients with HIV infection.(Wistuba *et al.*, 1998) In another study, HIV-infected patients easily developed pulmonary disease because of decreased glutathione and antioxidant levels, as well as increased lysosome and chemokine ligand 5 (CCL5) levels in broncho-alveolar lavage fluid.(Agostini *et al.*, 1995, Allard *et al.*, 1998, Buhl *et al.*, 1989, Gordon *et al.*, 2005) Chronic inflammation is associated with carcinogenesis in lung cancer.(Buhl *et al.*, 1989) (Fig. 1) Furthermore, downregulation of HIV Tat-interacting protein

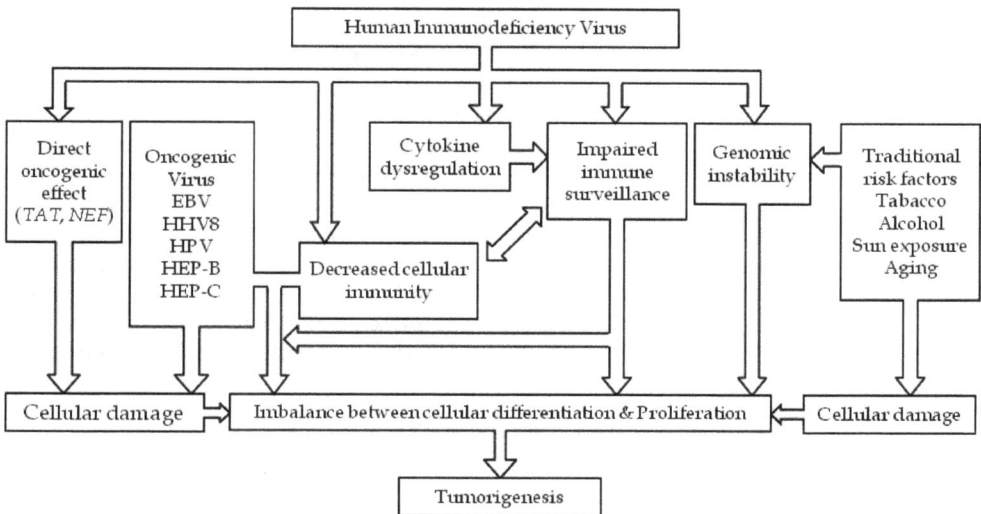

Fig. 1. Potential mechanisms for carcinogenesis in non-AIDS-defining cancer(Nguyen *et al.*)

30 (TIP30) has been verified to promote metastasis of lung cancer *in vitro* and in nude mice.(Baker *et al.*, 2000, Tong *et al.*, 2009) Thus, lung cancer in the HIV population tends to be aggressive with poor prognosis. Inhibiting HIV appears to inhibit carcinogenesis in lung cancer; however, there is no clear evidence of decreased incidence of lung cancer with the use of HAART. HAART reconstitutes immunity and decreases the risk of OIs.

4. Clinical manifestations

When compared to lung cancer in the general population, lung cancer in HIV-infected patients affects younger patients and is more aggressive. The median age of HIV-infected lung cancer patients is 45-50 years, while it is 62 years in the general population.(Spano *et al.*, 2004) With regard to the clinical stage of the lung cancer, 75-90% of all HIV-infected patients are advanced, 18-29% are in a locally advanced stage, and 50-68% are in the metastatic stage.(Lavole *et al.*, 2006) Adenocarcinoma is the most common (31-52%), followed by squamous cell carcinoma (17-39%), large cell carcinoma (3-16%), small cell carcinoma (SCLC) (1-14%), and bronchial alveolar carcinoma (less than 2%).(Tirelli *et al.*, 2000, Vyzula & Remick, 1996, Sridhar *et al.*, 1992, Alshafie *et al.*, 1997, D'Jaen *et al.*, 2010) This is similar to the distribution seen in the general population, as NSCLC accounts for 85% of all lung cancer patients in the general population. Comparing the pre-HAART era and the HAART era, the rate of adenocarcinoma was unchanged (48%), but the rate of squamous cell carcinoma was 21% in the pre-HAART era, as compared to 10% in the HAART era.(Brock *et al.*, 2006) Epidermal growth factor receptor (EGFR) mutation is a predictive factor for EGFR-tyrosine kinase inhibitors (EGFR-TKIs), and the incidence of harboring EGFR mutation among Asians is 30-35%, while it is ~10% among Caucasians.(Maemondo *et al.*, 2010, Mitsudomi *et al.*, 2009, Rosell *et al.*, 2009) A lung cancer patient harboring EGFR mutations with HIV infection has been reported.(Erickson *et al.*, 2008) CD4 cell counts at diagnosis range between 120 and 360 cells/μL,(Spano *et al.*, 2004, Tirelli *et al.*, 2000, Vyzula & Remick, 1996, Sridhar *et al.*, 1992, Brock *et al.*, 2006, Bedimo *et al.*, 2009, Tenholder & Jackson, 1993) while median CD4 cell counts in the HAART era are more than 300 cells/μL.

Overall, 25-50% of lung cancer patients with HIV infection had AIDS,(Alshafie *et al.*, 1997, Lavole *et al.*, 2006, Spano *et al.*, 2004, Sridhar *et al.*, 1992, Tirelli *et al.*, 2000, Vyzula & Remick, 1996) and 55% underwent HAART. The latency from diagnosis of HIV infection to the diagnosis of lung cancer differs by sex, being 4.1 years in women and 7.7 years in men (p=0.02). However, the gender-based difference has not been discussed.(Pakkala *et al.*, 2010) The frequency of metastatic organ involvement is uncertain. Release of interleukin-1 by intracerebral gp-120 components with HIV promotes brain metastasis *in vivo.*(Hodgson *et al.*, 1998) In the clinical setting, a patient with two intracerebral hemorrhages has been reported (the incidence of intratumoral hemorrhage in NSCLC is 0.52%).(Okuma *et al.*, 2010) Of note, HIV-infected patients have a higher risk of intracranial events(d'Arminio Monforte *et al.*, 2004); thus, careful follow-up is required for HIV-infected patients in clinical settings.

5. Multidisciplinary treatments & management

The fundamental modalities of treatment for lung cancer are surgery, radiotherapy, and chemotherapy.

SCLC is sensitive to both chemotherapy and radiotherapy; thus, radical concurrent chemoradiotherapy is indicated for limited-disease SCLC. When compared to NSCLC,

SCLC is characterized by higher grade, rapid progression with proliferation, and ease of metastasis to lymph nodes/distant organs in the early stage. Untreated, the median survival time is between 2 and 4 months. The response rate and median survival time in limited-disease SCLC are 70% and between 14 and 20 months, respectively. In extended-disease SCLC, chemotherapy is basic, and palliative radiotherapy is added according to the symptoms. The response rate in extended disease is 45-95%, and the median survival time is 7-10 months.(El Maalouf et al., 2007)

In NSCLC, radiotherapy or chemotherapy is less sensitive than SCLC. Radical surgery is limited in Stage I-III NSCLC, and palliative chemotherapy is indicated in Stage IV NSCLC, while surgery alone is for Stage IA, and surgery-based multidisciplinary treatment is required in Stage IB-III. A decision on the treatment strategy should take into account histology, age, performance status (PS), and co-morbidities. In Stage IV patients with poor PS (≥ 3) best supportive care is recommended. The 5-year survival is 50% in Stage IA, 43% in Stage IB, 36% in Stage IIA, 25% in Stage IIB, 19% in Stage IIIA, 7% in Stage IIIB, and 2% in Stage IV. The median survival time is 14 months in Stage III and 10 months in Stage IV.(Goldstraw et al., 2007)

In the period before the advent of HAART, HIV-infected patients were considered to have decreased immune competence of lymphocytes or CD4 cell counts because of accompanying complications or fragility to treatment. Toxicity and tolerance data in the treatment of other cancers are available. No fewer than 25% of advanced cancer patients with HIV infection were not treated,(Achenbach et al.) and among NSCLC patients with HIV infection, initial treatment consisted of chemotherapy in 31%, radiotherapy in 23%, and both in 15%.(D'Jaen et al., 2010)

5.1 Surgery

Surgery is a promising modality of treatment for Stage I and II NSCLC, and is the first-line choice of treatment for all operable patients. In previous reports, patients with CD4 cell counts of more than 500 cells/μL were considered operable, while in those with lower CD4 cell counts, the indication for surgery needed careful consideration. The treatment of HIV-infected lung cancer patients at present, however, should follow the standard of care for safety and efficacy, as their prognosis depends on their lung cancer, not their HIV status. Moreover, complications, such as cardiovascular diseases and interstitial pneumonia associated with cigarette smoking, need to be taken into account, because more of these patients have a history of smoking.(Aberg, 2009)

With surgery, a reported case series did not demonstrate an increased risk of postoperative complications because of CD4 cell counts or immunological status.(Massera et al., 2000) Thus, the indication for surgery in HIV-infected lung cancer patients should be determined based on pulmonary function, PS, and staging, as in the general population. Furthermore, the prognosis of such patients is good.(Spano et al., 2004) In addition, the clinician should consider the medical staff's perioperative risk for blood-borne infection and ensure that standard precautions are taken. The reported blood-borne infection rate associated with surgery ranges from 0.2-0.5%.(Bell, 1997)

In determining the clinical stage, 18F-fluorodeoxyglucose-positoron emission tomography-computed tomography (PET-CT) scan is a highly sensitive and specific examination. However, prudent assessment with regard to lymph nodal diagnosis is needed in the HIV population because of potential false positive to lymph nodes and upstaging in anal cancer.(Cotter et al., 2006)

With respect to adjuvant chemotherapy (postoperative chemotherapy) for patients with NSCLC, a 13% decrease in the risk of death was demonstrated with chemotherapy (HR 0.87, 95%CI 0.74-1.02, p=0.08) in 1995.(Non-small Cell Lung Cancer Collaborative Group, 1995) This rate is equivalent to a 5% improvement in the 5-year survival rate. In later studies, a 5-15% improvement in the 5-year survival rate was demonstrated (HR 0.89, 95%CI 0.82-0.96, p=0.005) in NSCLC patients with Stage II-IIIA with cisplatin-based chemotherapy.(Pignon *et al.*, 2008) However, as described later, toxicity, efficacy and prognostic factors for HIV-infected lung cancer patients are uncertain.

5.2 Radiotherapy

The role of radiotherapy in HIV-infected lung cancer patients is uncertain. In general, radiation therapy for ether ADCs or NADCs leads to severe mucosal toxicity in acute phase and late-phase disturbances, even when low-dose radiation is used. In KS patients who undergo thoracic irradiation, esophagitis occurs frequently and is often severe.(Chak *et al.*, 1988, Cooper *et al.*, 1984) The mechanism of the more severe mucositis is considered to be related to decreased mucosal restoration due to a shortage of glutathione antioxidant(Buhl *et al.*, 1989, Vallis, 1991) or to be related to OIs (Fungi, Candida species, herpes, cytomegalovirus, and Cryptococcus infections).(Boal *et al.*, 1979, Rodriguez *et al.*, 1989)

In the patient with good PS or without weight loss, unresectable locoregionally advanced NSCLC or limited-disease SCLC, the standard of care is concurrent chemoradiotherapy. The 3-year survival rate in unresectable locoregionally advanced NSCLC is around 10% with radiotherapy alone, and at present, the 3-year survival rate improves by more than 25% with concurrent platinum-based chemoradiotherapy.(Blackstock & Govindan, 2007) Concurrent chemoradiotherapy is more effective but more toxic than sequential chemoradiotherapy. At present, it is recommended that HIV-infected lung cancer patients be treated with the same standard care as the general population. However, aggressive treatment requires consideration of the risk of interactions between antiretroviral agents and antitumor agents, and fragility to treatment and safety of chemoradiotherapy are uncertain. A reported case having locally advanced squamous cell lung cancer, concurrently treated with nelfinavir and 5 species of HAART and intensity modulated radiotherapy, died of massive hemoptysis because of bronchial perforation, whereas pathological complete response (CR) was achieved with intensity modulated radiotherapy at a dose of 20 Gy.(Chapman *et al.*, 2009) In a phase I study involving pancreatic cancer patients with HIV infection, a radiosensitizing effect with nelfinavir was reported.(Brunner *et al.*, 2008)

Conformal radiotherapy is appropriate, as in the general population, because of narrowing of the irradiation fields. Palliative radiotherapy is indicated according to symptoms in Stage IV.

5.3 Chemotherapy

With regard to chemotherapy, adjuvant chemotherapy is used for Stage IB-IIIA NSCLC, concomitant chemoradiotherapy is given in locoregionally advanced NSCLC, and palliative chemotherapy is given in Stage IV.(Azzoli *et al.*, 2009) In the meta-analysis of Stage IV NSCLC, which accounts for 40% of all lung cancer, platinum doublet chemotherapy prolonged the median survival to 1.5-2.8 months and improved the 1-year survival rate to 10%.(Non-small Cell Lung Cancer Collaborative Group, 2008, Grilli *et al.*, 1993, Marino *et al.*, 1994, Souquet *et al.*, 1993) Chemotherapy significantly improved survival, with a HR of 0.73 (p<0.0001) in 1995.(Kivisto *et al.*, 1995) In 2008, the same group reported the results of a meta-analysis of 16 randomized studies, and chemotherapy showed a survival benefit with an HR of 0.73 (95% CI 0.71-0.83, p < 0.0001) again. On the other hand, the survival benefit is no different between 1995 and later studies (p = 0.77) (Non-small Cell Lung Cancer Collaborative Group, 2008). However, the survival time has gradually improved because of trials with novel antitumor drugs that were excluded from this meta-analysis and diversification of treatment strategies. As the population with HIV infection is excluded from clinical trials, information regarding the efficacy and safety of chemotherapy in these patients is limited to retrospective reports.

5.3.1 Chemotherapy for metastatic stage in patients with HIV infection

5.3.1.1 Front-line setting

Chemotherapy is more frequently used for advanced lung cancer in HIV-infected patients because 75-90% of lung cancer patients with HIV infection have advanced disease.(Lavole *et al.*, 2006, Lavole *et al.*, 2009, Cadranel *et al.*, 2006) However, the benefit of chemotherapy is questionable, as the prospective clinical benefits and toxicities have not been realistically evaluated. In a phase II prospective study with carboplatin and gemcitabine combination chemotherapy followed by paclitaxel maintenance therapy involving 47 patients consisting mainly of lung cancer patients with poor PS (2 or 3) and immunologically fragile patients, including HIV infection and post-bone marrow transplantation, tolerance and efficacy were demonstrated to be adequate.(Bridges *et al.*, 2008) Previous reports have concluded that the benefit of chemotherapy was controversial, but the prognosis of NSCLC patients with HIV infection treated with chemotherapy was reported to be the same as the prognosis of the general population with NSCLC. D'Jean *et al.* reported that, among HIV-infected lung cancer patients, 81% (taxanes 45%, gemcitabine 26%, vinca alkaloid 10%) were treated with platinum-doublet chemotherapy in the front-line setting. Patients treated with singlet chemotherapy or oral antitumor agents outside of standard regimens were 3% each.(Previous study, 2010) Elderly lung cancer patients and lung cancer patients with poor PS in the general population have a poorer prognosis with chemotherapy and singlet chemotherapy, not platinum-doublet chemotherapy, is generally recommended.(D'Addario *et al.*, 2009) Among lung cancer patients with HIV infection, PS is poor (before 1996, 37~57% of patients had PS of more than 2; after 1996, this decreased to less than 30% of patients)(Spano *et al.*, 2004) Thus, for treatment of fragile patients, chemotherapy would be applied to lung cancer patients with HIV infection.

Current standard chemotherapy for advanced NSCLC is based on platinum doublet (cisplatin or carboplatin) plus third-generation antitumor drugs (irinotecan, docetaxel, gemcitabine, vinorelbine, paclitaxel,(Schiller *et al.*, 2002, Kelly *et al.*, 2001, Ohe *et al.*, 2007) and pemetrexed(Scagliotti *et al.*, 2008)) or EGFR-TKIs; gefitinib(Maemondo *et al.*, 2010, Mitsudomi *et al.*, 2009) and erlotinib(Rosell *et al.*, 2009), and an antiangiogenic inhibitor (bevacizumab).(Sandler *et al.*, 2006) Maintenance therapy with pemetrexed(Ciuleanu *et al.*, 2009) and erlotinib(Cappuzzo *et al.*, 2010) is known to prolong survival. In SCLC, platinum and etoposide or irinotecan combination therapy is used.(Murray & Turrisi, 2006) For relapsed SCLC, amrubicin or topotecan is given. In locally advanced NSCLC and limited disease (LD) SCLC, thoracic irradiation is added. D'Jean *et al.* reported that, among HIV-infected lung cancer patients, the agents combined with platinum agents were topoisomerase in 67%, vinca alkaloid in 22%, and taxanes in 11%. The response rate to front-line chemotherapy was 39% in 41 patients. Of the treated patients, 63% had adverse events, and 34% were Grade 3/4. Treatment-related deaths were seen in 2 patients (0.05%); 1 with pneumonitis, and 1 from an unknown cause.(Previous study, 2010)

5.3.1.2 Second-line setting

Overall, 60% of lung cancer patients treated with front-line chemotherapy proceed to second-line chemotherapy. In NSCLC patients with good PS, the standard of care is docetaxel (Shepherd *et al.*, 2001, Fossella *et al.*, 2000), pemetrexed(Hanna *et al.*, 2004) and erlotinib.(Shepherd *et al.*, 2005) Docetaxel is indicated for all histological types of NSCLC. Pemetrexed is expected to be active for non-squamous cell histology.(Scagliotti *et al.*, 2009) Erlotinib is effective for both patients harboring EGFR mutation and EGFR wild-type,(Ciuleanu *et al.*, 2010) although the response rate and survival time differ between them. Platinum doublet chemotherapy or non-platinum doublet chemotherapy is not anticipated to have efficacy in the second-line setting.(Azzoli *et al.*, 2009) For SCLC, intravenous or oral topotecan,(Eckardt *et al.*, 2007, von Pawel *et al.*, 1999) amrubicin,(Inoue *et al.*, 2008, Onoda *et al.*, 2006) and carboplatin and paclitaxel, re-treatment for sensitive-relapse cases are considered.(Giaccone *et al.*, 1987, Postmus *et al.*, 1987, Groen *et al.*, 1999) In the HIV population, details concerning second-line chemotherapy in Stage IV are uncertain. The rates of HIV-infected lung cancer patients treated with second-line chemotherapy in HIV population were 32% (17/53) in NSCLC and 10% (1/9) in SCLC. The response rate in this study was 11%, as in the general population.(D'Jaen *et al.*, 2010)

5.3.1.3 Molecular targeted agents

The understanding of cancer at the molecular level is profound, and proteins playing significant roles in tumor proliferation, invasion, and metastasis have been identified. As a result, molecular targeted inhibitors or antibodies for these proteins have recently been developed. Of these, drugs targeting EGFR, vascular endothelial growth factor (VEGF), and echinoderm microtubule-associated protein-like 4-anaplastic lymphoma kinase translocation (EML4-ALK)(Kwak *et al.*, 2010) have been shown to be efficacious. EGFR-targeted drugs have particularly strong evidence supporting their use. In NSCLC harboring EGFR mutation in the general population, use of EGFR-TKIs doubles survival.(Mitsudomi *et al.*, 2009, Maemondo *et al.*, 2010, Rosell *et al.*, 2009) Thus, despite the potential for drug interactions, use of EGFR-TKIs is indicated in HIV-infected patients. Though no drug interactions are expected, prudence is required from the perspective of cost and safety.

5.3.2 Pharmacodynamic interactions between HAART & cytotoxic antitumor agents

HAART reconstructs immunity and decreases risk of OIs to inhibit HIV viral load and increase CD4 cell counts for patients infected with HIV. The goal for HAART is to continuously suppress the viral load to undetectable and maintain CD4 cell counts above 500 cells/μL.(Silverberg *et al.*, 2007) However, decreases in antiretroviral agent concentrations can exacerbate clinical status, and increased/decreased concentrations of antitumor agents lead to severe toxicity or reduced antitumor effects. Both increases and decreases in serum concentrations can occur for either/both antiretroviral agents and/or cytotoxic antitumor agents.(Kivisto *et al.*, 1995) Therefore, decreased effectiveness and increased toxicity of chemotherapy must be considered. In addition, failure of virological treatment may occur. Interactions between antiretroviral agents and chemotherapeutic agents must always be considered and are a cause for concern for oncologists in clinical settings.

	Expected chemotherapeutic concentration modifications based on antiretroviral drugs used						Expected interactions between HAART and chemotherapy
	NRTI	NNRTI	PI	INSTI	FI	MVC	
Platinum	→	→	→	→	→	→	Hematological toxicity with ZDV, Neuropathy, Nephropathy with TDF
Taxanes	→	↓	↑	→	→	→	Hematological toxicity with ZDV Neuropathy with d4T and DDI
Etoposide	→	↓	↑	→	→	→	Hematological toxicity with ZDV
Gemcitabine	→	→	→	→	→	→	Hematological toxicity with ZDV Nephropathy with TDF
Pemetrexed	→	→	→	→	→	→	Hematological toxicity with ZDV
Topotecan	→	→	→	→	→	→	Hematological toxicity with ZDV
Irinotecan	→	↓	↑	→	→	→	Hematological toxicity with ZDV
Gefitinib Erlotinib	→	↓	↑	→	→	→	None
Bevacizumab	→	→	→	→	→	→	None

INSTI: integrase strand transfar inhibitor; FI: fusion inhibitor; MVC: maraviroc; ZDV: zidovudine; TDF: tenofovir; ddI: didanosine

Table 3. Expected drug interactions between antiretroviral agents and antitumor agents commonly used in NSCLC and SCLC.(Makinson *et al.*, 2010)

However, the available pharmacokinetic data for antiretroviral drugs and antitumor agents are not predictive: 1. available pharmacokinetic data are limited to case reports, and limited individual data cannot be generalized; 2. antitumor agents of a similar class can have variable pharmacokinetics; and 3. unexpected drug interactions can occur because metabolism by CYP450 is associated with single nucleotide polymorphisms (SNPs).

Antiretroviral agents are classified into six categories: nucleoside reverse transcriptase inhibitors (NRTIs); non-nucleoside reverse transcriptase inhibitors (NNRTIs); protease inhibitors (PIs); integrase inhibitors; fusion inhibitor enfuvirtide; and C-C chemokine receptor type 5 (CCR5) coreceptor antagonists. Interactions among these during treatment for ADCs, such as PCNSL or KS, enhance adverse toxicities. For instance, KS patients with CD4 cell counts greater than 200 cells/μL are reported to have a good response to paclitaxel treatment, with the same prognosis as patients with a normal immunological status.

Drug interaction between antiretroviral agents and antitumor agents is assumed when the drug is metabolized by CYP450 pathway. Many PIs and NNRTIs are metabolized by this pathway, and competitive metabolism between antitumor drugs must be considered. (Table 3) Increases in toxicity between antiretroviral agents and antitumor agents have been reported. Among NNRTIs, efavirenz increases toxicity with concomitant use of vinka alkaloids and taxanes.(Makinson *et al.*, 2010) All NRTIs and most PIs have increased drug sensitivities *in vitro*, and this leads to increased toxicity. The NRTIs efavirenz, delavirdine, and nevirapine are primarily metabolized by CYP450.(Gulick, 1998, Flexner, 1998) In a study of patients with NHL undergoing treatment with concomitant antiretroviral agents and cyclophosphamide, doxorubicin, and etoposide, significantly lower nadir neutrophil counts were seen. As compared to the group with/without PIs, the group with PIs had greater toxicity (48% vs. 27%; p=0.0025). Drug interactions have also been confirmed *in vitro*; cultured cells that expressed P-glycoprotein (P-gp) accumulated increased concentrations of paclitaxel or vinblastine concomitant with PIs.(Washington *et al.*, 1998) PIs such as ritonavir and indinavir have a strong affinity for CYP450 and also strongly inhibit CYP3A4. These enzymes are used in metabolic pathways with ifosfamide, docetaxel, paclitaxel, irinotecan, vinka alkaloids, and etoposide.(Rowinsky & Donehower, 1997, Stebbing & Bower, 2006) Severe myelosuppression with atazanavir(Richman *et al.*, 1987, Tan & Ratner, 1997) and peripheral neuropathy with didanosine, stavudine, and zalcitabine occur.(Rowinsky & Donehower, 1997) Thus, their combined use with platinum or paclitaxel leads to increased toxicities. Combination treatment with irinotecan and atazanavir is also contraindicated. Cisplatin, the key drug in lung cancer chemotherapy,(Azzoli *et al.*, 2009, Barlesi & Pujol, 2005) is not metabolized by the CYP450 enzyme pathway. Thus, drug interactions with HAART do not occur, but accumulating toxicity, such as nephrotoxicity and neurotoxicity, must be considered. In addition, patients on antiretroviral agents having nephrotoxicity such as tenofovir disoproxil require careful follow-up.

Of the molecular targeted agents, EGFR-TKIs have been poorly evaluated, but they are known to be metabolized by CYP3A4, and ritonavir should be avoided. Raltegravir is metabolized by UGT1A1 (uridine diphosphate glucuronosyl transferase isoform 1) and does not induce or inhibit hepatic enzymes; thus, drug interactions appear to be absent. Maraviroc, a CCR5 antagonist, also does not interact with CYP3A4. As for PIs, indinavir and sequinavir inhibit cell proliferation or invasion by acting through matrix metalloprotease.(Toschi *et al.*, 2011) Due to the increased toxicity of such drug interactions, the drugs that are better to apply in HAART regimens with antiretroviral drug are those not associated with CYP450, such as NRTI, raltegravir, or enfuvirtide.

In the future, dose adjustments will be used to investigate Pharmacokinetic data via a prospective study; however, the prognosis of lung cancer patients with HIV infection is anticipated to be similar to that in the general population. Thus, conventional doses and regimens are adequate.

5.3.3 Prevention of opportunistic infections & potential complications

An increased risk of OIs is considered to be a complication of chemotherapy because of the associated decrease in CD4 cell counts. In lung cancer patients, changes in CD4 cell counts with chemotherapy are unclear. However, previous reports on treatment for ADCs provide information about changes in CD4 cell counts. CD4 cell counts in NHL on chemotherapy decreased to 50% of baseline at the nadir and recovered within a month. CD4 cell counts and viral load do not change with chemotherapeutic treatment.(Powles *et al.*, 2002) In addition, in ADCs, CD4 cell counts in patients receiving concomitant HAART or HIV viral load-negative patients are considered to recover sooner.(Powles *et al.*, 2002, Hakim *et al.*, 1997) OIs on chemotherapy occurred in 8 of 25 patients (32%), and their CD4 cell counts were less than 150 cells/μL. These patients also had poor PS, and half of the patients developed Grade 3 or 4 hematological toxicity.(Tirelli *et al.*, 2000) Recent few reports have discussed the occurrence of OIs during chemotherapy. Primary prevention of OIs is adequate; no specific preventive therapies are necessary in patients with a well-controlled viral load. Generally, in patients with less than 200 cells/μL, trimethoprim-sulfamethoxazole or pentamidine inhalation is used for pneumocystis pneumonia prevention, and in patients with less than 50 cells/μL, a macrolide is used for Mycobacteriaum avium complex (MAC) prevention. Thus, a monthly CD4 cell count check is preferred during chemotherapy and one month after treatment.

5.4 Supportive care

In supportive care, drug interactions between antiretroviral agents and other agents must be considered (Table 4). However, in clinical settings, physicians must administer palliative therapy. Interactions between morphine and some HAART drugs have been shown, but the benefit of morphine for palliation remains. In Stage IV NSCLC, early induction of palliative therapy after diagnosis significantly improves quality of life and mood, and prolongs survival by 2 months.(Temel et al., 2010) As in patients from the general population, early palliative therapy is indicated for HIV-infected patients, as well as psychological support at the end-stage. As for the lung cancer patients with bone metastasis, zoledronic acid, a new bisphosphonate, is an appropriate palliative treatment for skeletal-related events (SREs) and symptoms associated with bone metastases.(Rosen et al., 2003a, Rosen et al., 2003b) The efficacy and safety of zoledronic acid given concomitantly with HAART for the osteoporosis that is associated with long-term HAART administration have been evaluated in a clinical trial and found to be advantageous.(Bolland et al., 2008, Bolland et al., 2007, Huang et al., 2009) When SREs occur, they are associated with decreased activities of daily living and shorter survival.(Tsuya et al., 2007) Thus, zoledronic acid should be given to patients with bone metastases of lung cancer, even asymptomatic.

	Expected concentration modifications in drugs used supportive care based on antiretroviral drugs used					
	NRTI	NNRTI	PI	INSTI	FI	MVC
Dexamethasone	→	↓	↓	→	→	→
Lorazepam	→	↓	↑	→	→	→
Tricyclic antidepressants	→	→	↑	→	→	→
Fentanyl	→	→	↑	→	→	→
Carbamazepine	→	↓	↓	→	→	→

Table 4. Expected drug interactions between antiretroviral agents and frequently used supportive agents for chemotherapy.

6. Prognosis

Lung cancer patients with HIV infections are considered to have a poorer prognosis than the general population because of their younger age, immunodeficiency, aggressive extension, and more advanced stage at diagnosis. In a meta-analysis, the median survival time was 5-9 months.(Powles et al., 2003, Karp et al., 1993, Sridhar et al., 1992, Tirelli et al., 2000, Spano et al., 2004, Alshafie et al., 1997) The 1-year survival of HIV-infected lung cancer patients was 10% (0-15%), as compared to 40% (20-50%) in the general population.(Cadranel et al., 2006, Cinti et al., 2008, Grubb et al., 2006, Vyzula & Remick, 1996) Over the last 20 years, survival by histology was about 7 months in SCLC and 5 months in NSCLC.(Hakimian et al., 2007) Favorable prognostic factors are reported to be good PS and early stage at diagnosis. The concomitant use of HAART is controversial as a prognostic factor. The reason for these patients' poor prognosis is considered to be their more advanced stage at diagnosis.(Lavole et al., 2009)

CD4 cell count is sometimes considered to be a prognostic factor for chemotherapy. The prognosis for patients with a CD4 cell count greater than 200 cells/µL is 11.5 months, while that for patients with a CD4 cell count less than 200 cells/µL is 3.4 months.(Hakimian et al., 2007) At present, patients with CD4 cell counts greater than 200 cells/µL can be given chemotherapy, and they have been demonstrated to have the comparable survival to non-HIV patients. (Hakimian et al., 2007)

7. Future directions

Lung cancer has become common in HIV-infected patients and appears to be increasing in clinical settings, and NADCs have become the main cause of death. Thus, lung cancer has significant clinical meaning in the management of HIV-infected patients. Knowledge about its epidemiology, screening, risk factors, and intervention will reduce the incidence of lung cancer. In particular, aggressively promoting smoking cessation programs and screening for lung cancer for earlier detection will play important roles as strategies in preventing lung cancer.

HIV-infected patients should receive standard care for lung cancer, and it is anticipated that they will have the same prognosis as the general population. However, for these patients, we need to consider previously reported toxicities and fragility to treatment. In addition, increased intensity of treatment due to drug interactions and increased radiosensitization with HAART must be considered. As the clinical details of such patients have not been well reported, infectious disease physicians and oncologists must collaborate when treating HIV-infected lung cancer patients.

8. References

Aberg, J.A. (2009). Cardiovascular complications in HIV management: past, present, and future. *J Acquir Immune Defic Syndr*, Vol.50, No.1, pp. 54-64

Aberle, D.R., Berg, C.D., Black, W.C. et al. (2010). The National Lung Screening Trial: overview and study design. *Radiology*, Vol.258, No.1, pp. 243-253

Achenbach, C.J., Cole, S.R., Kitahata, M.M. et al. Mortality after cancer diagnosis in HIV-infected individuals treated with antiretroviral therapy. *AIDS*, pp.

Agostini, C., Sancetta, R., Cerutti, A. et al. (1995). Alveolar macrophages as a cell source of cytokine hyperproduction in HIV-related interstitial lung disease. *J Leukoc Biol*, Vol.58, No.5, pp. 495-500

Allard, J.P., Aghdassi, E., Chau, J. et al. (1998). Oxidative stress and plasma antioxidant micronutrients in humans with HIV infection. *Am J Clin Nutr*, Vol.67, No.1, pp. 143-147

Alshafie, M.T., Donaldson, B. & Oluwole, S.F. (1997). Human immunodeficiency virus and lung cancer. *Br J Surg*, Vol.84, No.8, pp. 1068-1071

Azzoli, C.G., Baker, S., Jr., Temin, S. et al. (2009). American Society of Clinical Oncology Clinical Practice Guideline update on chemotherapy for stage IV non-small-cell lung cancer. *J Clin Oncol*, Vol.27, No.36, pp. 6251-6266

Baker, M.E., Yan, L. & Pear, M.R. (2000). Three-dimensional model of human TIP30, a coactivator for HIV-1 Tat-activated transcription, and CC3, a protein associated with metastasis suppression. *Cell Mol Life Sci*, Vol.57, No.5, pp. 851-858

Barlesi, F. & Pujol, J.L. (2005). Combination of chemotherapy without platinum compounds in the treatment of advanced non-small cell lung cancer: a systematic review of phase III trials. *Lung Cancer*, Vol.49, No.3, pp. 289-298

Bedimo, R.J., Mcginnis, K.A., Dunlap, M. et al. (2009). Incidence of non-AIDS-defining malignancies in HIV-infected versus noninfected patients in the HAART era: impact of immunosuppression. *J Acquir Immune Defic Syndr*, Vol.52, No.2, pp. 203-208

Bell, D.M. (1997). Occupational risk of human immunodeficiency virus infection in healthcare workers: an overview. *Am J Med*, Vol.102, No.5B, pp. 9-15

Benard, A., Bonnet, F., Tessier, J.F. et al. (2007). Tobacco addiction and HIV infection: toward the implementation of cessation programs. ANRS CO3 Aquitaine Cohort. *AIDS Patient Care STDS*, Vol.21, No.7, pp. 458-468

Bertolaccini, L., Lybéris, P., Soncini, S. et al. (2008). Clinical characteristic lung cancer in HIV-infected patients. *Cancer Therapy*, Vol.6, pp. 903-906

Blackstock, A.W. & Govindan, R. (2007). Definitive chemoradiation for the treatment of locally advanced non small-cell lung cancer. *J Clin Oncol*, Vol.25, No.26, pp. 4146-4152

Boal, D.K., Newburger, P.E. & Teele, R.L. (1979). Esophagitis induced by combined radiation and adriamycin. *AJR Am J Roentgenol*, Vol.132, No.4, pp. 567-570

Bolland, M.J., Grey, A.B., Horne, A.M. et al. (2008). Effects of intravenous zoledronate on bone turnover and BMD persist for at least 24 months. *J Bone Miner Res*, Vol.23, No.8, pp. 1304-1308

Bolland, M.J., Grey, A.B., Horne, A.M. et al. (2007). Annual zoledronate increases bone density in highly active antiretroviral therapy-treated human immunodeficiency virus-infected men: a randomized controlled trial. *J Clin Endocrinol Metab*, Vol.92, No.4, pp. 1283-1288

Bonnet, F., Burty, C., Lewden, C. et al. (2009). Changes in cancer mortality among HIV-infected patients: the Mortalite 2005 Survey. *Clin Infect Dis*, Vol.48, No.5, pp. 633-639

Bower, M., Powles, T., Nelson, M. et al. (2003). HIV-related lung cancer in the era of highly active antiretroviral therapy. *AIDS*, Vol.17, No.3, pp. 371-375

Bridges, B.B., Thomas, L., Hausner, P.F. et al. (2008). Phase II trial of gemcitabine/carboplatin followed by paclitaxel in patients with performance status=2,3 or other significant co-morbidity (HIV infection or s/p organ transplantation) in advanced non-small cell lung cancer. *Lung Cancer*, Vol.61, No.1, pp. 61-66

Brock, M.V., Hooker, C.M., Engels, E.A. et al. (2006). Delayed diagnosis and elevated mortality in an urban population with HIV and lung cancer: implications for patient care. *J Acquir Immune Defic Syndr*, Vol.43, No.1, pp. 47-55

Brunner, T.B., Geiger, M., Grabenbauer, G.G. et al. (2008). Phase I trial of the human immunodeficiency virus protease inhibitor nelfinavir and chemoradiation for locally advanced pancreatic cancer. *J Clin Oncol*, Vol.26, No.16, pp. 2699-2706

Bruyand, M., Thiebaut, R., Lawson-Ayayi, S. et al. (2009). Role of uncontrolled HIV RNA level and immunodeficiency in the occurrence of malignancy in HIV-infected patients during the combination antiretroviral therapy era: Agence Nationale de Recherche sur le Sida (ANRS) CO3 Aquitaine Cohort. *Clin Infect Dis*, Vol.49, No.7, pp. 1109-1116

Buhl, R., Jaffe, H.A., Holroyd, K.J. et al. (1989). Systemic glutathione deficiency in symptom-free HIV-seropositive individuals. *Lancet*, Vol.2, No.8675, pp. 1294-1298

Cadranel, J., Garfield, D., Lavole, A. et al. (2006). Lung cancer in HIV infected patients: facts, questions and challenges. *Thorax*, Vol.61, No.11, pp. 1000-1008

Cappuzzo, F., Ciuleanu, T., Stelmakh, L. et al. (2010). Erlotinib as maintenance treatment in advanced non-small-cell lung cancer: a multicentre, randomised, placebo-controlled phase 3 study. *Lancet Oncol,* Vol.11, No.6, pp. 521-529

Chak, L.Y., Gill, P.S., Levine, A.M. et al. (1988). Radiation therapy for acquired immunodeficiency syndrome-related Kaposi's sarcoma. *J Clin Oncol,* Vol.6, No.5, pp. 863-867

Chapman, C.H., Shen, J., Filion, E.J. et al. (2009). Marked tumor response and fatal hemoptysis during radiation for lung cancer in a human immunodeficiency virus-positive patient taking nelfinavir. *J Thorac Oncol,* Vol.4, No.12, pp. 1587-1589

Cinti, S.K., Gandhi, T. & Riddell, J.T. (2008). Non-AIDS-defining cancers: should antiretroviral therapy be initiated earlier? *AIDS Read,* Vol.18, No.1, pp. 18-20, 26-32

Ciuleanu, T., Brodowicz, T., Zielinski, C. et al. (2009). Maintenance pemetrexed plus best supportive care versus placebo plus best supportive care for non-small-cell lung cancer: a randomised, double-blind, phase 3 study. *Lancet,* Vol.374, No.9699, pp. 1432-1440

Ciuleanu, T., Stelmakh, L., Cicenas, S. et al. (2010). LBOA5 - Erlotinib versus docetaxel or pemetrexed as second-line therapy in patients with advanced non-small-cell lung cancer (NSCLC) and poor prognosis: efficacy and safety results from the phase III TITAN study. *2010 Chicago Multidisciplinary Symposium in Thoracic Oncology,* Vol.*Abstract*, pp.

Clifford, G. & Franceschi, S. (2007). Immunity, infection, and cancer. *Lancet,* Vol.370, No.9581, pp. 6-7

Cooper, J.S., Fried, P.R. & Laubenstein, L.J. (1984). Initial observations of the effect of radiotherapy on epidemic Kaposi's sarcoma. *JAMA,* Vol.252, No.7, pp. 934-935

Cotter, S.E., Grigsby, P.W., Siegel, B.A. et al. (2006). FDG-PET/CT in the evaluation of anal carcinoma. *Int J Radiat Oncol Biol Phys,* Vol.65, No.3, pp. 720-725

Crum-Cianflone, N., Hullsiek, K.H., Marconi, V. et al. (2009). Trends in the incidence of cancers among HIV-infected persons and the impact of antiretroviral therapy: a 20-year cohort study. *AIDS,* Vol.23, No.1, pp. 41-50

D'addario, G., Fruh, M., Reck, M. et al. Metastatic non-small-cell lung cancer: ESMO Clinical Practice Guidelines for diagnosis, treatment and follow-up. *Ann Oncol,* Vol.21 Suppl 5, pp. v116-119

D'arminio Monforte, A., Cinque, P., Mocroft, A. et al. (2004). Changing incidence of central nervous system diseases in the EuroSIDA cohort. *Ann Neurol,* Vol.55, No.3, pp. 320-328

D'jaen, G.A., Pantanowitz, L., Bower, M. et al. (2010). Human immunodeficiency virus-associated primary lung cancer in the era of highly active antiretroviral therapy: a multi-institutional collaboration. *Clin Lung Cancer,* Vol.11, No.6, pp. 396-404

Eckardt, J.R., Von Pawel, J., Pujol, J.L. et al. (2007). Phase III study of oral compared with intravenous topotecan as second-line therapy in small-cell lung cancer. *J Clin Oncol,* Vol.25, No.15, pp. 2086-2092

El Maalouf, G., Rodier, J.M., Faivre, S. et al. (2007). Could we expect to improve survival in small cell lung cancer? *Lung Cancer,* Vol.57 Suppl 2, pp. S30-34

Engels, E.A., Biggar, R.J., Hall, H.I. et al. (2008). Cancer risk in people infected with human immunodeficiency virus in the United States. *Int J Cancer,* Vol.123, No.1, pp. 187-194

Engels, E.A., Brock, M.V., Chen, J. et al. (2006). Elevated incidence of lung cancer among HIV-infected individuals. *J Clin Oncol*, Vol.24, No.9, pp. 1383-1388

Erickson, T.M., Koeppe, J.R., Miller, Y.E. et al. (2008). Bronchioloalveolar carcinoma presenting as chronic progressive pulmonary infiltrates in a woman with HIV: a diagnosis worth making. *J Thorac Oncol*, Vol.3, No.11, pp. 1353-1355

Flexner, C. (1998). HIV-protease inhibitors. *N Engl J Med*, Vol.338, No.18, pp. 1281-1292

Fossella, F.V., Devore, R., Kerr, R.N. et al. (2000). Randomized phase III trial of docetaxel versus vinorelbine or ifosfamide in patients with advanced non-small-cell lung cancer previously treated with platinum-containing chemotherapy regimens. The TAX 320 Non-Small Cell Lung Cancer Study Group. *J Clin Oncol*, Vol.18, No.12, pp. 2354-2362

Friis-Moller, N., Weber, R., Reiss, P. et al. (2003). Cardiovascular disease risk factors in HIV patients--association with antiretroviral therapy. Results from the DAD study. *AIDS*, Vol.17, No.8, pp. 1179-1193

Frisch, M., Biggar, R.J., Engels, E.A. et al. (2001). Association of cancer with AIDS-related immunosuppression in adults. *JAMA*, Vol.285, No.13, pp. 1736-1745

Frisch, M. & Hjalgrim, H. (1999). Re: Nonmelanomatous skin cancer following cervical, vaginal, and vulvar neoplasms: etiologic association. *J Natl Cancer Inst*, Vol.91, No.6, pp. 565-566

Giaccone, G., Ferrati, P., Donadio, M. et al. (1987). Reinduction chemotherapy in small cell lung cancer. *Eur J Cancer Clin Oncol*, Vol.23, No.11, pp. 1697-1699

Goldstraw, P., Crowley, J., Chansky, K. et al. (2007). The IASLC Lung Cancer Staging Project: proposals for the revision of the TNM stage groupings in the forthcoming (seventh) edition of the TNM Classification of malignant tumours. *J Thorac Oncol*, Vol.2, No.8, pp. 706-714

Gordon, S.B., Janoff, E.N., Sloper, D. et al. (2005). HIV-1 infection is associated with altered innate pulmonary immunity. *J Infect Dis*, Vol.192, No.8, pp. 1412-1416

Grilli, R., Oxman, A.D. & Julian, J.A. (1993). Chemotherapy for advanced non-small-cell lung cancer: how much benefit is enough? *J Clin Oncol*, Vol.11, No.10, pp. 1866-1872

Groen, H.J., Fokkema, E., Biesma, B. et al. (1999). Paclitaxel and carboplatin in the treatment of small-cell lung cancer patients resistant to cyclophosphamide, doxorubicin, and etoposide: a non-cross-resistant schedule. *J Clin Oncol*, Vol.17, No.3, pp. 927-932

Grubb, J.R., Moorman, A.C., Baker, R.K. et al. (2006). The changing spectrum of pulmonary disease in patients with HIV infection on antiretroviral therapy. *AIDS*, Vol.20, No.8, pp. 1095-1107

Grulich, A.E., Van Leeuwen, M.T., Falster, M.O. et al. (2007). Incidence of cancers in people with HIV/AIDS compared with immunosuppressed transplant recipients: a meta-analysis. *Lancet*, Vol.370, No.9581, pp. 59-67

Gulick, R. (1998). Combination therapy for patients with HIV-1 infection: the use of dual nucleoside analogues with protease inhibitors and other agents. *AIDS*, Vol.12 Suppl 3, pp. S17-22

Hakim, F.T., Cepeda, R., Kaimei, S. et al. (1997). Constraints on CD4 recovery postchemotherapy in adults: thymic insufficiency and apoptotic decline of expanded peripheral CD4 cells. *Blood*, Vol.90, No.9, pp. 3789-3798

Hakimian, R., Fang, H., Thomas, L. et al. (2007). Lung cancer in HIV-infected patients in the era of highly active antiretroviral therapy. *J Thorac Oncol*, Vol.2, No.4, pp. 268-272

Hanna, N., Shepherd, F.A., Fossella, F.V. et al. (2004). Randomized phase III trial of pemetrexed versus docetaxel in patients with non-small-cell lung cancer previously treated with chemotherapy. *J Clin Oncol*, Vol.22, No.9, pp. 1589-1597

Herida, M., Mary-Krause, M., Kaphan, R. et al. (2003). Incidence of non-AIDS-defining cancers before and during the highly active antiretroviral therapy era in a cohort of human immunodeficiency virus-infected patients. *J Clin Oncol*, Vol.21, No.18, pp. 3447-3453

Hodgson, D.M., Yirmiya, R., Chiappelli, F. et al. (1998). Intracerebral HIV glycoprotein (gp120) enhances tumor metastasis via centrally released interleukin-1. *Brain Res*, Vol.781, No.1-2, pp. 244-251

Huang, J., Meixner, L., Fernandez, S. et al. (2009). A double-blinded, randomized controlled trial of zoledronate therapy for HIV-associated osteopenia and osteoporosis. *AIDS*, Vol.23, No.1, pp. 51-57

Inoue, A., Sugawara, S., Yamazaki, K. et al. (2008). Randomized phase II trial comparing amrubicin with topotecan in patients with previously treated small-cell lung cancer: North Japan Lung Cancer Study Group Trial 0402. *J Clin Oncol*, Vol.26, No.33, pp. 5401-5406

Irwin, L.E., Begandy, M.K. & Moore, T.M. (1984). Adenosquamous carcinoma of the lung and the acquired immunodeficiency syndrome. *Ann Intern Med*, Vol.100, No.1, pp. 158

James, J.S. (2006). Lung cancer: very high death rate with HIV, huge reduction possible with CT screening for early diagnosis. *AIDS Treat News*, No.420, pp. 5-6

Karp, J., Profeta, G., Marantz, P.R. et al. (1993). Lung cancer in patients with immunodeficiency syndrome. *Chest*, Vol.103, No.2, pp. 410-413

Kelly, K., Crowley, J., Bunn, P.A., Jr. et al. (2001). Randomized phase III trial of paclitaxel plus carboplatin versus vinorelbine plus cisplatin in the treatment of patients with advanced non--small-cell lung cancer: a Southwest Oncology Group trial. *J Clin Oncol*, Vol.19, No.13, pp. 3210-3218

Kirk, G.D., Merlo, C., P, O.D. et al. (2007). HIV infection is associated with an increased risk for lung cancer, independent of smoking. *Clin Infect Dis*, Vol.45, No.1, pp. 103-110

Kivisto, K.T., Kroemer, H.K. & Eichelbaum, M. (1995). The role of human cytochrome P450 enzymes in the metabolism of anticancer agents: implications for drug interactions. *Br J Clin Pharmacol*, Vol.40, No.6, pp. 523-530

Kwak, E.L., Bang, Y.J., Camidge, D.R. et al. (2010). Anaplastic lymphoma kinase inhibition in non-small-cell lung cancer. *N Engl J Med*, Vol.363, No.18, pp. 1693-1703

Lavole, A., Chouaid, C., Baudrin, L. et al. (2009). Effect of highly active antiretroviral therapy on survival of HIV infected patients with non-small-cell lung cancer. *Lung Cancer*, Vol.65, No.3, pp. 345-350

Lavole, A., Wislez, M., Antoine, M. et al. (2006). Lung cancer, a new challenge in the HIV-infected population. *Lung Cancer*, Vol.51, No.1, pp. 1-11

Levine, A.M., Seaberg, E.C., Hessol, N.A. et al. (2010). HIV as a risk factor for lung cancer in women: data from the Women's Interagency HIV Study. *J Clin Oncol*, Vol.28, No.9, pp. 1514-1519

Maemondo, M., Inoue, A., Kobayashi, K. et al. (2010). Gefitinib or chemotherapy for non-small-cell lung cancer with mutated EGFR. *N Engl J Med*, Vol.362, No.25, pp. 2380-2388

Makinson, A., Pujol, J.L., Le Moing, V. et al. (2010). Interactions between cytotoxic chemotherapy and antiretroviral treatment in human immunodeficiency virus-infected patients with lung cancer. *J Thorac Oncol,* Vol.5, No.4, pp. 562-571

Marino, P., Pampallona, S., Preatoni, A. et al. (1994). Chemotherapy vs supportive care in advanced non-small-cell lung cancer. Results of a meta-analysis of the literature. *Chest,* Vol.106, No.3, pp. 861-865

Massera, F., Rocco, G., Rossi, G. et al. (2000). Pulmonary resection for lung cancer in HIV-positive patients with low (<200 lymphocytes/mm(3)) CD4(+) count. *Lung Cancer,* Vol.29, No.2, pp. 147-149

Mitsudomi, T., Morita, S., Yatabe, Y. et al. (2009). Gefitinib versus cisplatin plus docetaxel in patients with non-small-cell lung cancer harbouring mutations of the epidermal growth factor receptor (WJTOG3405): an open label, randomised phase 3 trial. *Lancet Oncol,* Vol.11, No.2, pp. 121-128

Murray, N. & Turrisi, A.T., 3rd (2006). A review of first-line treatment for small-cell lung cancer. *J Thorac Oncol,* Vol.1, No.3, pp. 270-278

Nguyen, M.L., Farrell, K.J. & Gunthel, C.J. Non-AIDS-Defining Malignancies in Patients with HIV in the HAART Era. *Curr Infect Dis Rep,* Vol.12, No.1, pp. 46-55

Non-small Cell Lung Cancer Collaborative Group (1995). Chemotherapy in non-small cell lung cancer: a meta-analysis using updated data on individual patients from 52 randomised clinical trials. Non-small Cell Lung Cancer Collaborative Group. BMJ, Vol.311, No.7010, pp. 899-909

Non-small Cell Lung Cancer Collaborative Group (2008). Chemotherapy in addition to supportive care improves survival in advanced non-small-cell lung cancer: a systematic review and meta-analysis of individual patient data from 16 randomized controlled trials. J Clin Oncol, Vol.26, No.28, pp. 4617-4625

Ohe, Y., Ohashi, Y., Kubota, K. et al. (2007). Randomized phase III study of cisplatin plus irinotecan versus carboplatin plus paclitaxel, cisplatin plus gemcitabine, and cisplatin plus vinorelbine for advanced non-small-cell lung cancer: Four-Arm Cooperative Study in Japan. *Ann Oncol,* Vol.18, No.2, pp. 317-323

Okuma, Y., Hosomi, Y., Takagi, Y. et al. (2010). Long-term survival following metachronous intratumoral hemorrhage in an HIV-infected patient with lung cancer. *Int J Clin Oncol,* Vol.15, No.5, pp. 515-518

Onoda, S., Masuda, N., Seto, T. et al. (2006). Phase II trial of amrubicin for treatment of refractory or relapsed small-cell lung cancer: Thoracic Oncology Research Group Study 0301. *J Clin Oncol,* Vol.24, No.34, pp. 5448-5453

Pakkala, S., Chen, Z., Rimland, D. et al. (2010). HIV-associated lung cancer in the era of highly active antiretroviral therapy (HAART): Correlation between CD4 count and outcome. *J Clin Oncol,* Vol.28, No.15s, pp. suppl; abstr 7632

Parker, M.S., Leveno, D.M., Campbell, T.J. et al. (1998). AIDS-related bronchogenic carcinoma: fact or fiction? *Chest,* Vol.113, No.1, pp. 154-161

Patel, P., Hanson, D.L., Sullivan, P.S. et al. (2008). Incidence of types of cancer among HIV-infected persons compared with the general population in the United States, 1992-2003. *Ann Intern Med,* Vol.148, No.10, pp. 728-736

Petoumenos, K., Hui, E., Kumarasamy, N. et al. (2010). Cancers in the TREAT Asia HIV Observational Database (TAHOD): a retrospective analysis of risk factors. *J Int AIDS Soc,* Vol.13, No.1, pp. 51

Pignon, J.P., Tribodet, H., Scagliotti, G.V. et al. (2008). Lung adjuvant cisplatin evaluation: a pooled analysis by the LACE Collaborative Group. *J Clin Oncol*, Vol.26, No.21, pp. 3552-3559

Postmus, P.E., Berendsen, H.H., Van Zandwijk, N. et al. (1987). Retreatment with the induction regimen in small cell lung cancer relapsing after an initial response to short term chemotherapy. *Eur J Cancer Clin Oncol*, Vol.23, No.9, pp. 1409-1411

Powles, T., Imami, N., Nelson, M. et al. (2002). Effects of combination chemotherapy and highly active antiretroviral therapy on immune parameters in HIV-1 associated lymphoma. *AIDS*, Vol.16, No.4, pp. 531-536

Powles, T., Robinson, D., Stebbing, J. et al. (2009). Highly active antiretroviral therapy and the incidence of non-AIDS-defining cancers in people with HIV infection. *J Clin Oncol*, Vol.27, No.6, pp. 884-890

Powles, T., Thirwell, C., Newsom-Davis, T. et al. (2003). Does HIV adversely influence the outcome in advanced non-small-cell lung cancer in the era of HAART? *Br J Cancer*, Vol.89, No.3, pp. 457-459

Richman, D.D., Fischl, M.A., Grieco, M.H. et al. (1987). The toxicity of azidothymidine (AZT) in the treatment of patients with AIDS and AIDS-related complex. A double-blind, placebo-controlled trial. *N Engl J Med*, Vol.317, No.4, pp. 192-197

Rodriguez, R., Fontanesi, J., Meyer, J.L. et al. (1989). Normal-tissue effects of irradiation for Kaposi's sarcoma/AIDS. *Front Radiat Ther Oncol*, Vol.23, pp. 150-159

Rosell, R., Moran, T., Queralt, C. et al. (2009). Screening for epidermal growth factor receptor mutations in lung cancer. *N Engl J Med*, Vol.361, No.10, pp. 958-967

Rosen, L.S., Gordon, D., Kaminski, M. et al. (2003a). Long-term efficacy and safety of zoledronic acid compared with pamidronate disodium in the treatment of skeletal complications in patients with advanced multiple myeloma or breast carcinoma: a randomized, double-blind, multicenter, comparative trial. *Cancer*, Vol.98, No.8, pp. 1735-1744

Rosen, L.S., Gordon, D., Tchekmedyian, S. et al. (2003b). Zoledronic acid versus placebo in the treatment of skeletal metastases in patients with lung cancer and other solid tumors: a phase III, double-blind, randomized trial--the Zoledronic Acid Lung Cancer and Other Solid Tumors Study Group. *J Clin Oncol*, Vol.21, No.16, pp. 3150-3157

Rowinsky, E. & Donehower, R. 1997. Pharmacology of cancer chemotherapy-antimicrotubule agents. In *Cancer principles and practice of oncology, 5th ed.* (Ed. De Vitavt, H., Rosembersa, Editors), pp. 467-483. Lippincott-Raven Publishers, Philadelphia

Samet, J.M., Wiggins, C.L., Humble, C.G. et al. (1988). Cigarette smoking and lung cancer in New Mexico. *Am Rev Respir Dis*, Vol.137, No.5, pp. 1110-1113

Sandler, A., Gray, R., Perry, M.C. et al. (2006). Paclitaxel-carboplatin alone or with bevacizumab for non-small-cell lung cancer. *N Engl J Med*, Vol.355, No.24, pp. 2542-2550

Saves, M., Chene, G., Ducimetiere, P. et al. (2003). Risk factors for coronary heart disease in patients treated for human immunodeficiency virus infection compared with the general population. *Clin Infect Dis*, Vol.37, No.2, pp. 292-298

Scagliotti, G., Hanna, N., Fossella, F. et al. (2009). The differential efficacy of pemetrexed according to NSCLC histology: a review of two Phase III studies. *Oncologist*, Vol.14, No.3, pp. 253-263

Scagliotti, G.V., Parikh, P., Von Pawel, J. et al. (2008). Phase III study comparing cisplatin plus gemcitabine with cisplatin plus pemetrexed in chemotherapy-naive patients with advanced-stage non-small-cell lung cancer. *J Clin Oncol*, Vol.26, No.21, pp. 3543-3551

Schiller, J.H., Harrington, D., Belani, C.P. et al. (2002). Comparison of four chemotherapy regimens for advanced non-small-cell lung cancer. *N Engl J Med*, Vol.346, No.2, pp. 92-98

Sepkowitz, K.A. (2001). AIDS--the first 20 years. *N Engl J Med*, Vol.344, No.23, pp. 1764-1772

Shepherd, F.A., Fossella, F.V., Lynch, T. et al. (2001). Docetaxel (Taxotere) shows survival and quality-of-life benefits in the second-line treatment of non-small cell lung cancer: a review of two phase III trials. *Semin Oncol*, Vol.28, No.1 Suppl 2, pp. 4-9

Shepherd, F.A., Rodrigues Pereira, J., Ciuleanu, T. et al. (2005). Erlotinib in previously treated non-small-cell lung cancer. *N Engl J Med*, Vol.353, No.2, pp. 123-132

Silverberg, M.J., Chao, C., Leyden, W.A. et al. (2009). HIV infection and the risk of cancers with and without a known infectious cause. *AIDS*, Vol.23, No.17, pp. 2337-2345

Silverberg, M.J., Neuhaus, J., Bower, M. et al. (2007). Risk of cancers during interrupted antiretroviral therapy in the SMART study. *AIDS*, Vol.21, No.14, pp. 1957-1963

Souquet, P.J., Chauvin, F., Boissel, J.P. et al. (1993). Polychemotherapy in advanced non small cell lung cancer: a meta-analysis. *Lancet*, Vol.342, No.8862, pp. 19-21

Spano, J.P., Massiani, M.A., Bentata, M. et al. (2004). Lung cancer in patients with HIV Infection and review of the literature. *Med Oncol*, Vol.21, No.2, pp. 109-115

Sridhar, K.S., Flores, M.R., Raub, W.A., Jr. et al. (1992). Lung cancer in patients with human immunodeficiency virus infection compared with historic control subjects. *Chest*, Vol.102, No.6, pp. 1704-1708

Stebbing, J. & Bower, M. (2006). Comparative pharmacogenomics of antiretroviral and cytotoxic treatments. *Lancet Oncol*, Vol.7, No.1, pp. 61-68

Tan, B. & Ratner, L. (1997). The use of new antiretroviral therapy in combination with chemotherapy. *Curr Opin Oncol*, Vol.9, No.5, pp. 455-464

Temel, J.S., Greer, J.A., Muzikansky, A. et al. (2010). Early palliative care for patients with metastatic non-small-cell lung cancer. *N Engl J Med*, Vol.363, No.8, pp. 733-742

Tenholder, M.F. & Jackson, H.D. (1993). Bronchogenic carcinoma in patients seropositive for human immunodeficiency virus. *Chest*, Vol.104, No.4, pp. 1049-1053

Tirelli, U., Spina, M., Sandri, S. et al. (2000). Lung carcinoma in 36 patients with human immunodeficiency virus infection. The Italian Cooperative Group on AIDS and Tumors. *Cancer*, Vol.88, No.3, pp. 563-569

Tong, X., Li, K., Luo, Z. et al. (2009). Decreased TIP30 expression promotes tumor metastasis in lung cancer. *Am J Pathol*, Vol.174, No.5, pp. 1931-1939

Toschi, E., Sgadari, C., Malavasi, L. et al. (2011). Human immunodeficiency virus protease inhibitors reduce the growth of human tumors via a proteasome-independent block of angiogenesis and matrix metalloproteinases. *Int J Cancer*, Vol.128, No.1, pp. 82-93

Tsuya, A., Kurata, T., Tamura, K. et al. (2007). Skeletal metastases in non-small cell lung cancer: a retrospective study. *Lung Cancer*, Vol.57, No.2, pp. 229-232

Vajdic, C.M., Mcdonald, S.P., Mccredie, M.R. et al. (2006). Cancer incidence before and after kidney transplantation. *JAMA*, Vol.296, No.23, pp. 2823-2831

Vallis, K.A. (1991). Glutathione deficiency and radiosensitivity in AIDS patients. *Lancet*, Vol.337, No.8746, pp. 918-919

Von Pawel, J., Schiller, J.H., Shepherd, F.A. et al. (1999). Topotecan versus cyclophosphamide, doxorubicin, and vincristine for the treatment of recurrent small-cell lung cancer. *J Clin Oncol*, Vol.17, No.2, pp. 658-667

Vyzula, R. & Remick, S.C. (1996). Lung cancer in patients with HIV-infection. *Lung Cancer*, Vol.15, No.3, pp. 325-339

Washington, C.B., Duran, G.E., Man, M.C. et al. (1998). Interaction of anti-HIV protease inhibitors with the multidrug transporter P-glycoprotein (P-gp) in human cultured cells. *J Acquir Immune Defic Syndr Hum Retrovirol*, Vol.19, No.3, pp. 203-209

Wistuba, Ii, Behrens, C., Milchgrub, S. et al. (1998). Comparison of molecular changes in lung cancers in HIV-positive and HIV-indeterminate subjects. *JAMA*, Vol.279, No.19, pp. 1554-1559

4

Neuropsychiatric Manifestations of HIV Infection and AIDS

Victor Obiajulu Olisah

*Department of Psychiatry, Ahmadu Bello University Teaching Hospital, Zaria,
Nigeria*

1. Introduction

Acquired Immune Deficiency Syndrome (AIDS) was first reported in the United States in 1981 and has since become a major worldwide epidemic. AIDS is caused by the human immunodeficiency virus (HIV). By killing or damaging cells of the body's immune system, HIV progressively destroys the body's ability to fight infections and certain cancers. The term AIDS applies to the most advanced stages of HIV infection.

Statistics on the world epidemic of HIV/AIDS indicates that 39.5 million people are living with HIV/AIDS worldwide. Of these, 24.7 million (63%) live in Sub-Saharan Africa, a region that is home to just 10% of the world's population (UNAIDS/WHO report, 2006).

HIV is a retrovirus, which is immunosuppressive, predisposing the individual to opportunistic infections and certain neoplasm (Wiley, 1994). In addition to impairment in immune functions, evidence has suggested that HIV is neurotropic. It should therefore be anticipated that neuropsychiatric complication might be common in HIV positive individuals during all phases of HIV related illness.

Over the years, researchers have developed antiretroviral drugs to fight both HIV infection and its associated infections and cancers. Currently available drugs do not cure people with HIV infection or AIDS, and they all have side effects that can be severe. Because no vaccine for HIV is available, the only way to prevent infection is to avoid behaviours that put a person at risk of infection, such as sharing needles and unprotected sex.

It is believed that neuropsychiatric disorders account for over 15% of the world's disease burden. Due to the recent advances in antiretroviral therapy, the life expectancy of people living with HIV has increased, and thus clinicians are more likely to encounter the neuropsychiatric manifestations of the disease. In as many as 20% of HIV infected individuals, neurologic or neuropsychiatric symptoms may be the presenting features, prior to other medical symptoms of AIDS. Despite improvement in and combination of antiretroviral therapy, neuropsychiatric complications still occur in as many as 50% of people living with HIV and are mostly undiagnosed and untreated. Assessment and management of mental disorders is integral to an effective HIV/AIDS intervention program. Mental health professionals will increasingly be called upon to assist in the management of people living with HIV/AIDS. Thus psychiatrists will need to be familiar with disorders that are prevalent in HIV infection. It is now estimated that 40–70% of patients with AIDS develop clinical neurologic abnormalities. The most common neurologic manifestations are minor cognitive motor disorder (MCMD) and HIV-associated dementia (HAD). On the other hand, depression is the most common psychiatric condition in people living with

HIV/AIDS with estimated life time prevalence in the range of between 21% and 61% (Elliot et al, 1998). This category of psychiatric disorders presents diagnostic challenges because of the many neurovegetative confounding factors that are present in association with HIV illness. In both cases, the impact of these syndromes on seropositive patients is significant and appropriate intervention is required, the key to optimal treatment resting with early diagnosis and aggressive treatment.

Initially, the neuropsychiatric manifestations of HIV/AIDS were attributed to psychological reactions to a systemic illness, the effects of psychosocial stressors associated with the disease, or the consequences of opportunistic infections or neoplasms within the central nervous system (CNS). It is now recognized that the psychiatric sequelae of HIV infection and AIDS are numerous and have etiologies that involve neurobiological and psychosocial factors. These include the direct or primary effects of HIV on nervous tissue, the consequences of secondary viral and nonviral opportunistic infections, tumors, cerebrovascular disease, and the complications of systemic therapies for AIDS and associated disorders.

Some previous studies have indicated that Neuropsychiatric disorders in people living with HIV/AIDS are associated with disease progression, poor adherence to antiretroviral drugs, increased incidence of high risk sexual behavior with the potential for further HIV transmission, and deterioration in their quality of life.

Mental and neurological disorders have an intertwined relationship with HIV and AIDS, yet sadly are often overlooked when HIV interventions are planned and implemented. Several important aspects of HIV care and treatment place psychiatrists at the forefront of this epidemic, these include:

- psychiatric disorders (including substance use) can increase an individual's risk of acquiring sexually transmitted diseases, including HIV;
- pre-existing mental disorders (including substance use) can predate and/or complicate HIV-related illness;
- neuropsychiatric complications and psychiatric illness can affect adherence to antiretroviral therapy regimens;
- new antiretroviral treatments and combination therapies can affect the CNS and/or contribute to the development of   psychiatric side effects/symptoms;
- individuals with waning immunity and high viral loads may be at particular risk for the HIV-related CNS complications that can cause acute mental status changes;
- the proportion of mental health and/or substance abuse disorders among people living with HIV/AIDS is nearly 5 times greater than the proportion found in the general population;
- persons living with a severe mental illness are disproportionately vulnerable (as high as 23%) to infection with HIV and other sexually transmitted diseases;
- psychiatric syndromes can be especially challenging to recognize and accurately diagnose in the medically ill; and
- as HIV/AIDS becomes increasingly a chronic disorder with the improvement of treatments and longer survival times, the need for comprehensive psychiatric care and services is expected to rise.

2. Biology and pathophysiology of HIV infection

HIV is a lentivirus, a subgroup of retroviruses. As with other retroviruses, HIV has rapid rate of genetic mutation. This family of viruses is known for latency, persistent viremia, infection of the nervous system and weakening of the host immune responses. HIV-1 is the form of the virus that causes disease in most part of the world. HIV-2 discovered in 1986, causes a relatively small proportion of cases clustered in West Africa. HIV has high affinity for CD4 T lymphocytes and monocytes. When HIV binds to CD4 cells, it becomes internalized. The virus replicates itself by generating a DNA copy using reverse transcriptase enzyme. Viral DNA becomes incorporated into the host DNA, enabling further replication (Green, 1991, Stebbing et al, 2004). HIV causes the lysis of CD4 lymphocytes. These cells are critical in cell-mediated immunity. The course of HIV infection is characterized by latency. Unfortunately, profound immune deficiency eventually develops, as CD4 cell count drops below 200cells per mm3. At this point, the patient becomes vulnerable to opportunistic infections and malignancies (Centers for Disease Control, 1982). Progression from HIV to AIDS occurs at a median of 11years after infection. In the recent past, most patients would not survive more than 1 to 2 years after diagnosis of AIDS. However, since the introduction of antiretroviral drugs and prophylaxis against opportunistic pathogens, death rates from AIDS have begun to decline significantly.

3. Treatment of HIV infection

Treatment is accomplished through numerous combinations of antiretroviral agents belonging to the following groups: Nucleoside analogue reverse transcriptase inhibitors, nonnucleoside reverse transcriptase inhibitors, protease inhibitors and nucleoside analogues. In the mid-1990s, several investigators studied combination therapies of two reverse transcriptase inhibitors and a protease inhibitor. This therapy was later referred to as Highly Active Antiretroviral Therapy (HAART). HAART dramatically reduced viral load and often resulted in an increase in CD4 cell count. The current goal of treatment is to reduce viral load to undetectable levels and maintain such remission without interruption. Evidence suggests that the therapies suppress replication but do not eradicate HIV from all parts of the body, particularly lymphoid tissue and the brain. Not all patients who initiate antiretroviral therapy respond. The lack of clinical response is likely explained by problems with adherence, suboptimal antiretroviral treatment potency, and genetic mutation of HIV strains (Descamps et al, 2000). Many patients experience substantial side effects, and it is not uncommon for changes to be made in antiretroviral regimens because of such side effects. Adverse effects include lipodystrophy, hyperlipidemia, nephrotoxicity, bone marrow suppression, neuropathy and elevation of blood glucose to possibly diabetes mellitus levels (Deeks et al, 1997). Patients often experience nausea, vomiting, diarrhea, sleep disturbances and rashes.

Adherence is of utmost concern with antiretroviral treatment because even minor deviations from the prescribed regimen can result in viral resistance and permanent loss of efficacy for existing medications (Practice guidelines for HIV treatment, 2000). Studies of antiretroviral treatment continue to indicate that a near-perfect adherence is needed to adequately repress viral replication (Demasi et al, 2001).

As the world HIV epidemic spreads increasingly among disadvantaged persons with limited resources who have multiple comorbid disorders, significantly more psychosocial stressors, and less access to ongoing primary or mental health care, these individuals are at risk of not receiving the recommended treatment for HIV infection. Services for HIV patients must balance medical interventions with the emotional, economic, and social supports required for good quality of life and prevention of further transmission (Practice guidelines for HIV treatment, 2000).

4. Etiology of the neuropsychiatric manifestations of HIV/AIDS

4.1 Impact of HIV on the Central Nervous System (CNS)

Clinical evidence for direct infection of the CNS by HIV emerged in the mid- 1980s, when patients began to survive their presenting opportunistic infections but went on to develop neuropsychiatric syndromes that could not be attributed to CNS opportunistic infections and neoplasm. Additional evidence included signs of neuro-cognitive impairment in adults, loss or arrest of developmental milestones in children, ability to culture HIV from the cerebrospinal fluid, neuropathological lesions of the brain at autopsy, and abnormalities observed through brain imaging techniques, including cerebral atrophy (Deeks et al, 1997).

HIV invades the CNS early in the course of infection entering by way of macrophages, which along with microgial cells are largely responsible for HIV replication within the CNS. While HIV does not infect neurons in the CNS, it causes neuronal death by causing the elaboration of neurotoxins which in turn induce a variety of inflammatory factors that cause apoptosis, or programmed cell death of neurons (Swindells et al, 1999).

The pathogenesis of HIV infection within the brain and its relationship to neurologic and psychiatric complications remains obscure, but there is evidence that cellular and molecular components of the immune system are involved (Bloom & Rausch, 1997).

Several different mechanisms may explain the effects of HIV on the CNS. Researchers have hypothesized that pathogenesis begins with viral penetration of the CNS and associated loss of integrity of the blood-brain barrier. This may allow cellular and non-cellular inflammatory components of the immune system to enter the CNS, resulting in damage to neurons and non-neuronal support cells (Rabkin & Ferrando, 1997).

Some studies have examined viral load and CD4 cell counts, measures typically used to monitor immunologic function in patients with HIV infection, as potential markers of CNS injury and vulnerability to CNS complications. A study that followed viral loads and CD4 cell counts in a large cohort of HIV-infected men without AIDS found that relatively high plasma HIV RNA (> 3000 copies/ml) and low CD4 T-lymphocyte counts (< 500 x 106 cells/l) were predictive of both dementia and neuropathy (Childs et al., 1999).The authors suggested that effective suppression of HIV may reduce the risk of developing these neurological complications.

Based on evidence of basal ganglia dysfunction in HIV-associated dementia (Berger & Nath, 1997), some researchers proposed that microvascular abnormalities would be found in the basal ganglia of patients with this condition (Berger, 2000).Using time-course magnetic resonance imaging, these investigators observed increased enhancement, both immediate and late, in the basal ganglia of individuals with HIV infection and moderate-to-severe dementia, relative to HIV patients without dementia. These data suggested that increases in regional cerebral blood volume and disruption of the blood-brain barrier have an etiologic role in the development of HIV-associated dementia.

Most HIV DNA in the brain has been found in macrophages/microglia, often near apoptotic neurons, suggesting that cytokines produced by the infected cells might contribute to neuronal destruction (Shapshak et al., 1995). Macrophages may infiltrate the CNS by interacting with the endothelial cells that form the blood-brain barrier, causing endothelial cell damage and disrupting the barrier (Nottet, 1999). Chemokines (cytokines that act as macrophage attractants) and their receptors on neurons and glial cells appear to play a central role in HIV entry into the CNS and eventual cellular destruction (Gabuzda &Wang, 2000; Zheng, 1999).Synaptic damage, without neuronal loss, has been observed in patients with mild HIV-associated cognitive disorders. Using synaptic density as an indicator of damage in post-mortem brain samples from HIV-infected patients, Everall and colleagues found that reduced synaptic density correlated significantly with ante-mortem neuropsychological functioning, and stressed that early diagnosis and treatment could potentially reverse synaptic damage and prevent cognitive decline(Everall et al., 1999). Loss of subcortical neurons in the brain of people infected with HIV may be associated with the experience of depression.

Evidence is accumulating to suggest roles for several HIV proteins, including glycoprotein 120 (gp120), HIV-1 negative factor (Nef), and transactivating protein (Tat), in HIV-induced neuropathogenesis. For example, the viral envelope protein gp120 appears to bind to rat dorsal root ganglia and human neuroblastoma cells (Apostolski et al., 1993), and in rats exposure to gp120 has been shown to cause swelling and increase tumor necrosis factor in the sciatic nerve trunk, induce astrocyte and microglial infiltration into the spinal cord, and cause neuropathic pain behaviours (Herzberg & Sagen, 2001). *In vitro*, studies have shown that Nef induces macrophage chemotaxis (Koedel et al., 1999) and acts as a potent neurotoxin (Trillo-Pazos et al., 2000). Astrocytes treated with Tat *in vitro* produced pro-inflammatory cytokines and chemokines that may contribute to neuronal injury (Galey et al., 2001). Tat also stimulates macrophage production of metalloproteinases, enzymes that are expressed at increased levels in certain neurologic diseases and in the brain tissues of patients with AIDS (Johnston et al.2000). Although the significance of these laboratory findings for patients with HIV or AIDS remains to be clarified, it is probable that many of these mechanisms combine to produce the neurologic and psychiatric changes seen with HIV infection and AIDS. Identifying and characterizing the mechanisms involved may open new avenues for prevention and treatment.

4.2 Psychosocial factors

The psychosocial stress associated with a socially stigmatizing terminal illness and frequent infections carries with it tremendous emotional upheaval in vulnerable individuals. There is usually a sense or loss of health, financial security, independence and relationships in HIV infected persons. This is made worse when relevant social support is missing (Katalan et al, 1989).

Specific crisis points and psychosocial factors can precipitate psychiatric disorders especially anxiety and depression in HIV-infected persons. These crisis points includes- learning of HIV positive status, disclosure of HIV status to family and friends, introduction of medication, occurrence of any physical illness, recognition of new symptoms/ progression of disease, necessity for hospitalization, death of a partner, diagnosis of AIDS, changes in major aspects of lifestyle, necessity for making end of life and permanency decisions (HIV clinical guidelines, 2000).

5. Neurologic manifestations of HIV

HIV is classified among the lentiviruses, a family of viruses characterized in part by their tendency to cause chronic neurologic disease in their animal hosts. It is not surprising, then, that neurologic complications of HIV infection are common and not confined to opportunistic infections. All levels of the neuraxis can be involved, including the brain, meninges, spinal cord, nerve, and muscle. Neurologic disease is the first manifestation of symptomatic HIV infection in roughly 10-20% of persons, while about 60% of patients with advanced HIV disease will have clinically evident neurologic dysfunction during the course of their illness (Koppel et al., 1985). The incidence of subclinical neurologic disease is even higher: autopsy studies of patients with advanced HIV disease have demonstrated pathologic abnormalities of the nervous system in 75-90% of cases (De la Monte et al., 1987).

HIV has been cultured from brain, nerve, and cerebrospinal fluid (CSF) from persons at all stages of the disease, including those without neurologic signs or symptoms. Positive HIV cultures in CSF do not predict the presence or development of neurologic signs or symptoms later on. The development of neurologic manifestations of AIDS depends on a number of factors, such as antiretroviral treatment history, degree of immunosuppression, and the molecular biology of the viral strain, particularly its neurovirulence(McGuire & Greene, 1996) Host factors, including genetic makeup, undoubtedly play a role in selective vulnerability to neurologic manifestations.

The initial infection of the nervous system by HIV is usually asymptomatic, although acute aseptic meningitis, encephalitis, and inflammatory polyneuropathy have all occurred in this setting. Despite its potential to cause disease at all levels of the nervous system, HIV does not directly infect central or peripheral neurons, astrocytes, or oligodendroglial cells. Latent or low level HIV infection in the CNS is maintained by virus-infected cells of the monocyte/macrophage lineage. "Indirect effects" of macrophage activation--such as dysregulation of cytokines and chemokines, free-radical (oxidative stress) injury, and secretion of soluble factors that are potently neurotoxic, have been implicated as effectors of nervous Minor Cognitive system injury in HIV.

5.1 Minor cognitive impairment

Despite evidence of early infection of the CNS, symptoms of cognitive impairment typically occur late in symptomatic HIV disease, usually in the setting of severe immunosuppression (Miller et al., 1990).

Cognitive impairment has long been recognized as part of manifestation of human immune deficiency virus infection. These changes include loss of cognitive flexibility, difficulty in problem solving, mental slowness and difficulty in concentration. There are also difficulties in memory which manifest as delayed recall. Despite the wide spread use of highly active antiretroviral therapy (HAART), at least in developed nations and some developing nations, cognitive impairment and other neurological complications of HIV infection persist with devastating personal and socioeconomic consequences. Even though neurons are rarely infected by human immunodeficiency virus especially at early stage of the infection, neuronal loss is quite common in patient with HIV infection.

Although as many as 40% of patients with HIV/AIDS will have some form of cognitive impairment even before the development of full dementia, only a small percentage (5-10%) may go on to develop dementia itself. Various type of cognitive impairment in HIV infection has been documented and the American academy of Neurology (AAN) published a diagnostic criteria for HIV associated dementia (HAD) and minor cognitive motor disorder (MCMD); which include motor, affective and behavioural abnormalities, consistent with the early description of AIDS dementia complex.

5.2 AIDS Dementia Complex (ADC)

Some investigators hold that increased HIV proliferation in the brain is necessary for the development of ADC. Others propose that a macrophage-initiated cascade of events can lead to brain dysfunction and clinical dementia, even in the absence of high viral load in the brain. Activated macrophages, whether infected with HIV or not, are capable of secreting potent neurotoxins, inducing pro-inflammatory cytokines, and generating oxygen free radicals that can damage cells and lead to neuronal dysfunction or death (Glass et al., 1995). A particular subtype of monocyte/macrophages derived from the peripheral blood was found to be greatly increased among patients with AIDS dementia compared with both HIV infected and uninfected controls. Soluble factors from these macrophages were found to be highly neurotoxic--that is, they killed human brain cells in culture (Pulliam et al., 1997).

Although the incidence of nearly all nervous system opportunistic infections has declined dramatically in the era of potent antiretroviral therapy, the impact on the incidence and prevalence of HIV-associated cognitive impairment including frank ADC--has been low. The prevalence of ADC in HIV-infected individuals with higher CD4 counts (200-350 cells/µL) actually appears to have increased since 1996. Pathologically, the prevalence of HIV-associated brain disease, or encephalopathy, is rising despite suppressive antiretroviral therapy (Neuenburg et al., 2002). Poor penetration of the blood-brain barrier by many of the antiretroviral drugs, particularly the protease inhibitors, has been suggested as a reason for the persistence of ADC.

There is some evidence that, despite the poor CNS penetration of most antiretrovirals, effective antiretroviral therapy may attenuate the neurotoxicity of circulating monocytes/macrophages. Among individuals with ADC receiving effective antiretroviral regimens, macrophage-derived soluble factors were found to be less neurotoxic than observed prior to the availability of combination antiretroviral therapy (Pulliam et al., 1997).

The major difference between "HIV associated dementia complex" and "HIV associated minor cognitive/ motor disorder" is the severity of impairment in activities of daily living. That is, by definition, dementia must have cognitive impairment severe enough to interfere with occupational or social functioning. In "HIV associated minor cognitive/motor disorder," activities of daily living are generally intact with the possible exception of mild difficulties in the most demanding activities.

The initial features of HIV associated dementia include an overall slowing in cognition (i.e., bradyphrenia) and movement (i.e., bradykinesia) as well as difficulties in motor dexterity and coordination, forgetfulness, poor concentration, and marked apathy. Although dysphoric mood is not a common feature, the pronounced slowing and apathy may appear as if the patient is depressed. Furthermore, assessing other aspects of depression (e.g., weight loss, cognitive disturbance and insomnia) is difficult for patients with this disorder due to shared symptomatology that may be indistinguishable from the psychiatric symptoms.

Later in the course of HIV associated dementia, the patient may exhibit myoclonus, bowel and bladder incontinence, and, eventually, mutism and a vegetative state. Once these advanced features are present, death is typically imminent.

Because the above initial symptoms are similar to those seen in other patient groups with subcortical impairment (e.g., Parkinson's disease, progressive supranuclear palsy, multiple sclerosis) and because of the neuroimaging findings of subcortical neuropathology, HIV associated dementia was originally described as a subcortical dementia. However, in light of the more recent findings of cortical atrophy and higher cortical function deficits in AIDS patients, this characterization may not fully describe the spectrum of neuropsychiatric deficits associated with HIV infection and AIDS.

Antiretroviral therapy may be helpful in treating Minor Cognitive /Motor Disorder and HIV associated dementia and should be recommended for all patients, unless there are contraindications. The ability of particular antiretroviral drugs to penetrate the blood-brain barrier may be less important to treatment success than the overall potency of the regimen and the ability of the patient to adhere to it.

Studies from the 1980s showed that zidovudine monotherapy was beneficial in patients with HAD, so some clinicians include it in the ART regimen for anyone with neurocognitive impairment. Others suggest using at least 2 drugs that cross the blood-brain barrier (eg, zidovudine, stavudine, abacavir, lamivudine, and nevirapine). Efavirenz, didanosine, and lamivudine cross to a lesser degree. As a class, protease inhibitors (PIs) have poor blood-brain barrier penetration. Nevertheless, patients have shown neurocognitive improvement while taking PI-containing regimens, perhaps because of indirect effects on HIV activity in the CNS.

When present, depressive symptoms should be treated with low dosages of selective serotonin reuptake inhibitors (SSRIs).

Antipsychotic medications may be useful in treating agitation and hallucinations, but patients with these conditions are often extremely sensitive to anticholinergic adverse effects and extrapyramidal symptoms. Newer neuroleptic or antipsychotic agents, such as olanzapine and risperidone, have lower rates of significant side effects compared with older drugs. The starting dosage of olanzapine is 2.5 mg orally at bedtime; that for risperidone is 0.5-1 mg orally at bedtime. Note that these drugs may interact with antiretroviral medications, especially ritonavir, and can cause weight gain and other metabolic adverse effects. Avoid benzodiazepines, which tend to increase confusion and decrease concentration.

Psychostimulants such as methylphenidate (Ritalin) and dextroamphetamine (Dexedrine) have been used to improve attention, concentration, and psychomotor function. Dosages of methylphenidate start at 5 mg for a test dose, then 2.5-5.0 mg twice daily, increasing by doses of 5 mg every other day until the desired effect is achieved. Usual dosages are in the range of 20-30 mg per day. Monitor blood pressure, heart rate, and symptoms of restlessness, agitation, nausea, and psychosis.

For a patient who is knowledgeable about HIV, a dementia workup or diagnosis often precipitates a crisis, with an increased risk of suicide. Carefully screen for depression and suicidality, and treat these if they develop.

Behavioral management strategies may assist the patient with early manifestations of dementia to continue living with some degree of independence and safety in the home. Memory aids such as posted notes, calendars, alarmed pill-boxes, and other environmental cues may help.

It is critical to enlist the support of family members and significant others at an early stage of the illness. Because the disease is frightening and may be progressive, the patient and members of the support system need assistance in anticipating and planning for the future. Plans for assisted living or other in-home custodial care should be made early. Severe or late dementia causes fear, misunderstanding, and frustration for both the patient and care givers. All involved will require help from visiting nurses, social workers, hospice workers, and physicians. Recommend the preparation of an advance directive for the patient with early manifestations of dementia.

5.3 Overview of clinical neurologic disease
5.3.1 Cerebral symptoms and signs

Apart from dementia, HIV-infected patients are at risk for a wide range of neurologic diseases. Cerebral signs and symptoms are the most common. Global cerebral disease can present with altered mental status or generalized seizures, whereas focal disease often produces hemiparesis, hemisensory loss, visual field cuts, or disturbances in language use. Fungal, viral, and mycobacterial meningoencephalitides are the most common causes of global cerebral dysfunction, and progressive multifocal leukoencephalopathy (PML), primary CNS lymphoma, and toxoplasmosis account for the majority of focal presentations. As the epidemic has progressed, the epidemiology of CNS complications has changed. In general, availability of effective antiretroviral regimens has been associated with a dramatic decline in incidence and severity of opportunistic infections of the CNS. Even before the availability of these regimens, the incidence of CNS toxoplasmosis had declined among patients receiving trimethoprim-sulfamethoxazole prophylaxis against Pneumocystis. Unfortunately, antiretroviral regimens have not demonstrably decreased the prevalence of PML, and the incidence among individuals with higher CD4 counts may be increasing. However, the prognosis of this once uniformly fatal disease has improved dramatically, with long-term remissions now fairly common among patients receiving antiretroviral therapy (Berger et al., 1998).

5.3.2 Syndromes affecting cord, nerve roots, and muscle

Viral and, rarely, fungal and parasitic opportunistic infections can affect the spinal cord. Systemic lymphoma can infiltrate nerve roots and meninges, occasionally causing a mass lesion within the cord. In addition, HIV itself is associated with a spastic paraparesis similar to that seen with vitamin B12 deficiency. Peripheral nerve injury is very common, particularly a painful distal neuropathy seen late in HIV infection. About 35% of hospitalized patients with advanced HIV disease have peripheral neuropathy (Hall et al., 1991).

Although myalgias or muscle pains are a frequent complaint, frank muscle disease is less common. Both inflammatory myopathies and a toxic myopathy secondary to zidovudine have been observed. More recently, a syndrome of acute neuromuscular weakness, often associated with lactic acidosis, has been described in association with several nucleoside analogue reverse transcriptase inhibitors, including zidovudine (AZT), stavudine (d4T), didanosine (ddI), and lamivudine (3TC), either alone or in combination. Any patient on antiretroviral therapy presenting with a "Guillain-Barré-type" picture of ascending neuromuscular weakness should be tested for lactic acidosis and evaluated with electromyography and nerve conduction studies.

Among patients infected with HIV, serious neurologic disease may present with relatively trivial symptoms and signs. Therefore, a high index of suspicion must be maintained to detect disease early in these patients. A careful neurologic examination to attempt anatomic localization is necessary to guide further laboratory and imaging studies. Because multiple neurologic diseases often coexist in patients, close follow-up is needed even if a presumptive diagnosis has been made. A change in clinical condition often necessitates a thorough reevaluation.

5.3.3 Pain

There is growing awareness that pain from a variety of etiologies commonly complicates HIV disease. In general, patients with AIDS have pain comparable in prevalence and intensity to pain in patients with cancer, with similar mixtures of neuropathic and visceral-somatic etiologies. However, although efforts to improve malignant pain management have benefited many patients with cancer, pain in patients with AIDS is dramatically undertreated.

Aggressive pain treatment can be the single most important and most challenging intervention in the care of patients with HIV disease. In a recent U.S. study, only 15% of ambulatory AIDS patients with severe pain received adequate pain management. The principles of pain assessment and treatment in the patient with HIV/AIDS are not fundamentally different from those in the patient with cancer and should be followed.

These principles are described in the WHO analgesic ladder (WHO clinical guidelines, 1994), a well-validated, stepwise approach to pain management related to pain severity. Therapy ranges from nonopioid analgesics and adjuvants to systemic weak and strong opioids to intraspinal drug delivery for refractory severe pain. Opioids, except in quite high doses, can be ineffective in neuropathic pain; adjuvants (namely, tricyclics, anticonvulsants) are often more successful. Where neuropathic pain is refractory to such therapies, pain management specialists should be consulted.

5.4 Specific neurologic conditions
5.4.1 Neuromuscular disorders
A wide range of peripheral nervous system disorders develop in patients with HIV infection, leading to pain, sensory symptoms, and muscle weakness. Both "primary" HIV associated nerve disorders, and those secondary to opportunistic processes are well described. In addition, certain antiretroviral drugs may cause or exacerbate peripheral neuropathies.

Classification of Neuromuscular Disorders

Four types of neuropathy are important to recognize in clinical practice, either because of their high prevalence or their therapeutic implications, or both. They are:

1.   Distal symmetric polyneuropathy (DSPN)
2.   Mononeuropathy multiplex
3.   Chronic inflammatory demyelinating polyneuropathy
4.   Progressive lumbosacral polyradiculopathy

The incidence of neuropathy increases with declining CD4 cell count and advancing systemic HIV disease. Familiar causes of neuropathy, such as nutritional deficiency and diabetes mellitus, account for only a small percentage of the neuropathy in these patients. Toxicity of therapeutic drugs, notably zalcitabine (ddC) is responsible for some cases of neuropathy, or for progression; however, antiretroviral toxicity is probably overdiagnosed as a primary cause of HIV-associated neuropathy.

Proper recognition of the different types of peripheral nerve dysfunction is essential for patient management. Except for the few neuropathies with known causes, most of these disorders are characterized on the basis of clinical features alone. The rate of symptom progression, the degree of weakness relative to sensory loss, and the severity of immunosuppression guide the differential diagnosis. The electrophysiologic features of nerve conduction and electromyographic studies remain the gold standard for diagnosis, and may lead to different therapeutic options.

5.4.2 Myopathy
Symptomatic primary muscle disease is uncommon in patients with HIV infection. A polymyositislike syndrome occurs rarely, with few cases encountered even in large referral

centers. A secondary myopathy attributable to the muscle toxicity of AZT emerged in the latter half of the 1980s with widespread use of the drug. The hallmark of myopathy is diffuse, symmetric weakness of "proximal" muscles, hip or shoulder girdle muscles, with a sparing of sensory and autonomic functions. Difficulty with squatting, rising from a chair, or walking upstairs is often the presenting symptom of myopathy. Some patients have myalgia and muscle tenderness, but these complaints are also common in patients without myopathy. In patients receiving AZT, discontinuation of the drug may result in clinical improvement of myopathy. Muscle pain and serum creatine kinase levels decrease first, followed by a more delayed improvement in strength. Some patients may tolerate rechallenging with lower doses of AZT, although the use of other antiretroviral therapy is probably preferable (Dalakas et al., 1990).

5.4.3 Spinal cord disorders

Clinically significant spinal cord disorders are less common in HIV disease than are peripheral nervous system diseases. The neurologic signs of myelopathy such as increased tone and hyperreflexia in the legs and Babinski signs (extensor plantar responses) may be elicited even in the absence of subjective complaints. In most cases, such asymptomatic signs reflect mild HIV-associated spinal cord disease that may or may not progress. Patients with symptomatic myelopathy usually complain first of clumsy gait and urinary hesitancy. The clinical course is typically one of slow progression, and most patients remain ambulatory. A more fulminant course may be seen with wheelchair dependence within a few months. Upper extremities are affected very late, if at all. Baclofen (10-30 mg three times daily) or tizanidine (4 mg three times daily) may attenuate leg spasticity and reduce leg cramps. Painful dysesthesias may be treated with "neuropathic pain" adjuvants, such as lamotrigine or desipramine.

5.4.4 Intracranial disorders

The CNS disorders in the setting of HIV disease can be divided into four general categories: a) primary infection of the brain by HIV; b) opportunistic infections by parasitic, fungal, viral, and bacterial organisms; b) CNS neoplasms; and d) complications of systemic disorders.
Primary HIV Infection of the Brain: HIV Associated Dementia Complex has already been discussed above.

5.4.5 Intracranial opportunistic infections

CNS toxoplasmosis has been the most common cause of intracerebral mass lesion in HIV-infected patients. Its incidence has declined dramatically among patients receiving PCP prophylaxis, and further declined among patients treated with effective antiretroviral therapy. Earlier reports described frequencies of 3-40%, reflecting the considerable regional variation in exposure to the parasite. CT scan of the brain usually shows multiple ring-enhancing lesions with predilection for cortex and deep gray-matter structures such as the basal ganglia. The cerebellum and brain stem are less commonly involved. Radiologic appearance can vary markedly; single lesions and lesions with diffuse enhancement, as well as nonenhancing lesions can appear.

5.4.6 Aseptic meningitis

Patients with aseptic meningitis often present initially with headache and occasionally with altered mental status or cranial neuropathies. Many patients with this syndrome probably have primary HIV meningoencephalitis. In investigating symptoms such as headache, altered mental status, and cranial neuropathy, aseptic meningitis must be a diagnosis of exclusion.

5.4.7 Viral encephalitis
Among the opportunistic viral infections of the CNS, the most important are the herpes viruses: herpes simplex types 1 and 2 (HSV-1 and -2), herpes varicella-zoster (VZV), and CMV. Each can cause a meningoencephalitis with mental status changes and focal neurologic findings. Diagnosis is complicated by the low yield of CSF viral cultures in herpesvirus encephalitis in general. In general, the onset of headache, fever, and seizures should, in the absence of other clear etiologies, prompt empiric treatment for herpes simplex encephalitis with acyclovir (10.0 to 12.5 mg/kg intravenously every 8 hours).

5.4.8 Fungal encephalitis
Candida Albicans, which commonly infects the oral mucosa of patients with HIV disease, can cause a meningoencephalitis, usually in the setting of fungemia. Microabscesses are the usual pathologic findings in the brain. Mucormycosis, especially among injection drug users, and aspergillosis have been reported causes of meningoencephalitis in patients with advanced HIV disease.

5.4.9 Systemic neoplasms
Although Kaposi sarcoma (KS) is the most common systemic neoplasm in HIV disease, it rarely spreads to the CNS. Among the systemic cancers, non-Hodgkin lymphoma is the most important cause of neurologic dysfunction in HIV disease and invades the CNS by spreading along the leptomeninges. Common signs and symptoms include cranial nerve palsies and polyradiculopathy and less commonly, myelopathy due to epidural metastasis with spinal cord compression.

5.4.10 Central nervous system lymphoma
Primary CNS lymphoma (PCNSL) is a fairly common cause of cerebral mass lesions in patients with advanced HIV disease. The most common signs and symptoms are confusion, lethargy, and personality changes, usually with focal deficits, such as hemiparesis, hemisensory loss, ataxia, and aphasia. Seizures are less common, but not rare.

5.4.11 Metabolic encephalopathy
Metabolic encephalopathy occurs frequently in patients with advanced HIV disease. Adverse reactions to therapeutic drugs, hypoxia, electrolyte imbalance, and multiorgan failure are common etiologies. Efavirenz can cause a transient encephalopathy for a few weeks after initiation of therapy. In the cachectic patient or in patients with significant liver disease or history of protracted vomiting, Wernicke encephalopathy due to thiamine deficiency should be considered.

5.4.12 Stroke
Cerebral infarction and transient ischaemic attacks are seen infrequently in HIV infected patients, with a reported incidence ranging from 0.5% to 8.0%. Based on a case control

study, this incidence is less than that among age-matched young adults with other terminal illnesses. Among patients with advanced HIV disease, cerebral ischemic disease is more common than hemorrhagic stroke.

6. Psychiatric manifestations of HIV infection

Recognizing the psychiatric manifestations of HIV disease can be complicated by the complex biologic, psychologic and social circumstances associated with this illness, and psychiatric symptoms often go unrecognized and untreated(Evans et al., 1999). The significance of these findings is magnified by emerging evidence that certain symptoms, such as depression, may be associated with an increase in mortality rate among HIV-seropositive women and with disease progression in HIV-seropositive men.

The psychiatric sequelae of HIV infection and AIDS are numerous and have etiologies that involve neurobiological and psychosocial factors. These include the natural and expected grief response to being diagnosed with a terminal illness, later reactions to disability and illness, exacerbation of preexisting psychiatric illness, development of new primary psychiatric symptoms and syndromes, and the neuropsychiatric manifestations of HIV associated neurological illness.

It is understandable that individuals who receive notification of positive HIV test results will be emotionally distressed as they adjust to the knowledge of their HIV serostatus. The severity of the acute distress will vary from individual to individual. Whereas some individuals may react with little distress, others may be at increased risk of suicide. Thus, it appears that although individuals are often distraught after receiving positive HIV test results, after an adjustment period lasting weeks to a few months, most will cope well and will show a reduction in anxiety and depressive symptoms. Consequently, it appears that symptoms of depression and anxiety should not be considered "normal" in asymptomatic HIV infection. Rather, significant symptoms should warrant careful clinical evaluation.

6.1 Depressive disorder in patients with HIV/AIDS

Depressive symptoms are the commonest psychiatric complication of chronic medical illnesses (Practice guidelines for HIV treatment, 2000). Studies have shown that the prevalence of depression in people living with HIV/AIDS is 2 to 3 times higher than that in the general population (Bing et al, 2001). Depressive disorder is the most common psychiatric condition in people living with HIV/AIDS with estimated life time prevalence in the range of between 21% and 61% (Elliot et al, 1998). A recent meta-analysis of data from ten studies examining the prevalence of depression among HIV-infected individuals reveal a two-fold increase in rates of depression compared with HIV-negative individuals (Ciesla et al, 2001).The current estimates may represent an underestimation as there is evidence that depression may be under diagnosed in the context of HIV medical care (Steven et al, 2003). Previous research has also shown that depression in patients with HIV/AIDS may be associated with disease progression (Cook et al, 2004), reduced compliance with antiretroviral treatment (Rabkin et al, 2002), and as a result of additional illness burden, lead to a reduction in the quality of life (Sherbourne et al, 2000). Depressed individuals with HIV use significantly more health care and related services (Williams et al, 2005). Despite all of these important evidences, depression remains underrecognized, underdiagnosed and undertreated in medical clinics. Thus, recognizing and treating depression is important because of its association with poor self-care and worse health outcomes in those with HIV (Paterson et al, 2000).

The relationship between depression and HIV/AIDS may be complex. Firstly, populations at risk for HIV infection have elevated rates of major depression. High rates of major depression have been found in homosexual men (Sittirai et al, 1993) and patients with substance use disorders (Mc Kinon et al, 1996). Secondly, major depression is a risk factor for HIV infection by virtue of its impact on behavior, intensification of substance abuse, exacerbation of self-destructive behaviors, and promotion of poor partner choice in relationships. In this way, depression can be seen as a vector of HIV transmission. Patients with depression have also been shown to be at increased risk for disease progression and mortality. Thirdly, HIV increases the risk of developing major depression through a variety of mechanisms, including direct injury to subcortical areas of the brain, chronic stress, stigma, worsening social isolation, bereavement, debilitation and intense demoralization (Zisook et al, 1998). Although direct evidence for a relationship between worsening HIV disease and the development of depression is limited, there are several studies that support this link, particularly the study based on the Multicenter AIDS Cohort Study showing that there is a two and half fold increase in rates of depression as patients CD4 cell count falls below 200cells per mm[3.]

Symptoms of depression include persistent sadness, loss of interest, decreased energy and appetite, low concentration, sleep problems, guilt/worthlessness feelings, psychomotor retardation or agitation, and suicidal ideations. In addition to significant distress, symptoms of depression can also cause other health-related functional and quality of life impairments.

6.2 Mania

Higher rates of mania have also been noted with progression of HIV infection. In early HIV infection, 1%-2% of patients experience manic episodes (Lyketsos &Treisman, 2001), which is only slightly higher than the rate in the general population. However, after the onset of AIDS, 4%-8% of patients appear to experience mania (Lyketsos et al., 1993). This increased frequency of mania around the time of onset of AIDS has been closely associated with cognitive changes or dementia and is thought to be a secondary manic syndrome due to HIV infection of the CNS. In a 17-month chart review, among the 8% of patients with manic episodes, counts of helper/inducer lymphocyte (CD3+/CD4+) cells were significantly higher in those with a history of mood disorder, suggesting that mania may be a direct effect of HIV on the CNS (Lyketsos et al., 1993).In a case–control study of 19 patients with HIV-associated mania and 57 HIV-seropositive controls, AIDS dementia was significantly more common in patients with mania, which suggests a strong association between HIV neuropathology and manic symptoms(Mijch et al., 1999). Sometimes referred to as "AIDS mania," this condition is phenomenologically different from the typical manic syndrome of bipolar disorder in both its symptom profile and severity, and it is often characterized by irritability rather than euphoria.

6.3 Anxiety

Anxiety is common in patients with HIV seropositivity. Individuals with pre-existing disorder may be at increased risk for exacerbation of symptoms, due to the numerous stresses of HIV positivity. Concern over possible progression of HIV disease, the impact of illness on social status, friends, family and work, as well as existential concerns all may result in significant anxiety.

6.4 Psychosis

Psychosis is a recognized, but relative to the mood disorders, an uncommon psychiatric manifestation of AIDS. Even less commonly, antiretroviral therapy may precipitate psychosis. For example, there have been anecdotal reports of psychosis associated with ganciclovir and efavirenz. Paranoid delusions, and auditory hallucination have been reported most frequently and manic symptoms and catatonia have also been described. Psychosis has been found more frequently in patients with AIDS-related neurocognitive impairments and can be a manifestation of psychiatric conditions such as delirium, affective disorders, or schizophrenia, but it also may occur in the absence of these conditions. Estimates of the prevalence of new-onset psychosis in patients with HIV range from 0.5 to 15% (which is considerably higher than would be expected in the general population).

6.5 Delirium

Delirium is a frequent consequence of the severe medical illnesses or treatment that occurs over the course of AIDS. Behavioural manifestations include agitation, psychosis, aggressive behaviour, mutism and marked withdrawal. The delirium in AIDS is usually indistinguishable from the delirium resulting from any other serious acute medical illness.

6.6 Substance abuse

Abuse of variety of substances, including alcohol, and other illicit drugs may be common in groups at high risk of HIV infection. Continued abuse of substances may have many adverse consequences, including interference with patients adherence to needed medical treatment, increased risk of behaviour that could result in further transmission of HIV (such as unsafe sex while intoxicated, sharing needles etc.), as well as morbidity related directly to the use of the substance. It is therefore necessary to do a careful assessment for an existing substance use disorder in HIV positive patients.

6.7 Suicide

Several epidemiological studies suggest that AIDS patients are at increased risk of death by suicide. The relative prevalence is estimated to range from 7 to 36 times the rate in demographically similar control populations. Other studies, however, have not found patients with AIDS to have higher suicidal ideation, especially when comparing persons with AIDS to other medically or neuropsychiatrically ill patients.

HIV infection may exacerbate psychiatric conditions, including major depression, bipolar disorder, and schizophrenia. One study of patients who had schizophrenia before they were diagnosed with HIV infection found that the patients had more severe depressive episodes and reduced tolerance to psychopharmacologic medications (including benzodiazepines and neuroleptics) after infection than before. Although methodological issues make such studies difficult, more research is needed to understand better the role of HIV infection in worsening pre-existing psychiatric disorders.

Various complications of HIV infection including opportunistic infections of the CNS, tumors, systemic disease, and adverse effects of medications may mimic psychiatric illnesses, producing symptoms that resemble mania, depression, psychosis, or drug intoxication. In all cases, any underlying medical problem should be addressed. The acute onset of psychiatric symptoms in a patient with no such prior history should prompt a complete neuropsychiatric evaluation, toxicology and laboratory screens, and when appropriate, neuroimaging studies and lumbar puncture to help identify possible causes.

7. Assessment and treatment of psychiatric disorders in people living with HIV/AIDS

A comprehensive history from the patient and/or caregiver is needed. There should be special focus on the history of the current complaint, past psychiatric history, past and present substance abuse history, full medical history and sexual risk history and the patient's adherence to previous treatment regimens. Of equal importance is identification of social support systems.

A mental status examination (MSE) of the patient's level of cognitive (knowledge-related) ability, appearance, emotional mood, and thought patterns at the time of evaluation should be conducted. In the psychotic patient one needs to focus specifically on the behaviour and appearance of the patient. His or her speech and speed of thoughts should be assessed, and mood symptoms, affect, suicidality and neuro-vegetative symptoms evaluated. Perceptual disturbances, thought form, thought content and finally insight and judgment also need to be assessed.

A comprehensive and meticulous physical and neurological examination should be performed to exclude any organic causes for the presenting psychiatric symptoms. One should first examine for signs of delirium and rule out HIV-associated cognitive disorders. Medical diagnoses should first be considered and only after that should a psychiatric diagnosis be entertained.

Differential diagnosis needs to consider the presence of a pre-existing psychiatric illness, use of illicit substances and the presence of cognitive impairment.

Assessment and treatment of psychotic disorders in people living with HIV/AIDS (PLWHA) can be very challenging. A useful delineation may be to divide psychosis in the PLWHA into: (i) psychiatric disorders predating HIV infection; (ii) new-onset psychotic disorders; and (iii) disorders associated with medical conditions (delirium) or substance intoxication or withdrawal, and those that are likely to be complications of treatment (i.e. antiretrovirals or antituberculosis drugs). A good history, mental state and physical examination is usually important in making this delineation. Laboratory investigations are crucial in the assessment of delirium and substance intoxication.

The choice of antipsychotic drugs depends largely on the patient, presenting symptoms, past response, potential side-effect profile, possible drug interactions, cost, and pill burden of the chronically ill patient. Many patients with new-onset psychosis or psychosis associated with various medical conditions may only require short-term treatment with antipsychotic medication. However, some patients may require long-term maintenance treatment with antipsychotic agents, and here special attention must be paid to the following factors. The typical antipsychotics are commonly used in resource-constrained settings. Here low doses of haloperidol or chlorpromazine can be used. Vigilance is required with regard to extrapyramidal side effects. Newer atypical antipsychotics such as Risperidone or Olanzepine are now widely used in the treatment of psychotic disorders in HIV/AIDS. They have lower propensity to cause extrapyramidal side effects.

The impact of depression on the course of HIV has initiated the application of specific psychosocial and pharmacologic treatments targeting individuals with HIV and comorbid depression. Pharmacotherapy is the mainstay of treatment of moderate to severe depression. Several studies have demonstrated efficacy of various antidepressant agents in HIV patients, but no single antidepressant has been found superior in treating HIV-infected patients as a group (Olatunji et al, 2006).

Aside from how well the pharmacology of the antidepressant matches a patient's disease, the engine that drives effectiveness is patient adherence. The general rule is to start at low doses of any medication and titrate up to a therapeutic dose slowly, so as to minimize early side effects that may act as obstacles to adherence. Patients who show partial response to antidepressant after adequate dosage and duration should be offered an augmentation strategy. The choice of an antidepressant is largely based on their side effect profile. Some of the antidepressant drugs that are useful in treatment of depression in patients with HIV/AIDS include Amitriptyline, Imipramine, Clomipramine, Fluoxetine, Paroxetine, Sertraline, Fluvoxamine and Venlafaxine (Elliot et al, 1998). The use of psychostimulants such as Methylphenidate and Dextroamphetamine has also been found effective (Wagner et al, 2000).

Some clinicians often wonder about the interaction of antidepressants and HAART. Some interactions may occur but two points deserve emphasis. Firstly, because depression is associated with reduction in adherence to HAART, untreated depression may be equally or more detrimental to disease progression than any medication interaction. Secondly, experience in working with comorbid HIV and depression has not shown clinical significance to antidepressant-HAART interaction.

Psychosocial intervention is an integral part of treatment for depression in patients with HIV/AIDS. A combination of psychosocial intervention and medication was shown to be more effective for patients than either modality alone. Among the individual psychotherapies, interpersonal psychotherapy, cognitive-behavioral psychotherapy and supportive psychotherapy are effective in treatment of depression in patients with HIV/AIDS (Markowitz et al, 1995). A social intervention such as social support group therapy is also effective (Kelly et al, 1993).

Identifying and treating depression in patients with HIV/AIDS could result in substantial improvement in quality of life and potentially increase medication adherence, which would in turn affect illness severity and progression.

Treatment of anxiety disorders in HIV/AIDS also requires a combination of psychosocial intervention and medication. Adequate counseling and relaxation techniques are sufficient to treat mild anxiety associated with the various crisis points in the course of HIV/AIDS. For the more severe anxiety disorders, antidepressants and cognitive behavioural techniques are useful.

Every patient with HIV/AIDS presenting with psychiatric disorder must also be assessed for suicidal risk and cases where risk is high, patients should be hospitalized for detailed evaluation and appropriate treatment.

Substance abuse is a common problem in patients with HIV/AIDS. Physicians should have a high index of suspicion while assessing patients. When present, motivational interviews are important. Patients with severe problems who are motivated should be hospitalized for detoxification and appropriate pharmacological and psychosocial treatment.

8. Neurologic and psychiatric complications of antiretroviral drugs

Much progress has been made in treating HIV infection in the last several years and people infected with HIV are now living longer, healthier lives. What was once considered a progressive, ultimately fatal disease has become, in developed countries, a chronic condition that often can be managed long term.

In large part, this change has resulted from the introduction of protease inhibitors (PI), nucleoside reverse transcriptase inhibitors (NRTI), and non-nucleoside reverse transcriptase inhibitors (NNRTI) in highly active antiretroviral treatment (HAART) regimen. Now, carefully selected combinations of these agents can bring viral loads below detectable levels, increase CD4 T-lymphocyte counts, and improve immune function.

Investigators have realized that HIV cannot be completely eradicated with the treatments that are currently available and that long-term HAART may have side-effects that are severe or health- complicating enough to require modification or temporary cessation of treatment. Even when the virus is virtually undetectable in the blood, it appears to remain sequestered in host reservoirs that are inaccessible to HAART and may provide a source for viral rebound if therapy is withdrawn. With the treatments currently available, HAART will probably need to continue for the patient's lifetime, and clinicians need a thorough understanding of the health implications associated with long-term HAART, the potential complications of HIV infection even in the absence of overt illness, and the strategies for maintaining treatment adherence and minimizing treatment side-effects.

Unfortunately, complications of HAART and complications of HIV infection, particularly in patients with advanced disease and AIDS, overlap significantly. Among health risks that may be associated with HIV or HAART are neurologic complications (such as myelopathy, neuropathy and neuropathic pain, changes in cognition, and dementia), and psychiatric complications (such as mania, depression, schizophrenia, and substance abuse and dependence). CNS complications in patients with HIV, including psychiatric syndromes, delirium, seizures, and cognitive impairment, may in some cases reflect consequences of treatment with antiretroviral drugs that penetrate the CNS. For example, zidovudine and efavirenz, both considered attractive choices for patients with CNS complications because they have good CNS penetration, are themselves associated with potentially significant neuropsychiatric complications. Peripheral neurologic complications including neuropathic pain, neuropathic weakness, and denervation syndromes have been attributed to various toxic and metabolic factors in association with antiretroviral treatment. In managing neurologic complications, it is important to distinguish, when possible, between symptoms related to the HIV disease process and side-effects of HAART. To make such distinctions, clinicians need to understand which antiretroviral agents may cause neurologic and psychiatric symptoms.

Zidovudine, a nucleoside analogue that inhibits replication of HIV by interfering with viral reverse transcriptase, was the first agent to significantly reduce mortality and opportunistic infections in HIV-infected patients. Zidovudine has been found effective at high doses in slowing the progression of AIDS dementia, and can penetrate the blood-brain barrier. Zidovudine is therefore an attractive choice in HAART regimens targeting dementia and other CNS complications of HIV. However, its CNS penetration may also explain the confusion, agitation, and insomnia in up to 5% of people who took zidovudine for one year. In addition, there are anecdotal reports of psychiatric symptoms, including mania and depression, in patients treated with zidovudine. Several case reports document manic episodes in association with zidovudine treatment, even in patients with no previous psychiatric history. In some patients, mania was severe enough to necessitate hospitalization. In recent years, fewer problems have been reported, in part because zidovudine is now used in lower doses‹approximately of 600 mg/day (or 300 mg twice a day) versus the up to 2000 mg/day doses used in the pre-HAART era.

The mechanisms involved in zidovudine-associated psychiatric effects are unknown. For some patients, dose reduction is beneficial, but for others, discontinuation may be necessary. Discontinuing zidovudine treatment has been shown to rapidly reduce manic symptoms (and symptoms returned upon reintroduction of the drug, suggesting a causal relationship). However, patients have been able to resume zidovudine treatment if they also received treatment for mania.

Other adverse neurologic effects of zidovudine treatment are insomnia, myalgia, and severe headaches. Zidovudine also has been associated with seizures, particularly in cases of overdose, which have on rare occasions been fatal. Because HIV infection is associated with similar neurological problems, it is important to exclude other causes before attributing them to zidovudine treatment. However, the severity of these side-effects suggests the need to closely monitor patients taking this drug.

Neurologic symptoms associated with other NRTI may include headache, malaise, and fatigue; for most patients, these symptoms are not severe enough to discontinue HAART. A more serious side-effect is peripheral neuropathy and may be seen with didanosine, zalcitabine, or stavudine treatment but not with zidovudine treatment. The mechanism is unknown, but in vitro studies have shown that zalcitabine, stavudine, and didanosine but not zidovudine - inhibit nerve growth factor (NGF)-stimulated differentiation of a neuronal cell line.

For patients with peripheral neuropathy, symptomatic treatment with ibuprofen or topical analgesic creams can sometimes be effective. Tricyclic antidepressants have been used to manage pain in patients with HIV-associated peripheral neuropathy. In clinical practice, we have found that Tricyclic antidepressants can be partially effective, but for many patients, the pain of neuropathy can be severe, irreversible, and debilitating. Therefore, patients with HIV who develop neuropathy require careful evaluation to determine the risks and benefits of continuing NRTI treatment. In some cases, decreasing dosage may help, but in others, the contributing drug must be discontinued.

Three NNRTIs - efavirenz, delavirdine, and nevirapine - are currently available for the treatment of HIV infection. They are usually prescribed in combination with NRTI. Clinical trials of delavirdine and nevirapine revealed few adverse events affecting the CNS; therefore, the relatively more substantial CNS side-effects seen in clinical trials of efavirenz were unexpected.

CNS side-effects observed with efavirenz include dizziness, headache, confusion, stupor, impaired concentration, agitation, amnesia, depersonalization, hallucinations, insomnia, and abnormal or vivid dreams. For most patients, these side-effects resolve within 6-10 weeks of starting treatment, but for some patients, symptoms seem to wax and wane over a long term. For most patients, these disturbances diminished or resolved within 2 months. Neither dose reduction nor dose splitting shortened or reduced the intensity of symptoms.

Psychiatric effects also have been noted with efavirenz, though they occur less frequently than neurologic effects.When efavirenz-associated psychiatric effects occur, they may be serious and may include anxiety, depression, and suicidal ideation.

Clinicians should advise patients of possible CNS effects of efavirenz, and should watch for changes in behavior, cognition, or mood. If side-effects persist or patients find them intolerable, a switch in HAART regimen may be appropriate. Although efavirenz is often a first-line treatment, many patients receive it after experiencing treatment failure on earlier HAART regimens. Therefore, patients who switch to efavirenz and then experience neurologic or psychiatric side-effects may have limited options for future antiretroviral treatment. It is important to carefully consider risks and treatment alternatives for these patients.

The combination of HIV Protease Inhibitor with the older antiretroviral agents brought about substantial decreases in viral loads and opportunistic infections with concomitant increases in CD4 T-cell counts. As a result, HIV-associated morbidity and mortality has declined dramatically in recent years.

Although PI may have neurologic side-effects, they tend to be variable and less prominent than those seen with NRTI or NNRTI. Neurologic symptoms may occur more often with ritonavir or ritonavir/saquinavir combination treatments than with indinavir treatment.

9. Consequences of neuropsychiatric problems in patients with HIV/AIDS

Some previous studies have indicated that Neuropsychiatric disorders in people living with HIV/AIDS are associated with disease progression, poor adherence to antiretroviral drugs, increased incidence of high risk sexual behavior with the potential for further HIV transmission, and deterioration in their quality of life. Thus, the place of psychiatrists in the treatment and care of patients with HIV/AIDS is crucial.

There is a consistently strong evidence from high income countries that adherence to Highly Active Antiretroviral Therapy is lowered by depression, cognitive impairment, alcohol use and substance use disorders. A study in Ethiopia showed that depression was associated with less than 95% self reported adherence (Ambebir et al., 2008). Previous research has also shown that depression in patients with HIV/AIDS may be associated with reduced adherence with antiretroviral treatment (Byakika-Tusuiime et al., 2009; Dimatteo et al., 2000; Mugavero et al., 2000; Phyllips et al., 2002; Rabkin & Goetz 2002)and disease progression(Cook 2004; Paterson 2000).They concluded that identifying and treating depression in these patients may improve medication adherence.

In a study of women who were medically eligible to receive Highly Active Antiretroviral Therapy (HAART), its non receipt was associated with substance use. Furthermore, other epidemiological studies indicate that the presence of drug use disorder can complicate the management of HIV illness and compromise adherence to HIV medication and secondary preventive efforts (HIV clinical resource 2009).

HIV-infected subjects in several studies reported "forgetting" as one of the most common reasons for poor adherence to antiretroviral drugs. It is also possible that HIV-associated neurocognitive disturbances, which are common and more prominent as the disease advances, might be responsible for some of the cases of poor medication adherence. Other studies have reported a significantly greater risk of poor adherence to HAART in HIV-infected persons with neurocognitive impairment (Hinkin et al. 2002).

Depression has been associated with immune suppression and other health outcomes in studies of individual with and without chronic disease (; Herbert & Cohen 1993; Rover et al., 1991). Studies have documented association between depression and HIV progression (Lesserman et al., 1997; Lesserman et al, 1999), HIV-related symptoms (Leketsos et al., 1993) and mortality (Lesserman et al., 1997). Some studies found that HIV-sero-positive gay men who reported depressive symptoms demonstrated immunological changes associated with HIV activity and progression, for example CD4, CD8 cell count proliferate.

Some studies have compared pattern of neuropsychiatric disorder especially the neurocognitive impairment at various level of CD4 cell counts namely 200, 250, 300, 350 and 400 cells /ml and found that there is generally worsening trend of neurocognitive impairment as the CD4 cell count decreases and therefore recommended the serial determination of CD4 cell count in HIV infected patient and screening for neuropsychiatric syndromes in those with CD4 count values of less than 350 cell/ml(Bornstein et al., 1992; Heaton et al., 1995; Miller et al., 1990).

Research has shown that neuropsychiatric disorders in patients with HIV/AIDS complicates help seeking, diagnosis, quality of care provided, treatment and its outcome and adherence(World Health Organization report, 2008). Regardless of aetiology, the co morbidity of mental illness and HIV poses special challenge for HIV care. Individual with these co morbidity face even greater barriers to care than those with HIV alone. Once in care, their treatment is more complex (Francine et al., 2009). Mental and substance use disorders in HIV/AIDS affects help seeking behaviour or uptake of diagnostic and treatment services for HIV and AIDS.

People with alcohol use disorders are more likely than the general population to contract HIV. Similarly, rates of alcohol problems are high among HIV/AIDS patients (Petry, 1999). Lifetime prevalence rates of alcohol use disorders ranging from 29% to 60% have been found among HIV positive populations (Bryant, 1998). This is 2 to 4 times higher than in the general population. Alcohol use is associated with high-risk sexual behaviors and intravenous drug use which are two major modes of HIV transmission.

In persons already infected, the combination of heavy drinking and HIV has been associated with increased medical and psychiatric complications, delays in seeking treatment (Samet et al., 1998), difficulties with HIV medication adherence (Cook et al., 2001; Wagner et al., 2001), and poorer HIV treatment outcomes (Lucas et al., 2002). Decreasing alcohol use in people who have HIV or who are at risk for becoming infected reduces the spread of HIV and the diseases associated with it.

People who abuse alcohol are more likely to engage in behaviors that place them at risk for contracting or transmitting HIV. A history alcohol use has been correlated with a lifetime tendency toward high-risk sexual behaviors, including multiple sex partners, unprotected intercourse, sex with high-risk partners (e.g., injection drug users, prostitutes), and the exchange of sex for money or drugs (Avins et al., 1994; Boscarino et al., 1995; Malow et al., 2001; Windle, 1997).There may be many reasons for this association. For example, alcohol can act directly on the brain to reduce inhibitions and diminish risk perception (Cooper, 2002; Fromme et al., 1999; MacDonald et al., 2000).

Decreasing alcohol use among HIV patients not only reduces the medical and psychiatric consequences associated with alcohol consumption but also decreases other drug use and risky sexual behavior and hence reduces HIV transmission (Lucas et al., 2002). Thus, alcohol and other drug abuse treatment can be considered primary HIV prevention as well (Metzger et al., 1998).

With improved treatments and longer survival times for persons with HIV infection, the maintenance and improvement of their functioning and well-being (collectively referred to as "health-related quality of life") have become major goals of treatment. The World Health

Organization (WHO) defined quality of life (QOL) as an individual's perception of their position in life in the context of the culture and value systems in which they live and in relation to their goals, expectations, standards and concerns. It is a broad-ranging concept affected in a complex way by the person's physical health, psychological state, level of independence, social relationships and their relationship to salient features of their environment (WHOQOL Group, 1995).

We know from studies of patients and general populations that mood disorders, particularly depression, have a substantial negative impact on a person's health-related quality of life (Jia et al, 2004). In fact, for most domains of functioning and well-being, depression is more debilitating than most medical conditions (Sherbourne et al, 2000). In a study conducted by Sherbourne et al (2000) to assess the impact of psychiatric conditions on health related quality of life, they recruited a national probability sample of persons with HIV, receiving medical care in the United States. Subjects were screened for psychiatric conditions and their health-related quality of life was assessed. They found that 36% of subjects screened positive for a current depressive disorder and 26% for dysthymia. Subjects with a probable diagnosis of any mood disorder had significantly worse functioning and well-being than those without a mood disorder diagnosis on all health-related quality of life measures, including the physical and mental health composites. These findings substantiate the considerable additional illness burden associated with mood disorders in HIV infected people.

This chapter is intended to help create awareness about mental health problems and its consequences in patients with HIV/AIDS, so as to facilitate routine screening of mental disorders and mental health integration in the comprehensive care of people living with HIV/AIDS.

10. References

Ambebir A, Woldemicheal K, Getachew S, Girma B & Deribe K.(2008). Predictors of adherence to antiretroviral therapy among HIV infected persons: a prospective study in Southwest Ethiopia. *BMC Public Health*, 30(8): 265.

Apostolski S,McAlarney T,Quattrini A, Steven WL, Rosoklija G, Lugaressi A, Cobo M, Sadiq SA, Lederman S, Hays AP & Latov N. (1993). The gp120 glycoprotein of human immunodeficiency virus type 1 binds to sensory ganglion neurons. *Annals of Neurology*, 34:855-863.

Avins, A.L., Woods, W.J., Lindan, C.P., Hudes, E.S., Clark, W., & Hulley, S.B. (1994). HIV infection and risk behaviors among heterosexuals in alcohol treatment programs. *Journal of the American Medical Association*, 271(7), 515–518.

Berger JR & Nath A.(1997). HIV dementia and the basal ganglia. *Intervirology*, 40:122-131.

Berger JR, Levy RM, Flomenhoft D & Dobbs M. (1998). Predictive factors for prolonged survival in acquired immunodeficiency syndrome-associated progressive multifocal leukoencephalopathy. *Annals of Neurology*. 44(3):341-9.

Berger JR,Nath A, Greenberg RN, Anderson AH, Greene RA, Bognar A & Avison MJ. (2000). Cerebrovascular changes in the basal ganglia with HIV dementia. *Neurology*, 54:921-926.

Bing EG, Burnam MA, Longshore D, Fleishman JA, Sherbourne CD, London SA, Turner BJ, Eggan F, Beckman R, Vitiello B, Morton SC, Orlando M, Bozzette SA, Ortiz-Borron L & Shapiro M. (2001). The estimated prevalence of psychiatric disorders, drug use and dependence among people with HIV disease in the United States. *Archives of General Psychiatry*, 58 : 721-28.

Bloom FE & Rausch DM.(1997). HIV in the brain: pathology and neurobehavioral consequences. *Journal of Neurovirology*, 3:102-109.

Bornstein RA, Nasrallah HA & Para MF. (1992). Neuropsychological performance in asymptomatic HIV infection. *Journal of Neuropsychiatry and clinical Neuroscience*, 4:386-394.

Boscarino, J.A., Avins, A.L., Woods, W.J., Lindan, C.P., Hudes, E.S. & Clark, W. (1995). Alcohol-related risk factors associated with HIV infection among patients entering alcoholism treatment: Implications for prevention. *Journal of Studies on Alcohol*, 56(6), 642–653.

Bryant, K. (1998).Alcohol and AIDS: A Guide to Research Issues and Opportunities: *National Institute on Alcohol Abuse and Alcoholism.*

Byakika-Tusuiime J, Crane J, Oyugi JH, Ragland K, Kayume A, & Musoke P.(March, 2009). Longitudinal antiretroviral adherence in HIV +ve Ugandan parents and their children initiating HAART in the MTCT-Plus family treatment model: role of depression in declining adherence over time. *AIDS Behaviour.* (Epub ahead of print) Pubmed PMID: 19301113

Centers for Disease Control (1982): Undifferentiated non-Hodgkins Lymphoma among homosexual males in United States. *MMWR* 31: 227 – 30.

Childs EA,Lyles RH,Selnes OA, Chen B, Miller EN, Cohen BA, Becker JT, Mettors J & Mc Arthur JC. (1999). Plasma viral load and CD4 lymphocytes predict HIV-associated dementia and sensory neuropathy.*Neurology*,52:607-613.

Ciesla MA & Robert JE.(2001). Meta-analysis of the relationship between HIV infection and risk for depressive disorders. *American Journal of Psychiatry*, 158, 5 : 725-30.

Cook, R.L., Sereika, S.M., Hunt, S.C., Woodward, W.C., Erlen, J.A. & Conigliaro, J. (2001). Problem drinking and medication adherence among patients with HIV infection. *Journal of General Internal Medicine*, 16(2), 83–88.

Cook J. (2004). Depressive symptoms increase AIDS-related death. *American Journal of Public Health*, 150 {10}: 85-94.

Cooper, M.L. (2002). Alcohol use and risky sexual behavior among college students and youth: Evaluating the evidence. *Journal of Studies on Alcohol*, 14,101–117.

Dalakas MC, Illa I, Pezeshkpour GH, Laukaitis JP, Cohen B & Griffin JL.(1990). Mitochondrial myopathy caused by long-term zidovudine therapy. *New England Journal of Medicine*, 322(16):1098-105.

Deeks SG, Smith M, Holodniy M & Kahn JO.(1997). HIV-1 Protease inhibitor: A review of clinicians. *JAMA*, 277: 145 – 53.

de la Monte SM, Ho DD, Schooley RT, Hirsch MS & Richardson EP. (1987). Subacute encephalomyelitis of AIDS and its relation to HTLV-III infection. *Neurology*, 37(4):562-9.

Demasi RA, Graham MN, Tolson JM, Pham SV, Capuano GA, Fisher RL, Shaefer MS, Pakes GE, Sawyerr GA & Eron JJ. (2001). Correlation between self reported adherence to highly active antiretroviral therapy and virologic outcome. *Advances in Therapy*, 18(4): 163 – 73.

Descamps D, Flandre P, Calvez V, Pentavin G, Meiffredy V, Collin G, Delangerre C, Robert-Delmas S, Bazin B, Aboulker JP, Pialoux G, Raffi F & Brun-Vezinet F. (2000). Mechanisms of virologic failure in previously untreated HIV-infected patients from a trial of Induction-Maintenance Therapy. *JAMA*, 283: 205 – 19.

Dimatteo MR, Lepper HS, & Croghan TW.(2000). Meta-analysis of the effects of anxiety and depression on patient adherence. *Archives of Internal Medicine*, 160:2101-07.

Elliot AJ & Roy-Byrne PP.(1998). Major depressive disorder and HIV-1 infection. *Seminars in Clinical Neuropsychiatry*, 3:137-50.

Evans DL, Staab JP, Petitto JM, Morrison MF, Szuba MP, Ward HE, Wingate B, Luber MP, & O'Reardon JP. (1999). Depression in the medical setting: biopsychological interactions and treatment considerations. *Journal of Clinical Psychiatry*, 60(Suppl 4):40-55.

Everall IP,Heaton RK,Marcotte TD, Ellis RJ, McCutchan JA, Atkinson JH, Grant I, Mallory M & Mastiah E. (19999). Cortical synaptic density is reduced in mild to moderate human immunodeficiency virus neurocognitive disorder.HNRC Group. HIV Neurobehavioral Research Center.*Brain Pathology*, 9:209-217.

Francine C, Karen M & Milton W. (2005). Official journal of the world psychiatry association. Pmcid: pmci414758 [online] 2005 Oct [cited 2009 Nov 16]; Available from: URL:http://www.unaids.org/en/default.asp

Fromme, K., D'Amico, E. & Katz, E.C. (1999).Intoxicated sexual risk taking: An expectancy or cognitive impairment explanation? *Journal of Studies on Alcohol*, 60(1), 54–63.

Gabuzda D & Wang J.(2000). Chemokine receptors and mechanisms of cell death in HIV neuropathogenesis. *Journal of Neurovirology*, 6(Suppl 1):S24-S32.

Galey D, Woodward J & Nath A.(2001). Regulation of cytokines and chemokines by HIV, Tat, and gp120 in astrocytes. *Eighth Conference on Retroviruses and Opportunistic Infections*. Chicago, February 2001 [abstract 70].

Glass JD, Fedor H, Wesselingh SL & McArthur JC.(1995). Immunocytochemical quantitation of human immunodeficiency virus in the brain: correlations with dementia. *Annals of Neurology*, 38(5):755-62.

Green WC. (1991). The molecular biology of HIV-1 infection. *New England Journal of Medicine*, 324: 308 – 16.

Hall CD, Snyder CR, Messenheimer JA, Wilkins JW, Robertson WT, Whaley RA & Robertson KR.(1991). Peripheral neuropathy in a cohort of human immunodeficiency virus-infected patients. Incidence and relationship to other nervous system dysfunction. *Archives of Neurology*, 48(12):1273-4.

Heaton RK, Grant I & Butters N.(1995). The HNRC 500-Neuropsychology of HIV in function at different disease stages. *Journal of international neuropsychological Society*, 1:231-251.

Herbert TB & Cohen S.(1993). Depression and immunity: a meta-analytical review. *Psychology Bulletin*, 113:472-486.

Herzberg U & Sagen J.(2001). Peripheral nerve exposure to HIV viral envelope protein gp120 induces neuropathic pain and spinal gliosis. *Journal of Neuroimmunology*,116:29-39.

Hinkin CH, Castellon SA, Durvasula RS, Hardy DJ, Lam MN, Mason KI, Thrasher D, Goetz MB & Stefaniak M.(2002). Medication adherence among HIV+ adults: effects of cognitive dysfunction and regimen complexity. *Neurology*, 59:1944–1950.

HIV clinical guidelines for the primary care practitioner. Mental health care for people with HIV infection. Published by the AIDS Institute, New York State department of health, 2000. Pg. 2.

HIV clinical resource. Depression and mania in patient with HIV/AIDS. [online] 2008 Jun [cited 2009 Nov16]; Available from: URL:http://www.hivguidelines.org/guideline.aspx?guidelineid=13

Jia H, Uphold CR, Wu S, Reid K, Findley K & Duncan PW. (2004). Health-related quality of life among men with HIV infection: effects of social support, coping and depression. *AIDS Patient Care STDS*, 18: 594 – 603.

Johnston J, Zhang K & Silva C. (2000). HIV-1 Tat induction of matrix metalloproteinases causes neuronal damage. Seventh Conference on Retroviruses and Opportunistic Infections. San Francisco, [abstract 439].

Katalan J. (1989). HIV disease and Psychiatry practice. *Psychiatric Bulletin*, 13: 316 – 22.

Koedel U,Kohleisen B,Sporer B, Lahrtz F, Ovod V, Fontana A, Erfle V & Pfister H. (1999). HIV type 1 Nef protein is a viral factor for leukocyte recruitment into the central nervous system. *Journal of Immunology*, 163:1237-1245.

Koppel BS, Wormser GP, Tuchman AJ, Maayan S, Hewlett D Jr & Daras M.(1985). Central nervous system involvement in patients with acquired immune deficiency syndrome (AIDS). Acta Neurology Scandinavica, 71(5):337-53.

Lesserman J, Petitton JM, Perkins DO, Folds TD, Golden RN & Evans DL.(1997). Severe stress, depressive symptoms and changes in lymphocytes subsets in HIV- infected men: a 2-year follow –up study. *Archives of General Psychiatry*, 54:279-285.

Lyketsos CG, Hoover DR & Guccione MS.(1993). Depressive symptoms as predictors of medical outcomes in HIV infection. *JAMA*, 270:2563-2567.

Lyketsos CG, Hanson AL, Fishman M, Rosenblatt A, McHugh PR & Treisman GJ. (1993). Manic syndrome early and late in the course of HIV. *American Journal of Psychiatry*, 150:326-7.

Lyketsos CG & Treisman GJ.(2001). Mood disorders in HIV infection. *Psychiatry Annals*, 31:45-50.

MacDonald, T.K., MacDonald, G., Zanna, M.P. & Fong, G.T. (2000).Alcohol, sexual arousal, and intentions to use condoms in young men: Applying alcohol myopia theory to risky sexual behavior. *Health Psychology*, 19(3), 290–298.

Malow, R.M., Dévieux, J.G., Jennings, T.E., Lucenko, B.A. & Kalichman, S.C. (2001). Substance-abusing adolescents at varying levels of HIV risk: Psychosocial characteristics, drug use, and sexual behavior. *Journal of Substance Abuse*, 13,103–117.

Markowitz JC, Klerman GL, Clougherty KF, Spielman LA, Jocobsberg LB, Fishman B, Frances AJ, Kocsis JH & Perry SW. (1995). Individual Psychotherapies for depressed HIV-positive patients. *American Journal of Psychiatry*, 152: 1504 – 9.

McGuire D & Greene WC.(1996). Neurological damage in HIV infection: the Molecular Biology of HIV/AIDS. *New York: John Wiley & Sons*,127-142.

Mc Kinon K, Cournos F, Sugden R, Guido JR & Herman R.(1998). The relative contributions of psychiatric symptoms and AIDS knowledge to HIV risk behaviours among people with severe mental illness. *Journal of Clinical Psychiatry*, 57(11): 506 – 13.

Metzger, D.S., Navaline, H. & Woody, G.E. (1998). Drug abuse treatment as HIV prevention. *Public Health Reports*, 113(1), 97–106.

Miller EN, Selnes OA & McArthar JC.(1990). Neuropsychological performance in HIV-1 infected homosexual men; the multicenter AIDS cohort study. *Neurology*, 40 197-203.

Mijch AM, Judd FK, Lyketsos CG, Ellen S & Cockram A.(1999). Secondary mania in patients with HIV infection: Are antiretrovirals protective? *Journal of Neuropsychiatry Clinical Neuroscience*, 11:475-80.

Mugavero M, Ostermann J, Whetten K, Leserman J, Swartz M, Stangl D & Thielman. (2006). Barriers to antiretroviral adherence: the importance of depression, abuse, and other traumatic events. *AIDS Patient Care STDS*, 20(6):418-28.

Neuenburg JK, Brodt HR, Herndier BG, Bickel M, Bacchetti P, Price RW, Grant RM & Schlote W.(2002). HIV-related neuropathology, 1985 to 1999: rising prevalence of HIV encephalopathy in the era of highly active antiretroviral therapy. *Journal of Acquired Immune Deficiency Syndrome*, 31(2):171-7.

Nottet HS. (1999). Interactions between macrophages and brain microvascular endothelial cells: role in pathogenesis of HIV-1 infection and blood - brain barrier function. *Journal of Neurovirology,5:659*-669.

Olatunji BO, Mimiaga MJ, O'cleirigh C & Safren SA.(2006). Review of treatment studies of depression in HIV. *Top HIV Medicine* , 14(3): 112 – 24.

Paterson DL, Swindells S, Mohr J, Brester M, Vergis EM, Squier C, Wagener MM & Singh N. (2000). Adherence to protease inhibitor therapy and outcomes in patients with HIV infection. *Annals of Internal Medicine*, 133: 21 – 30.

Petry, N.M. (1999). Alcohol use in HIV patients. *International Journal of STD and AIDS*, 10(9), 561–570.

Phyllips KD, Moneyham L, Murdaugh C, Boyd MR, Tavakoli A, Jackson K & Vyavaharkar M. (2005). Sleep disturbance and depression as barriers to adherence. *Clinical Nursing Research*, 14:273-293.

Practice guidelines for the treatment of patients with HIV/AIDS. American Psychiatric Association 2000. www.psych.org

Pulliam L, Gascon R, Stubblebine M, McGuire D & McGrath MS.(1997). Unique monocyte subset in patients with AIDS dementia. *Lancet*, 349(9053):692-5.

Rabkin JG & Ferrando S.(1997). A 'second life' agenda. Psychiatric research issues raised by protease inhibitor treatments for people with the human immunodeficiency virus or the acquired immunodeficiency syndrome. *Archives of General Psychiatry*, 54:1049-1053.

Rabkin JG & Goetz RR.(2002). Effects of depressive symptoms and mental health quality of life on use of highly active antiretroviral therapy among HIV sero-positive women. *AIDS Journal*, 30: 401-9.

Rover BW German PS, Brant LJ, dark R, Burton L & Folstein MF. (1991). Depression and mortality in nursing homes. *JAMA*, 265:993-996.

Samet, J.H., Freedberg, K.A., Stein, M.D., Lewis, R., Savetsky, J., Sullivan, L, Levenson SM & Hingson R. (1998). Trillion virion delay: Time from testing positive for HIV to presentation for primary care. *Archives of Internal Medicine,* 158(7), 734–740.

Shapshak P,Nagano I,Xin K, Bradley W, McCoy CB, Sun NC, Stewart RV, Yoshioka M, Petito C & Goodkin K. (1995). HIV-1 heterogeneity and cytokines. Neuropathogenesis.*Advances in Experimental Medicine & Biology,* 373:225-238.

Sherbourne CD, Hays RD, Fleishman JA, Vitiello B, Magruder KM, Bing EG, McCaffrey D, Burnam A, Longshore D, Eggon F, Bozzette SA & Shapiro MF. (2000). Impact of psychiatric conditions on health related quality of life in persons with HIV infection. *American Journal of Psychiatry,* 157 {2} 248-54.

Sittirai W, Brown T & Sakondhavat C.(1993). Level of HIV risk behavior and AIDS knowledge in Thai men having sex with men. *AIDS Care,* 5(3): 261 – 71.

Stebbing J, Gazzard B & Douck DC.(2004). Where does HIV live? New England Journal of Medicine, 350 (24) 2487 – 98.

Steven MA, Kilbourne AM, Gifford AL, Burnam MA, Turner B et al. (2003). Underdiagnosis of depression in HIV. *Journal of General Internal Medicine,* 18(6): 450-60.

Swindells S, Zheng J & Gendelman HE.(1999). HIV associated dementia: new insight into disease pathogenesis and therapeutic interventions. *AIDS Patient Care STDS ,* 3: 153 – 63.

Trillo-Pazos G,McFarlane-Abdulla E,Campbell IC,Pilkington GJ & Everall IP.(2000). Recombinant nef HIV-IIIB protein is toxic to human neurons in culture.*Brain Research,* 864:315-326.

UNAIDS/WHO report on Global HIV/AIDS statistics. November 2006.

Wagner GJ & Rabkin R.(2000). Effects of Dextroamphetamine on depression and fatigue in men with HIV: a double-blind, placebo-controlled trial. *Journal of Clinical Psychiatry,* 61: 436 – 40.

Wagner, J.H., Justice, A.C., Chesney, M., Sinclair, G., Weissman, S. & Rodriguez-Barradas, M. (2001). Patient and provider-reported adherence: Toward a clinically useful approach to measuring antiretroviral adherence. *Journal of Clinical Epidemiology,* 54(1), 91–98.

Wiley AC. (1994). Pathology of neurologic diseases in AIDS. *Psychiatric Clinics of North America,* 17: 1 – 15.

Williams P, Narciso L, Browne G, Roberts J, Weir R & Gafni A. (2005). The prevalence, correlates, and cost of depression in people living with HIV/AIDS in Ontario: Implications for service directions. *AIDS Education and Prevention,* 17: 119 – 30.

World Health Organization. Clinical practice guidelines. Washington DC: U.S. Department of Health and Human Services AHCPR Pub. #94-0592. 1994;14.

World Health Organization. HIV/AIDS and mental health. [online] 2008 Nov [cited 2009 Nov]; 24th session.

WHOQOL Group.(1995). *Social Science Medicine,* 41(10): 1403 – 9.

Zheng J,Ghorpade A,Niemann D, Shapiron MF & Bozzette SA. (1999). Lymphotropic virions affect chemokine receptor-mediated neural signaling and apoptosis: implications for human immunodeficiency virus type 1-associated dementia. *Journal of Virology*, 73:8256-8267.

Zisook S, Peterkin J, Goggin KJ, Sledge P, Atkinson JH, Cotter RL, Thylin MR, Epstein L, Swartz JM, Shepard RB, Liu X, Nukuna A & Gendelman HE. (1998). Treatment of major depression in HIV positive men. *Journal of Clinical Psychiatry*, 59: 217 – 24.

5

Cutaneous Manifestations of HIV/AIDS in Sub-Sahara African

Innocent Ocheyana George[1] and Dasetima Dandison Altraide[2]
[1]*Department of Paediatrics, University of Port Harcourt Teaching Hospital, Port Harcourt,*
[2]*Department of Medicine, University of Port Harcourt Teaching Hospital, Port Harcourt,*
Nigeria

1. Introduction

The burden of skin disease is high in developing countries particularly the sub-Saharan Africa. The HIV/AIDS epidemic does not make it any better. More than 90% of HIV positive patients may develop mucocutaneous problems at one stage of the disease or the other with significant morbidity and mortality.

The aim is to highlight common cutaneous manifestations of HIV/AIDS in sub-Sahara Africa. A good knowledge of these cutaneous lesions may aid in early diagnosis and appropriate treatment of HIV infection.

2. Cutaneous manifestations of HIV/AIDS

Cutaneous manifestations are common in patients with HIV infection in the sub-Saharan Africa and can be broadly classified into infection/infestation, malignancy, and cutaneous hypersensitivity. It may be the sentinel event that brings the patient to the physician. Majority of HIV-infected patients will have dermatologic problem at some time during their illness. This may provide a more accurate measure of the disease progression than other organs because the skin is much accessible (Johnson, 1999).

Skin disorders are mostly attributable to the alterations in immune function. Some of the skin diseases are unique to HIV infection, while some are really not new diseases (Aftergut and Cockerell , 1999; Olumide, 2002). The later diseases may be more widespread, have an unusual character or a more prolonged course and may be resistant to therapy. The affected individuals have a significantly increased incidence of skin complaints which rises as HIV infection progresses (Wiwanitkit, 2004). In the asymptomatic stage of HIV infection, cutaneous manifestations are non-specific. Common cutaneous disorders present with atypical features for instance, shingles (VZV) may be severe, recurrent, haemorrhagic or affect more than one dermatome; warts may be multiple and large. Seborrhoeic dermatitis, pityrosorum folliculitis, eosinophilic pustulosis and bacilliary angiomatosis are all well recognized. In the later symptomatic stages, in addition to those infections mentioned above, the following should also be remembered: mycobacterium tuberculosis and atypical mycobacteria, candida species; *Trichophyton rubrum, Malassezia furfur*, chronic herpes simplex, florid molluscum contagiosum. Neoplastic processes, especially Kaposi's sarcoma make their appearance at this time.

2.1 Mycobacteria

These organisms are important causes of systemic infection in HIV disease, but cutaneous lesions have also been recognized, both direct infection and papulonecrotic tuberculide. Cutaneous lesions of mycobacterium avium complex (MAC) include nodules (Fig 1), ulcerations, pustules abscesses, folliculitis and lymph adenitis. Cutaneous lesions of mycobacterium tuberculosis (TB) include scrofuloderma, papules, vesicles, necrotic ulcerations, subcutaneous nodules and pustules. Bacillus calmette – Guerin (BCG) vaccine may cause local and systemic infection in HIV patients especially after signs of defective immunity have appeared, it is regarded as contra-indicated except for children as yet asymptomatic in areas of high risk for tuberculosis.

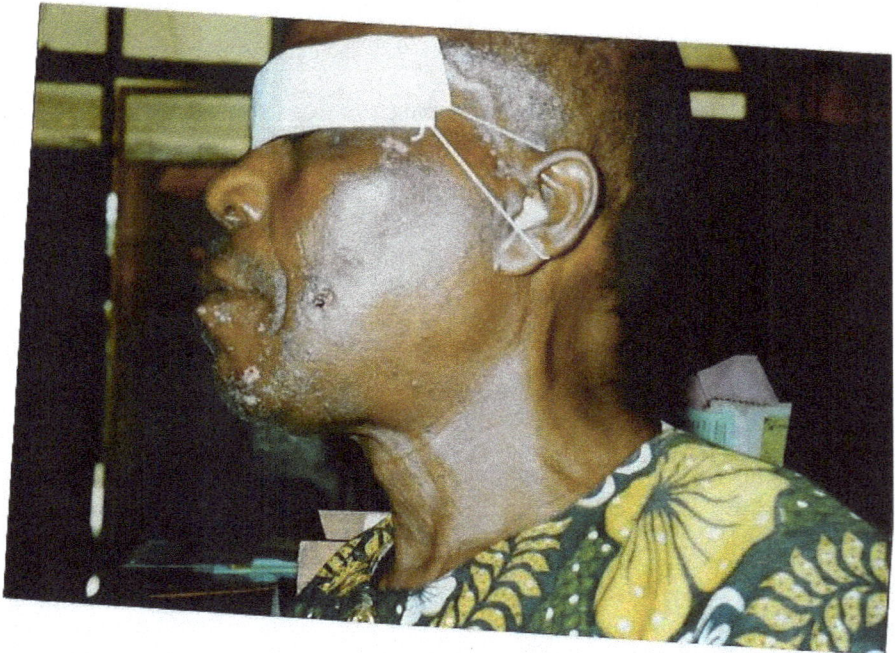

Fig. 1. Cutaneous nodule of Tuberculosis in HIV

The treatment of mycobacterium tuberculosis is the conventional DOTS using rifampicin, isonazid, ethambutol and pyrazinamide. It is recommended that for MAC treatment regimen should include at least 2 agents, with ethambutol being one of the agents.

2.2 Syphilis

Syphilis is a sexually transmitted disease due to infection with *Treponema pallidum*. Both syphilis and HIV infection are sexually transmitted diseases and so could occur concurrently (Olumide; 2002).

Unusual courses of syphilis have been reported in HIV infections. Not only may the serological response to *T. pallidum* be impaired but also syphilis may progress much more rapidly to advanced stages than in individuals without HIV. Moreover syphilis in patients with HIV infection may not respond to conventional treatment. Skin signs of syphilis in HIV infected patients are usually similar to that of HIV – negative patients but are often extensive and atypical.

A severe form of secondary syphilis or lues, 'syphilis maligna' can occur in HIV patients with papular, papulovesicular, pustular and necrotizing lesions which may form thick crusts and painful ulcers accompanying severe systemic symptoms . Tertiary gummata and neurosyphilis also appear more common.

Recommended treatment is benzathine penicilin 2.4 million units intramuscularly in a single dose given as 1.2 million units in each buttock. The treatment is repeated in a week. If there is central nervous system involvement 2.4 million units of aqueous penicillin is given intravenously every 4 hours for 10 – 14 days. This is because intramuscular benzathine penicillin does not give therapeutic levels in the CSF.

2.3 Staphylococcus aureus

Skin infections with *Staph aureus* are quite common in HIV infected patients and the frequency increases with progression of immune-deficiency. Not only is *Staph aureus* the most common bacterial pathogen in HIV infected patients but also a large percentage of patients become chronic carriers. Apart from the types of skin lesions commonly associated with *Staph aureus* in patients without HIV such as folliculitis, impetigo, ecthyma, abscesses and cellulitis, more unusual manifestations such as atypical plaque – like folliculitis, pyomyositis or botryomycosis are frequently encountered during HIV diseases.

Botryomycosis is characterized by chronic, Suppurating, granulomatous lesions which may present as inflammatory nodules, discharging ulcers, sinuses and fistulae. The lesions usually solitary can occur in the skin, liver, bones, etc, and on gross examination of the pus, pinhead – sized whitish yellow granules are evident. The granules simply contain a central mass of bacteria surrounded by a capsule and can be demonstrated on biopsy or smear of the purulent focus. The capsule is usually periodic – Acid – Schiff (PAS) positive. Botryomycosis is caused by bacteria with *Staph aureus* usually the major causal agent and *Pseudomonas aeruginosa* ranking second in frequency. The therapy of choice is surgical excision in conjunction with antibiotics.

2.4 Bacillary angiomatosis

These angioma-like lesions may affect skin, mucosal surfaces and internal organs, Cutaneous lesions typically begin as tiny pinpoint papules, resembling Campbel de Morgan sports, often in large numbers and very widespread. They enlarge rapidly both outwards and inwards, looking like pyogenic granulomas and subcutaneous nodules. They may resemble some forms of AIDS-related Kaposi's sarcoma (and indeed the two may coexist but can generally be distinguished by their faster growth, bright red color and rounder shape, with no elongation along skin crease). If injured, lesions bleed profusely. Visceral lesions may occur and deaths from laryngeal obstruction and disseminated intravascular obstruction are recorded. Bacillary angiomatosis has been seen mainly in HIV disease, but also in other immunodeficient patients and rarely in the otherwise healthy. It is caused by *Bartonella henselae* or occassional *B. quintana*, argyrophilic bacilli. Confirmation of diagnosis is by recognition of histological features or by PCR amplification of the organism's nucleic acid obtained from biopsy tissue.

Treatment – the recommended treatment for bacillary angiomatosis is erythromycin 500mg qds. If the patient has severe disease or can not tolerate orally, intravenous erythromycin can be given. Alternative to erythromycin include doxycline 100mg bid; minocycline 100mg bid or tetracycline 50mg qid, treatment should continue for 8-12 weeks and in case of systematic disease 3-4 months.

2.5 Demodicidosis
Folliculitis due to *Demodex folliculorum* may cause an itchy papular eruption in HIV patients. Affected areas include head and neck, and trunk and arms Microscopy of smears or scrapings, or histology confirms the presence of numerous mites. There is a rapid response to topical treatment with insecticides such as y-benzene hexachloride.

2.6 Viral infection
Viruses other than HIV-1 are common pathogens in HIV-1 disease and are probably important infectious co-factors for disease progression (Sterling and Kurtz, 1998). These opportunistic infections range from relatively benign disorder such as cosmetically disfiguring molluscum contagiosum to severe infections of the skin and mucus membranes such as ulcerating herpes simplex and oral hairy leukoplakia, which is attributed to Epstein Barr virus infection.

2.7 Herpes simplex
Chronic painful, non-healing ulcers found in herpes simplex virus (HDV) infections are commonly located at the junction between skin and mucous membranes, mainly in the perioral and perianal areas. Chronic ulcerating herpes simplex must first be differentiated from conventional recurrent HSV infection. Whereas the latter can occur at any stage of HIV-1 disease and is clinically and morphologically indistinguishable from the blistering eruptions commonly seen in patients without HIV-1 infection, the former heralds profound immunodeficiency. Chronic ulcerating herpes simplex is one of the AIDS-defining opportunistic infection according to Centers for Disease Control and Prevention. Systemic antiviral treatment is essential since these lesions show no tendency to resolve spontaneously. The differential diagnosis, which depends on the location of the lesions, includes pyoderma gangrenosum, bacterial and fungal infection, and cutaneous manifestation of lymphomas.

The recommended treatment for primary or recurrent HSV injection is oral acyclovir. In severe infections, intravenous acyclovir can be used. Other alternatives include famciclovir and fascarnet.

2.8 Varicella-zoster
Clinical manifestation of infection with the varicella-zoster virus (VZV), another member of the herpes virus family, depends largely on the age of the patient. Primary VZV infection in HIV-1 infected children is often severe, with dissemination and pneumoina, encephalitis, or pancreatitis. As with adult patients, epidemiological studies indicate that the frequency of reactivation of latent VZV, leading to herpes zoster, is greatly increased, with a relative risk in one study of 16.9 for HIV-1 infected person over non-infected

persons. 8-13% of patients with AIDS have experienced at least one episode of herpes zoster and recurrent herpes zoster is observed more frequently in HIV-1 seropositive patients than in sero-negative individuals. However, herpes zoster is not a reliable sign of profound immunodeficiency because it can occur at any state of HIV infection. Clinical manifestations range from an uneventful vesicular eruption in a dermatomal pattern, similar to that in non-HIV-1 infected individuals, to severe haemorrhagic and necrotic lesions that may extend over several dermatomes, followed by cutaneous dissemination. In contrast to the high frequency of systemic dissemination associated with primary VZV infection, dissemination is infrequent in conventional herpes zoster. Nevertheless, chronic verrucous or ecthymatous VZV infections may persist for months.

2.9 Molluscum contagiosum
Poxvirus infection causing Molluscum contagiosum is ordinarily self-limited in immunocompetent individuals, occurring mainly in children. However, during HIV-1 disease molluscum contagiosum is seen in up to 20% of patients, and is usually associated with established immunodeficiency.

Characteristics lesions, which appear commonly on the face and in the genital regions, include skin-coloured umbilicated papules with one or more central hyperkeratotic pores. Individual lesions can grow to more than 1 cm in size and, if located on the face, may be disfiguring. If multiple nodular lesions become confluent they are difficult to treat, commonly recurring after conventional local destruction. The differential diagnosis includes basal-cell carcinoma, common warts, keratacanthoma, atypical mycobacterial infections, and, especially, cutaneous manifestations of systemic infections with *Cyptococcus neoformans*, *Histoplasma capsulatum*, or *Penicillium marneffei*. Since differentiation of molluscum contagiosum from these important fungal infections is often uncertain clinically, histopathological confirmation should always be sought.

Human Papilloma virus- Common warts may occur in unusual locations, with unusual severity, and with high frequency in HIV-1 infected patients but they are seldom serious. With respect to genital involvement in women (Fig2), both frequency of human papilloma virus (HPV) infection and the progression of HPV-associated cervical lesions correlate with the level of immune suppression. Moderate to severe cervical dysplasia and carcinoma-in-situ are part of category B symptomatic conditions in the revised classification system for HIV infection. In men, the rate of anogenital HPV infection is high in HIV-1 sero-positive and sero-negative homosexuals. However, as for women, HPV prevalence and symptoms tend to increase with disease progression.

3. Fungal infections

3.1 Dematophyte Infection
Tinea infections of varying sites do occur and may be chronic and widespread in HIV positive patient (Fig 3). The overall frequency is higher in non-infected control population. Nail involvement is common and can cause diffuse whitening. Proximal nail whitening or proximal subungual onychomycosis, unusual in immunocompetent individuals is regarded by some as characteristic of HIV-associated nail infection.

Treatment is standard with the use of topical and systemic anti-fungal agents.

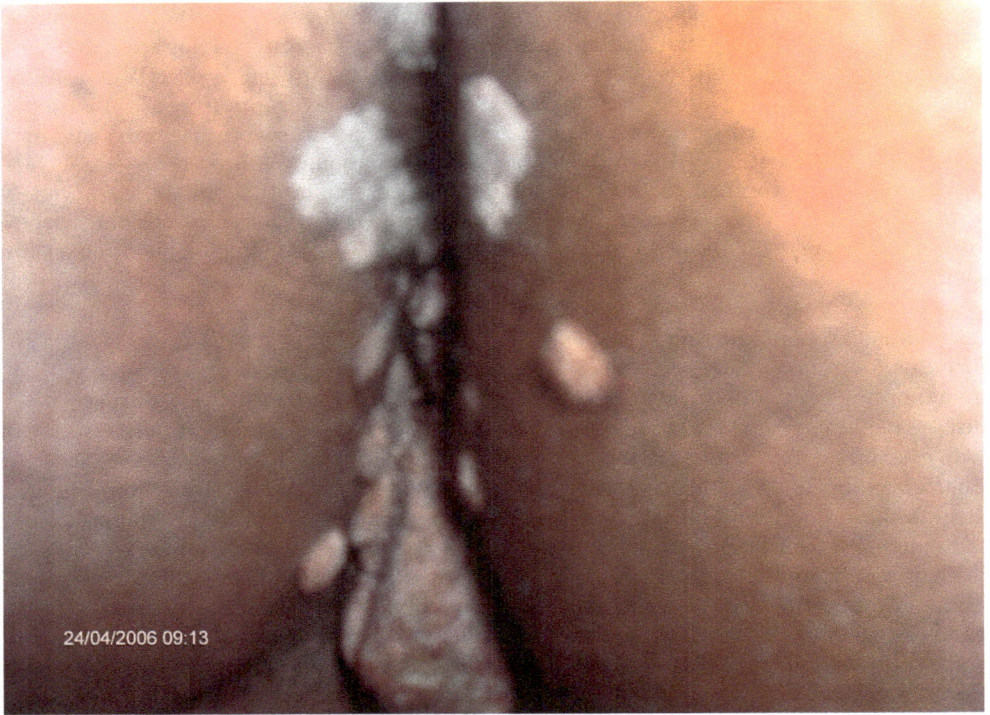

Fig. 2. Genital warts in HIV

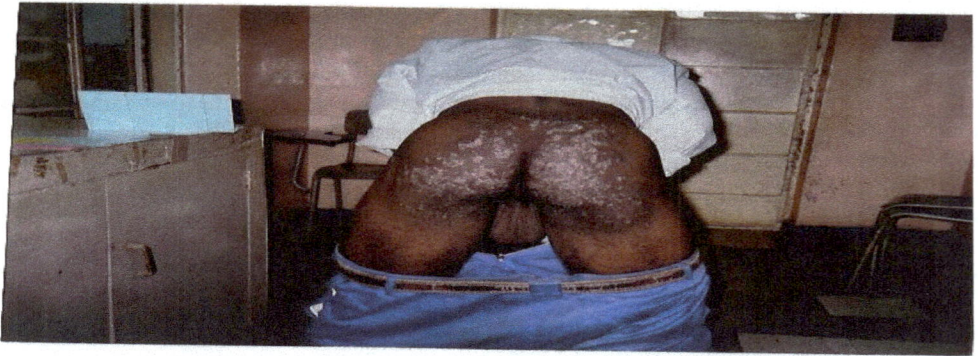

Fig. 3. Extensive tinea cruris and corporis

3.2 Candidiasis

This is common in all stages of HIV infection affecting the skin, nail, genitals and oral mucosa.Cutaneous lesions are often located in the intertriginous areas/ skin folds as highly pruritic inflamed areas with satellite lesions and/or follicular pustules. In addition to HIV, other risk factors are diabetes mellitus, obesity, malignancy, use of immunosuppressive therapy and cytotoxic drugs, use of systemic and topical corticosteroids and antibiotic therapy, hot humid environment, occlusion e.g. diapers, casts and dressings, blood malignancies and neutropenia and skin disease which disturb the cutaneous barrier e.g. psoriasis and contact dermatitis.

Nail lesions affect the proximal nail fold and nail plate. Nail fold lesions (paronychia) present as painful, erythematous swellings which may discharge purulent material. Genital lesions present as pruritic vulvo-vaginitis with discharge of a creamy white material. There may be involvement of the perineum with erythematous and satellite lesions. In severe cases, the oral mucosa may show extensive white plagues or widespread erythema, and esophageal involvement may give rise to dysphagia and retrosternal pain.

Standard topical therapy will suffice but in severe cases and nail involvement systemic therapy may be needed. Fluconazole (50mg daily) has a higher cure rate than ketoconazole (20mg daily) and intermittent administration of fluconazole (150mg) also proved effective.

3.3 Cutaneous malignancies

Persons infected with Human Immunodeficiency Virus (HIV) are at higher risk for the development of certain types of cancers. The AIDS was first reported in the summer of 1981 in Los Angeles among young homosexuals who were observed to have had a disseminated type of Kaposi's sarcoma and pneumocystis carini infection.

3.4 Kaposi's sarcoma

Kaposi's sarcoma (KS), the most common tumor in patients with AIDS, is strongly associated with immunosuppression (Schwartz et al., 2008). KS is a vascular neoplasm affecting the endothelial cell and that affects the skin, and the mucosa, less commonly involves other organs like the gastrointestinal tracts, lungs and lymph nodes. KS can occur in HIV-negative patients where it typically has a chronic indolent course. In HIV infected patients KS has a more aggressive course and may have systemic involvement.

Epidemiological data suggest that the cause is a sexually transmitted infectious agent and this has recently been supported by the finding of herpes virus nucleic acid in Kaposi's sarcoma lesions (Schwartz et al., 2008) .However, this virus called Kaposi's sarcoma associated herpes virus (or human herpes virus type 8) has also been detected in classical KS; Gut lymphomas and other skin lesions of AIDS patients. The role of HHV-8 in the pathogenesis of Kaposi's sarcoma is yet to be clearly defined.

The mucocutaneous lesions of KS are usually asymptomatic vary from the earliest pink macules to the thickened papules and plaques which later develop to nodules. Diffuse lesions may manifest mainly as oedema. The lesions initially may appear benign-looking and may be misdiagnosed as pigmented naevi, Spitz naevi, dermatofibroma, bruises, pyogenic granulomas, malignant melanoma, ecchymosis, molluscum contagiosum or lichen planus. The lesions may appear any where on the skin but the tip of the nose and the hard palate are common sites. Lesions in the feet may occasionally become warty. Lesions may develop at the site of trauma (Kobner Phenomenon).

Unlike the metastatic behavior of other malignant tumors, KS is a multifocal neoplasm in which each lesion seems to develop de novo from endothelial cells that line lymphatic or blood vessels into skin or visceral.

Progression of lesions depends upon the immune status. If the CD4+ cell count rises, either with or without treatment lesion may regress at least temporary.

Treatment: This is not curative. Palliative therapy is indicated for lesions that are disfiguring, causing pains or with systemic symptoms.

Local therapy would include:

a. Surgery for large lesions. This would include the use of excision and laser.
b. Cryosurgery
c. Intralesional chemotherapy using vinblastine
d. The tumor is sensitive to radiotherapy.

Systemic therapy would include the following:

a. Chemotherapy including vinblastine, bleomycin, Doxorubicin
b. Biology response modifiers which include IFN-a, interleukin-2 and intravenous immunoglobulin
c. Antiretroviral therapy
d. Photodynamic therapy.

3.5 Other malignancies

AIDS-related lymphomas are not uncommon and are usually high grade of the immunoblastic or small-cell type.

3.6 Cutaneous hypersensitivity

This is a group of eruptions in patients with HIV disease. The pathophysiology of some of them is not well defined and therapeutic responses have been disappointing. However, some explanations have been advised based on some immunologic findings. Monocytes, macrophages, epidermal langerhans cells and dendritic cells of the dermis have CD4 antigen and are potential targets for infection by HIV. The decrease in langerhans cells as in AIDS may lead to altered cell mediated immunity.

3.7 Xeroderma

Dry skin is common in HIV/AIDS especially if chronic diarrhea is a masked feature and may be related to malabsorption. There is associated prutitus. In more severe cases with changes you have acquired ichthyosis. Icythuosis is a disorder of keratinization characterized clinically by dry scaly skin. It should be noted that acquired ichthyosis can also be found in lymphomas, lepromatous leprosy and sarcoidosis which are conditions with reduced immunity. Treatment is the use of emollients.

3.8 Pruritic Papular Eruption (PPE) of HIV

PPE of HIV is a unique manifestation of HIV which has not been seen in seronegative patients (Eisman, 2006, Machtinger et al., 2004). Clinically, the lesions are red or skin coloured papules that are symmetrically disseminated in the trunk, buttocks and extremities (Fig 4). The lesions are extremely pruritic. The lesions heal with post inflammatory hypopigmentation with new hyperpigmented lesions. The eruptions wax and wane during the course of the illness. The cause of the lesion is not known but most people think that it is a hypersensitivity reaction to antigens or a direct effect of the HIV.

Treatment with antihistamines, phototherapy and photochemotherapy may be used but of limited success.Patient education as to the cause of the illness is important.

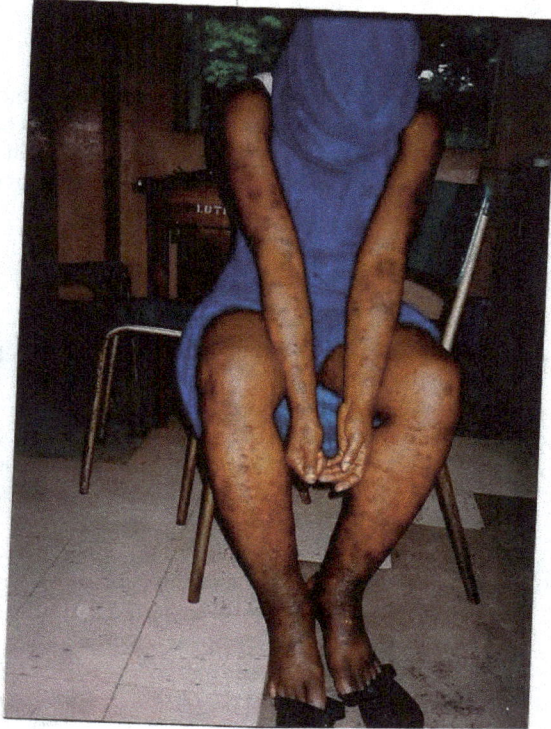

Fig. 4. Pruritic papular of HIV infection

3.9 Seborrheic Dermatitis

Seborrheic dermatitis (SD) is a chronic papulosquamous disorder characterized by distinctive morphology (red, sharply marginated lesion covered with greasy looking scales and hypopigmentation which is usually seen in dark skinned people) and a distinctive distribution in areas with a rich supply of sebaceous glands namely the scalp, forehead, eyebrows, lashline, nasolabial folds, beard and post auricular skin. Other areas include presternal region, inter scapular area, axillae, groin and gluteal crease.

The prevalence of seborrheic dermatitis is around 1-3% in the general population and 40-83% in HIV/AIDS patients.

The aetiology of SD is unclear. It has been suggested that the yeast *Pityrosporum ovale* is important in the aetiology of SD. Clinically, a wide spectrum of lesions exist but characteristic distribution; hypopigmented nummular patches which may coalesce to form polycyclic lesion on the back and presternal area; diffuse erythematous hypopigmented macules involving the scalp margins and butterfly areas of the face and trunk; scalp and facial involvement presenting as   dandruff and blepharitis; flexural, petaloid and pityrosporum folliculitis.

In Africa, hypopigmentation is a prominent feature which has been explained as a result of dicarboxylic acids produced by malassezia causing competitive inhibition of tyrosinase and perhaps a direct cytotoxic effect on hyperactive melanocytes (Altraide et al., 2010).

Seborrheic dermatitis in HIV/AIDS patients occur in varying severity (Altraide et al; 2010). It is usually characterized by thick micaceous scales and usually hyperkeratotic and inflammatory and more widespread and generalized.

Conclusion: Skin disorders are common in sub-Saharan African and may present with early, severe, unusual and atypical manifestations in the course of HIV infection. Awareness of the varied pattern of these manifestations would help in the early diagnosis and management of HIV infection, which would in turn decrease the morbidity and improve the quality of life of HIV-infected patients.

4. References

Aftergut K., Cockerell CJ (1999). Update on the cutaneous manifestations of HIV infection. Clinical and pathologic features. Dermatol. Clin. Vol.17, No.3, pp. 445-71.

Altraide DD, Olumide YM, Mohammed TT (2010). Predictive value of seborrheic dermatitis for HIV infection in Lagos Nigeria. Port Harcourt Medical Journal. 5(1): 30-36.

Eisman S (2006). Pruritic papular eruption in HIV. Dermatol. Clin. Vol.24, pp.449-457.

Johnson RA (1999). Cutaneous manifestations of human immunodeficiency virus disease.In: Friedberg IM, Eisen AZ, Wolf K, et al., eds . Fitzpatrick's Dermatology. McGraw- Hill, pp. 2138-2150.

Machtinger EL, Van Beek M, Furmanski L, et al(2004).Etiology of pruritic papular eruption with HIV infection in Uganda. JAMA. ; vol292, pp.2614-2621.

Olumide YM (2002). A self–instructed textbook of acquired immune deficiency syndrome (HIV/AIDS) for medical students, resident doctors and medical practioners. Longman Nigeria PLC pp.22-80.

Schwartz RA, Micali G, Nasca MR, Scuderi L (2008). Kaposi sarcoma: a continuing conundrum. J Am Acad Dermatol. Vol.59, No. 2, pp. 179-206.

Sterling JC, Kurtz JB. Viral infections: In. Champion RH, Burton JL, Burns DA, Breathnach SM eds Rookwdkinson/Ebling, Textbook of dermatology 6th edition. London 1998: Blackwell science LTD 2: 1057-1079.

Tschachler E, Bergstresser PR, Stingl G (1996) . HIV-related skin diseases. Lancet Vol. 348, pp. 659-63.

Wiwanitkit V. Prevalence of dermatological disorders in Thai HIV-infected patients correlated with different CD4 lymphocyte count statuses: a note on 120 cases. Int JDermatol 2004; 43 (4): 265-8.

6

Sexual Dysfunctions

Marco de Tubino Scanavino
Institute of Psychiatry, University of São Paulo
Brazil

1. Introduction

Although HIV-positive individuals kept a central role in the maintenance of the epidemic, only from the 12th World AIDS Conference, held in Geneva in 1998, the sexuality of people living with HIV/AIDS received more systematic attention (Schiltz and Sandfort 2000). After receiving the diagnosis of HIV infection is common for people to become involved in a state of negative mood and decrease the frequency of sexual activity and those who remain with sexual practices most likely do so without adequate protection (Rosser, Gobby and Carr 1999). The adhesion to safe sex practices after diagnosis of HIV infection may have a negative impact on sexual functioning of most subjects (Newshan, Taylor and Gold 1998). The individuals that have partnership are significantly more likely to maintain sexual activity than those without (Stein et al. 2005). On the professionals, the sexual functioning is often overlooked among the care of HIV positive patients. Generally, information about the relationship between hormonal factors, psychological factors, drug effects, disease stage, and sexual functioning are not spoken by health professionals (Newshan et al. 1998). In addition, one must consider that individuals who acquire HIV through sexual or parenteral (excluding blood transfusions) are already part of a population at higher risk for sexual dysfunction, as many risk factors for HIV are also to the occurrence of sexual dysfunction, such as conflicts with the orientation or sexual identity, depression, and psychological problems related to self-image (Hijazi, Nandwani and Kell 2002).

Several factors may modify the sexual response. Beginning in youth, sexual dysfunctions are highly prevalent in all age groups. Symptoms of sexual dysfunction include erectile dysfunction, loss of libido, premature or delayed ejaculation, orgasmic disturbances, arousal difficulties, and dyspareunia, among others (Lewis et al. 2004).

For the Diagnostic and Statistical Manual of Mental Disorders, Fourth Edition, Text Revision (DSM-IV-TR) ((APA) 2000), the fundamental concepts of the principals sexual dysfunctions are: *Dyspareunia* is recurrent or persistent genital pain associated with sexual intercourse in men or women. *Female orgasmic disorder* is the delay of orgasm following normal excitement and sexual activity. Due to the widely varied sexual response in women, it must be judged by a clinician to be significant taking into account the person's age and situation. *Female sexual arousal disorder* is inability to attain or maintain until completion of sexual activity adequate lubrication in response to sexual excitement. *Hypoactive sexual desire disorder* is deficient or absent sexual fantasies and desire for sexual activity. This judgment must be made by a clinician taking into account the individual's age and life circumstances. *Male erectile disorder (impotence)* is recurring inability to achieve or maintain an erection until completion of the sexual activity. *Male orgasmic disorder* is delay or absence of orgasm following normal excitement and sexual activity. Due to the widely varied sexual response in men, it must be judged by a clinician to be significant, taking into account the person's age and situation. *Premature ejaculation* is the ejaculation with minimal sexual stimulation before or shortly after penetration and before the person wishes it. The condition is persistent or occurs frequently and causes significant distress (APA, 2000).

Factors such as lack of ability, poor sex education, and psychological conflicts play an important role in the development of sexual dysfunction at the start of sexual activity (Lewis et al. 2004). Life habits and morbid conditions become important risk factors for sexual dysfunction during aging; these factors include hypertension, diabetes, depression, heart disease, sex hormone deficiency, smoking, sedentary life style, and drug addiction (Moreira et al. 2001). Socioeconomic factors, such as education, employment and marital status, have also been related to sexual difficulties (Nicolosi et al. 2003).

Highly active antiretroviral therapy (HAART) has previously been shown to provide the best clinical management for HIV-infected patients, as it decreases the prevalence of hypogonadism and advanced HIV disease, which are principal causes of sexual dysfunction in people infected with HIV (Danoff 1996, Collazos 2007). However the prevalence on sexual dysfunctions in the HAART years show high rates (Collazos 2007). In this chapter we analyze the etiologic factors involved on sexual dysfunctions of HIV/AIDS people. We also describe the most prevalent sexual dysfunctions in males, and females. We propose steps for assessment, and diagnosis of the sexual dysfunction in HIV/AIDS people. We talk about the principal therapeutic strategies for recover healthy sexual function of this people. Finally, we comment on the prognostic factors.

2. Epidemiology

The prevalence rates of sexual dysfunctions in HIV/AIDS patients were reviewed: 46% presented with erectile dysfunction   (range 9-74%), 39% with ejaculatory disturbances (range 36-42%), 44% with decreased libido   (range 24-73%), and 27% with orgasmic disorders (range 7-49%). The high interval of range is because so much different designs and methods used in the HIV sexual dysfunctions studies (Collazos 2007). There are differences on the most prevalent sexual dysfunctions among men, and women.

The most prevalent female sexual dysfunctions are low sexual desire, orgasmic dysfunction, and dyspareunia (Hijazi et al. 2002, Luzi et al. 2009). A higher frequency (36%) of sexual inactivity during the last 12 months in female with AIDS has been reported by a Brazilian study (de Tubino Scanavino and Abdo 2010), which is in according with another study of females with HIV/AIDS, of which 28% reported having no sexual partners for an average of 69 months (Lambert, Keegan and Petrak 2005). We already know that HIV/AIDS females that has partners keep more the sexual activity than who does not have. But in the Brazilian study the female also does not maintain sexual arousal until the end of the sex, and probably this may partly explain the sexual inactivity because these women seem to find sex unsatisfactory (de Tubino Scanavino and Abdo 2010).

On men infected by HIV the most prevalent sexual dysfunctions are erectile dysfunction and premature ejaculation. In Brazil, a case-control study nested in a cross-sectional population study with people who reported AIDS found that almost 50% of the male reported ejaculatory symptoms, and 33% of the men living with AIDS reported erectile dysfunction (de Tubino Scanavino and Abdo 2010). In this study 12% of men with AIDS also reported dyspareunia, while no men without AIDS reported it (de Tubino Scanavino and Abdo 2010). Male dyspareunia is not commonly reported in the literature, possibly because it is not regularly investigated in studies of male sexual function.

3. Etiology

There are four important factors associated with sexual dysfunctions in HIV/AIDS patients: mental, hormonal, pharmachological, and other morbid conditions.

3.1 Mental factors

At the first moment, the condition of being HIV seropositive may cause feelings of loss of sexual attractiveness, reduction of sexual desire and sexual satisfaction. Moreover, they may be confronted with the absence of sexual partners, particularly when revealing their serological status. In addition, the sexual response may be undermined by fear or guilt in coming to contaminate partnerships (Newshan et al. 1998, Schiltz and Sandfort 2000).

A representative French study with HIV outpatients showed association among sexual difficulties and the discrimination by friends and partners, suffering by lipodystrophy, very disturbing HIV related symptoms. The authors recommend psychological support for HIV experience for improves the sexual life (Bouhnik et al. 2008). Feelings of guilt by have acquiring the HIV on sexual transmission may become a psychogenic factor and influence negatively the sexual response. Maybe because of this point, sexual dysfunctions are more prevalent on homosexual men than intravenous drug users (Sollima et al. 2001). In fact, gay and bisexual men have higher rates of sexual dysfunctions (Catalan and Meadows 2000) or just complaint more to the physicians on the disorder due to valorize more the sexual function than others.

Depression is one of the most important mental factors associated with sexual dysfunctions (Ciesla and Roberts 2001). A study on 300 HIV infected men found the older age and depression were associated with erectile dysfunction, and current higher CD4 account was protective (Crum-Cianflone et al. 2007).

The most common factors associated with female sexual dysfunction are the psychosocial aspects of HIV infection and the negative body image associated with use of medications that cause lipodystrophy (Bell et al. 2006, Hijazi et al. 2002, Luzi et al. 2009).

3.2 Hormonal factors

Hypogonadism was one of the most frequent causes of sexual dysfunction before HAART. Currently, HIV infected individuals may have testosterone levels higher than non infected individuals. Moreover, estradiol is often higher in men (50% of them) on HAART possibly because the augmentation of the peripheral conversion of the androgens to estrogens in lipid tissues (Bell et al. 2006, Goldmeier et al. 2002). But the role of estradiol in HIV sexual dysfunctions is not clear. The expected decrease in blood of the gonadotropin hormones was not confirmed (Collazos et al. 2002a), and one study observed improving on sexual function despite higher blood levels of estradiol (Collazos et al. 2002b). On the other side, an study on rabbits found estrogen receptors in cavernous body, and found pathophysiological changes in erectile function when rabbits are under continuous estrogen intake (Srilatha and Adaikan 2004). Another study with older men found that the balance between testosterone (decreased) and oestradiol (higher) are associated with erectile dysfunction (Srilatha, Adaikan and Chong 2007).

Hyperprolactinemia may be associated with sexual dysfunction as it decreases the gonadotropin releases and have been found in part of the HIV individuals, but one study does not found difference in prolactin levels between patients with and without sexual difficulties (Collazos et al. 2002b).

3.3 Pharmacological factors

HAART era shows high rates of sexual dysfunction despite the improvement of health conditions. Anedotical report from studies suggest association among protease inhibitors and sexual dysfunctions, but just a few studies found a kind of evidence on it. These studies have found a possible effect on testosterone receptor by protease inhibitors (Yang et al. 2005, Baker, Vaughn and Fanestil 1978). Other evidences to explain sexual dysfunction by an effect of HAART are scarce. Future studies on pharmacological issues may specify the etiologic role of antiretrovirals to sexual dysfunction.

It has been reported ejaculatory dysfunction associated by use of didanosine (Hijazi et al. 2002). The neuropathy is a possible complication by use of some antiretrovirals and may be a sexual dysfunction factor for some patients (Rogstad et al. 1999).

However, HIV infected individuals use a lot of other medications that are associated with decrease on sexual response. Medications such as ketoconazole, fluconazole, ganciclovir, megestrol, methadone and cimetidine may decrease the level of testosterone and cause sexual dysfunction (Newshan et al. 1998, Daniell 2002). Antihypertensives, diuretics, hypolipemics, benzodiazepines, antidepressants, and antipsychotics are also associated with sexual dysfuncitons (Asboe et al. 2007, Lue 2000, Daniell 2002, Bruckert et al. 1996).

3.4 Comorbid conditions

Some morbid conditions are common in HIV people and some of them are often associated with sexual dysfunction as hepathopathy, diabetes, hyperlipidemia, hypertension, vascular disease, alcohol dependence (Moreira et al. 2001).

4. Diagnosis

When a patient comes for receiving care on sexual function, he needs time and more than one meeting with the health professional, to bind and reveal your intimate life problems.

But if a patient seeks medical care for other reasons but also has sexual problems, difficultly he will talk about spontaneously. Moreover, sexual life is poored investigated by practitioners, indeed in mental health settings. It also occurs on HIV/AIDS clinical context. In a research in the United Kingdom on HIV clinics, 60% of the physicians do not ask on sexual functioning of female HIV infected (Bell et al. 2006) despite the sexual difficulties are very prevalent on HIV women.

For this reason, in order to investigate sexual function of HIV people, the first point to consider is an appropriate doctor patient relationship (Lawlor and Braunack-Mayer 2004), which is basic to investigate clinical and sexual symptoms of the patients. It is important an attitude of open minded and free of judgments by the professional.

The diagnosis of sexual dysfunctions follows some steps for diagnosis: consistent doctor-patient relationship, investigation of clinical history and physical examination, investigation of the sexual life history, assessment on sexual response, and check the hormonal serum levels.

4.1 Clinical history and physical examination

The clinical history compreends the assessment on the immunological conditions, comorbidities, and medications. Severe immunological damage may indicates AIDS diagnosis. The poor health condition undermine physical and sexual response. Nevertheless the hypogonadism should be investigated. On the physical examination the gynecomaestia and testicular atrophy may indicates hypogonadism (Rosen et al. 2006). Hypogonadism is defined as low levels of testosterone (< 300 nh/dL) in early morning, with associated clinical manifestations, including sexual dysfunction, weight and muscle mass loss, fatigue, depressed mood, and anemia (Crum et al. 2005).

We already spoke on the most frequent comorbidity and the use of some medications which also influence the sexual response.

4.2 Sexual history

The sexual history should starts investigating the concepts on sexuality of the family (father and mother), following to the patient's sexual history, finishing with focus about some specific gender issues.

4.2.1 Sexuality on origin family

When sexuality is very repressed, it could undermine to live a broad experience of sex and love in adolescence and young adult life (Basson 2008), which are fundamental to sexual maturing process. The non psychological and sexual maturing and possible internal conflicts influence the sexual response. When somebody lives in a dysfunctional family in childhood and has early contact with the erotic experience (sexual abuse or permissive family ambience), it could be traumatic and harm the personality development, as the children experience feelings of being unprotected, unsafety, shame or guilt. Then, this person could presents sexual problems (aversion, excessive drive, sexual difficulties) later in your life (Noll, Trickett and Putnam 2003).

On sexual violence suffered during childhood and adolescence many studies have reported serious psychological effects and sexual consequences (Gwandure 2007, Greenberg 2001, Whetten et al. 2006). Victims of violence often have a high frequency of the stress post-traumatic disorder, depression, suicidal ideation and low self-esteem (Gwandure 2007) (Greenberg 2001, Whetten et al. 2006). This psychopathological issues are risk factors for HIV / AIDS in adult life, as negative moods promote sexual practices without the use of condoms and, therefore, exposure to virus (Gwandure 2007). Thus, research has documented the association between childhood sexual abuse and higher frequency of sexual risk behavior in adult life (Gwandure 2007, Greenberg 2001, Whetten et al. 2006, Sikkema et al. 2008). At the same time, in several studies of HIV-positive individuals is described childhood sexual abuse, which frequency varies between 24% and 76% (Whetten et al. 2006, Bedimo, Kissinger and Bessinger 1997, Kalichman et al. 2002, Liebschutz et al. 2000, Segurado et al. 2008).

4.2.2 Own sexual history

The own sexual history is very important. The first sexual experiences with boys or girls, the first complete sexual relationship, the exercise of masturbation are all significant steps in sexual maturing process, which compreend gaining knowledge on your body (erogenous zones) and of the others. When somebody has sexual difficulties in early sexual experiences and are not prepared to deal with, it could promote negative attitude regarding sex, and new experiences will be avoided, undermining the sexual maturing (Lewis et al. 2004). A person with sexual inexperiece is under higher risk for sexual dysfunction (Lewis et al. 2004), and, in turn, a person with sexual dysfunction is under higher risk for unsafe sex behavior (Rosen et al. 2006), even if become infected by HIV.

4.2.3 Gender issues

Some specific gender issues are also important to be investigated. For men, homosexual orientation presents a special vulnerability for sexual dysfunction, maybe because the process to accept the sexual orientation, the difficulties to deal with low acceptance by family and society, and the problems with gender identity (Coleman, Rosser and Strapko 1992). Some studies have reported higher rates of sexual dysfunction in HIV infected men who have sex with men (Cove and Petrak 2004).

For women, the mental health is a strong point to be investigated. Depression is a strong risk factor for sexual dysfunction (Cyranowski et al. 2004) and when treated can improve substancially the sexual dysfunction symptoms (Clayton et al. 2007).

Less investigated but so important is self-image and body image. Self-image compreends the perception from herself of the female issue, and the erotic issue. They are steps of sexual developing and are determinant to woman fells secure to engage in sexual experiences in adult life. The prejudice on body image by lipodystrophy has been considered the most important factor for sexual dysfunction in HIV infected women (Luzi et al. 2009) and could also influence to women do not engage in sex with partners.

Another important point on female sexual function is the presence of positive feelings for the partner (Basson 2008) and the sexual partner hability, as we know a lot of women just have positive sexual experiences when they are estimulated by a partner in an appropriate context, which involve affect and foreplay (Basson 2008).

4.2.4 Difference between organic and psychogenic sexual dysfunction

It is also relevant in sexual history to distinguish between characteristcs of organic or psychogenic sexual dysfunction (Table 1) (Speckens et al. 1993, Hatch, de la Peña and Fisher 1987). The psychogenic occurs more often in younger individuals, the onset is rapid, it could be related with adverse life events (when it appears soon after HIV diagnosis, e.g.) or problematic onset sex lives, the presentation is not constant and it changes depending on the partners, or the situations, and could not be presented in masturbation. Moreover, the organic occurs more often in older men, the onset is insidious, it does not have relation with life adverse events, the presentation is constant, and it also occurs in masturbation. For men, when the nocturnal penile erection is present it is suggestive of psychogenic etiology. Considering HIV infection we could think that individuals just seropositive with good health conditions probably presents sexual dysfunction by psychogenic etiology, and individuals with poor imunological conditions or AIDS diagnosis probably presents sexual dysfunction by organic factors.

Characteristics	Organic	Psychogenic
Age of onset	Older	Younger
Onset	Insidious	Quick
Pattern	Constant	Variable
Masturbation	Yes	No
Adverse life events and/or problems on the onset of sex life	No	Yes
Men: penile nocturnal Erection	No	Yes

Table 1. Clinical difference between organic and psychogenic sexual dysfunction

4.3 Assessment on sexual response

Some standardized instruments for quick assessment of sexual response can be used, as the health practitioners often find it difficult to investigate the sex lives of patients. For female we can use The Female Sexual Function Index (FSFI) to assess female sexual function. The FSFI is a self-responsive questionnaire with 19 multiple choice questions divided into six main domains. The questionnaire evaluates phases of the sexual cycle (desire, excitement and orgasm), sexual satisfaction and dyspareunia in the last four weeks (Rosen et al. 2000). For male there is The International Index of Erectile Function (IIEF) which addresses the relevant domains of male sexual function (erectile function, orgasmic function, sexual desire, intercourse satisfaction, and overall satisfaction), is psychometrically tested, readily self-administered in research or clinical settings (Rosen et al. 1997).

The Figure 1 shows generally items for investigating sexual function (de Tubino Scanavino and Abdo 2010).

In general items evaluating sexual function involves the follows (de Tubino Scanavino and Abdo 2010): "Did you have sexual intercourse during the last 12 months?", "Do you need to be stimulated by your partner to begin sexual intercourse?", "Is stimulation (foreplay) necessary for you for a long time before sexual intercourse?", "If there is no previous reciprocal stimulation (foreplay), do you and your partner proceed to genital sexual intercourse?", "Do you masturbate regularly?", "Do you usually have sexual desire?", "Do you feel pain during sexual intercourse?". Items evaluating female sexual function involves the follows: "When you kiss and hug during sexual intercourse, do you feel sexual arousal and does the vagina become wet?", "Do you maintain sexual arousal and a wet vagina until the end of sexual intercourse?", "Do you reach orgasm during sexual activity (inside the vagina or outside on the clitoris)?". Items evaluating male sexual function involves the follows: "Do you feel the pleasure of getting an erection and keeping it until the end of sexual intercourse?", "Do you always manage to maintain an erection (hard penis) until the end of sexual intercourse?", "Do you ejaculate (expel white liquid through the penis) quicker than you want?", "Do you ejaculate (expel white liquid through the penis) later than you want?", "Do you ejaculate (expel white liquid through the penis) at the desired time for you?".

Items for men and women	"Did you have sexual intercourse during the last 12 months?", "Do you need to be stimulated by your partner to begin sexual intercourse?", "Is stimulation (foreplay) necessary for you for a long time before sexual intercourse?", "If there is no previous reciprocal stimulation (foreplay), do you and your partner proceed to genital sexual intercourse?", "Do you masturbate regularly?", "Do you usually have sexual desire?", "Do you feel pain during sexual intercourse?".
Items specifically for women	"When you kiss and hug during sexual intercourse, do you feel sexual arousal and does the vagina become wet?", "Do you maintain sexual arousal and a wet vagina until the end of sexual intercourse?", "Do you reach orgasm during sexual activity (inside the vagina or outside on the clitoris)?".
Items specifically for men	"Do you feel the pleasure of getting an erection and keeping it until the end of sexual intercourse?", "Do you always manage to maintain an erection (hard penis) until the end of sexual intercourse?", "Do you ejaculate (expel white liquid through the penis) quicker than you want?", "Do you ejaculate (expel white liquid through the penis) later than you want?", "Do you ejaculate (expel white liquid through the penis) at the desired time for you?".

Fig. 1. Items for assessment the sexual function (de Tubino Scanavino and Abdo 2010).

4.4 Laboratory assessment

Laboratory assessment may involve a sexual hormones screening including testosterone, estrogen, estradiol, prolactin, gonadotropin. It is important check the serum free testosterone or the levels of sex hormone-binding globulin because it usually is increased in HIV infected individuals (Hofbauer and Heufelder 1996). When organic etiology is suspected, more profound evaluations can take place, such as Doppler ultrasonography (arterial obstruction) or nerve conduction study (neuropathy).

The Figure 2 summarizes the steps for the diagnosis.

5. Treatment

The treatment of sexual dysfunctions on HIV/AIDS patients involves pharmacotherapy, psychotherapy interventions, and psychoeducational approaches on safer sex.

5.1 Pharmacotherapy

For pharmacologycal management may be considered the changing of the antiretroviral used, the association of phosphodiesterase-5 inhibitors, testosterone replacement when hypogonadism was diagnosed, and letrozole if estradiol is increased.

1. Consistent doctor-patient relationship			
2. Clinical history and physical examination	Immunological Co-morbidities Hypogonadism		
3. Sexual history	Family	Repression Sexual abuse	
	Own sexual history	The onset Masturbation exercise First complete intercourse	
	Gender issues	Men who have sex with men	Sexual orientation Gender issues
		Women	Mental health Self-image Body image Feelings for the partner Hability of the partner
	Characteristics of the dysfunction	Organic Psychogenic	
4. Assessment on sexual response	Desire Arousal Orgasm Resolution Satisfaction		
5. Laboratory assessment	Hormonal	Testosterone Estradiol Gonadotropin Prolactin Estrogen Sex hormone-binding globulin	
	Metabolic	Carbohydrate Lipid profile	

Fig. 2. Steps for the diagnosis

5.1.1 Antiretrovirals

If medication is the principal factor you can try another drug that has poor influence on sexual response, such as nevirapine (Collazos 2007, Collazos et al. 2002c) or atazanavir (Bernal et al. 2005).

5.1.2 Phosphodiesterase-5 inhibitors

The use of phosphodiesterase-5 inhibitors is highly recommended in male sexual dysfunction, but one should be careful about drug interactions with antiretrovirals, particularly with protease inhibitors (especially ritonovir) because both are metabolized by the cytochrome P-450 system. Because the increases of serum concentration of phosphodiesterase-5 inhibitors when associated with protease inhibitors and cetoconazol, the dosage should be reduced (Merry et al. 1999, Rosen et al. 2006). The phosphodiesterase-5 inhibitors most often used are sildenafil, tadalafil and vardenafil.

Poppers (amyl nitrate) are contraindicated by men user of phosphodiesterase-5 inhibitors because lowers blood pressure especially in combination with phosphodiesterase-5 inhibitors.

5.1.3 Testosterone replacement

If the patient reaches the diagnostic criteria for hypogonadism there is some options for testosterone replacement.

On the other side, testosterone replacement is not prescribed for HIV patients without decreases on free testosterone blood levels because does not improve sexual dysfunctions have been reported in this condition, and they will be exposed to the adverse effects (Collazos 2007). Sometimes testosterone replacement could be problematic even to hypogonadal male, as in the report of three HIV infected patients with erectile dysfunction whose present low testosterone and SHBG despite are receiving long-term oxandrolone in addition to testosterone replacement therapy, beyond HAART. Discontinuation of oxandrolone led to the normalization or improvement of testosterone levels in all three patients with symptomatic improvement in one patient. The authors hypothesized the first pass metabolism of orally administered oxandrolone may decrease hepatic synthesis of SHBG, allowing exogenously supplied testosterone to be excreted (Wasserman, Segal-Maurer and Rubin 2008).

By the way, the testosterone replacement shows good results in sexual dysfunction of most of hypogonadal HIV infected individuals (Cofrancesco, Whalen and Dobs 1997, Rabkin, Rabkin and Wagner 1997, Rabkin, Wagner and Rabkin 1999, Rabkin, Wagner and Rabkin 2000, Seftel et al. 2004) and the replacement by testosterone gel topic shows good benefits (Schrader et al. 2005).

5.1.4 Letrozole

Finally, some improvement in sexual desire has been reported in a few patients on HAART who were treated with letrozole, an aromatase inhibitor that inhibits the conversion of testosterone to estradiol. Thirteen men who have sex with men on HAART with low sexual desire as well as raised estradiol levels were randomly allocated to receive either parenteral testosterone or letrozole for six weeks. Standardized instruments pointed out improvement in desire, and frequency of sexual acts in both treatment arms (Richardson et al. 2007).

5.2 Psychotherapy

The psychotherapic approaches on sexual dysfunction of HIV infected people involve supportive, processual, psychosexual, and psychoeducational therapies.

5.2.1 Supportive

If the most important factor is the psychogenic can use supportive therapy in early period after HIV diagnosis. It should foccuses in demystify the stigmas from HIV/AIDS as mortal disease and as associated to non conventional sex behavior. The supportive approach would diminish the fear and guilt.

A structured supportive approach could be necessary for the women who suffered sexual violence could overcoming and retake sexual life.

5.2.2 Processual

People who have severe sexual conflicts because grown in a family with high sexual repression or suffered childhood sexual abuse, a processual approach could be recomended as psychoanalysis.

5.2.3 Psychosexual

Psychosexual therapy such as sensitive focus or masturbation training are indicated when the acceptance of HIV seropositivity is solved and the sexual dysfunctions remains.

5.2.4 Psychoeducational

As most of the population did not receive sexual education, the psychoeducational approach is always useful involving anatomy concepts, the differences between male and female sexual response, e.g.

5.3 Psychoeducational approach on safer sex

Psychoeducational approach on safer sex is offered concomitant with the treatment of the sexual dysfunction. Always the approach involves the patient and his or her partner. Safer sex counseling is fundamental for explaining the risk for contact with different strains of HIV, and favouring the development of the resistence to antiretrovirals.

Finally, psychoeducational approach should stimulate lifestyle modification including safer sex, exercise, recreational drugs information, modifications of cardiovascular risk factors (Rosen et al. 2006).

The Figure 3 summarizes the treatment.

6. Prognosis

The sexual function before HIV diagnosis, the current physical and mental health, and the psychosocial support are important factors to improve sexual response. A medical team updated with knowledge on human sexuality is essential for diagnosis, and treatment of the sexual dysfunctions. When these conditions are preserved the results on therapeutics are good (Wasserman et al. 2008, Richardson et al. 2007, Schrader et al. 2005).

The problem is that in many times the sexual issues are not investigated by health professionals, and just a few of patients will talk about sexual problems spontaneously. As sexual dysfunction is so prevalent in general population and in people living with HIV, a lot of them, keep without caring on sexual difficulties. On addiction, sexual dysfunction has impact on quality of life, very often influencing negative attitudes by the individual, including bad adherence to antiretroviral regimens, and to safer sex strategies (Trotta et al. 2007, Trotta et al. 2008). Moreover, HIV infected people with sexual dysfuntion have

Intervention	Problem	Management strategy
1. Pharmacotherapy	Antiretrovirals	Change medication
	Association with Phosphodiesterase-5 inhibitors	Reduce the dosage Does not use with poppers
	Hypogonadism	Testosterone replacement
	Estradiol increased (low sex desire)	Letrozole
2. Psychotherapy	Early period after HIV diagnosis	Supportive therapy
	Women who suffered sexual violence	Supportive therapy
	Severe sexual repression Childhood sexual abuse Dysfunctional family	Psychoanalysis
	Poor sexual education Poor knowledge on human sexuality	Psychoeducational therapy
3. Psychoeducational on safer sex	Poor knowledge on sexual health	Strategies for safer sex to the patient and to the partner

Fig. 3. Interventions

increased risk of transmission of drug-resistant strains because the higher sexual risk behavior, and inadvertent use of phosphodiesterase-5 inhibitors without medical recommendations with higher likelihood of negative interaction with antiretrovirals (Trotta et al. 2007, Trotta et al. 2008).

Another important point is on the scarcity of health professional team with expertise in human sexuality. A so private issue needs professionals with hability to approach on these intimate issues of the patients. Otherwise the patients do not open your sexual problems to them.

When the patient receives attention on your sexual life, he feels valuable, and will be more open to engage in positive ways as on adherence to medications as on safer sex strategies.

7. Conclusion

Sexuality is a very important point to quality of life. A person who becomes infected by HIV particularly by sexual contact could be extremely confused about continuing engaging in sexual intercourses. The consequences mostly are negative attitudes toward life, harm on quality of life, sexual risk behaviors, and bad adherence to antiretrovirals. People who are living with HIV/AIDS are extremely important to epidemia control. Take care of your sexual life may improve your self steam and your protective behaviors.

By the way, the approach on sexual dysfunction in HIV infected people involves multiple variables and includes the assessment on clinical history (morbid conditions, medications), sexual history (family and own), sexual function (male and female), and laboratory studies (hormonal, metabolic). The management strategies by health professionals with expertise in human sexuality involves pharmacology and psychotherapy interventions. Always the psychoeducational approach on safer sex will be developed in parallel with others interventions. The recovery of the sexual function, associated with a good adherence to safe sex practices, will improve the quality of life of the people living with HIV/AIDS and help controlling the epidemic.

8. References

American Psychiatric Association (APA) (2000): Diagnostic and Statistical Manual of Mental Disorders, Fourth Edition, Text Revision. Washington, DC: American Psychiatric Association.

Asboe, D., J. Catalan, S. Mandalia, N. Dedes, E. Florence, W. Schrooten, C. Noestlinger & R. Colebunders (2007) Sexual dysfunction in HIV-positive men is multi-factorial: a study of prevalence and associated factors. *AIDS Care*, 19, 955-65.

Baker, M. E., D. A. Vaughn & D. D. Fanestil (1978) Inhibition by protease inhibitors of binding of adrenal and sex steroid hormones. *J Supramol Struct*, 9, 421-6.

Basson, R. (2008) Women's sexual function and dysfunction: current uncertainties, future directions. *Int J Impot Res*, 20, 466-78.

Bedimo, A. L., P. Kissinger & R. Bessinger (1997) History of sexual abuse among HIV-infected women. *Int J STD AIDS*, 8, 332-5.

Bell, C., D. Richardson, M. Wall & D. Goldmeier (2006) HIV-associated female sexual dysfunction - clinical experience and literature review. *Int J STD AIDS*, 17, 706-9.

Bernal, E., M. Masiá, S. Padilla & F. Gutiérrez (2005) Unexpected improvement of sexual dysfunction during atazanavir therapy. *AIDS*, 19, 1440-1.

Bouhnik, A. D., M. Préau, M. A. Schiltz, Y. Obadia, B. Spire & V. s. group (2008) Sexual difficulties in people living with HIV in France--results from a large representative sample of outpatients attending French hospitals (ANRS-EN12-VESPA). *AIDS Behav*, 12, 670-6.

Bruckert, E., P. Giral, H. M. Heshmati & G. Turpin (1996) Men treated with hypolipidaemic drugs complain more frequently of erectile dysfunction. *J Clin Pharm Ther*, 21, 89-94.

Catalan, J. & J. Meadows (2000) Sexual dysfunction in gay and bisexual men with HIV infection: evaluation, treatment and implications. *AIDS Care*, 12, 279-86.

Ciesla, J. A. & J. E. Roberts (2001) Meta-analysis of the relationship between HIV infection and risk for depressive disorders. *Am J Psychiatry*, 158, 725-30.

Clayton, A., S. Kornstein, A. Prakash, C. Mallinckrodt & M. Wohlreich (2007) Changes in sexual functioning associated with duloxetine, escitalopram, and placebo in the treatment of patients with major depressive disorder. *J Sex Med*, 4, 917-29.

Cofrancesco, J., J. J. Whalen & A. S. Dobs (1997) Testosterone replacement treatment options for HIV-infected men. *J Acquir Immune Defic Syndr Hum Retrovirol*, 16, 254-65.

Coleman, E., B. R. Rosser & N. Strapko (1992) Sexual and intimacy dysfunction among homosexual men and women. *Psychiatr Med*, 10, 257-71.

Collazos, J. (2007) Sexual dysfunction in the highly active antiretroviral therapy era. *AIDS Rev*, 9, 237-45.

Collazos, J., E. Martinez, J. Mayo & S. Ibarra (2002a) Sexual hormones in HIV-infected patients: the influence of antiretroviral therapy. *AIDS*, 16, 934-7.

Collazos, J., E. Martínez, J. Mayo & S. Ibarra (2002b) Sexual dysfunction in HIV-infected patients treated with highly active antiretroviral therapy. *J Acquir Immune Defic Syndr*, 31, 322-6.

Collazos, J., J. Mayo, E. Martínez & S. Ibarra (2002c) Association between sexual disturbances and sexual hormones with specific antiretroviral drugs. *AIDS*, 16, 1294-5.

Cove, J. & J. Petrak (2004) Factors associated with sexual problems in HIV-positive gay men. *Int J STD AIDS*, 15, 732-6.

Crum, N. F., K. J. Furtek, P. E. Olson, C. L. Amling & M. R. Wallace (2005) A review of hypogonadism and erectile dysfunction among HIV-infected men during the pre- and post-HAART eras: diagnosis, pathogenesis, and management. *AIDS Patient Care STDS*, 19, 655-71.

Crum-Cianflone, N. F., M. Bavaro, B. Hale, C. Amling, A. Truett, C. Brandt, B. Pope, K. Furtek, S. Medina & M. R. Wallace (2007) Erectile dysfunction and hypogonadism among men with HIV. *AIDS Patient Care STDS*, 21, 9-19.

Cyranowski, J. M., J. Bromberger, A. Youk, K. Matthews, H. M. Kravitz & L. H. Powell (2004) Lifetime depression history and sexual function in women at midlife. *Arch Sex Behav*, 33, 539-48.

Daniell, H. W. (2002) Hypogonadism in men consuming sustained-action oral opioids. *J Pain*, 3, 377-84.

Danoff, A. (1996) Endocrinologic complications of HIV infection. *Med Clin North Am*, 80, 1453-69.

de Tubino Scanavino, M. & C. H. Abdo (2010) Sexual dysfunctions among people living with AIDS in Brazil. *Clinics (Sao Paulo)*, 65, 511-9.

Goldmeier, D., G. Scullard, M. Kapembwa, H. Lamba & G. Frize (2002) Does increased aromatase activity in adipose fibroblasts cause low sexual desire in patients with HIV lipodystrophy? *Sex Transm Infect*, 78, 64-6.

Greenberg, J. B. (2001) Childhood sexual abuse and sexually transmitted diseases in adults: a review of and implications for STD/HIV programmes. *Int J STD AIDS*, 12, 777-83.

Gwandure, C. (2007) Sexual assault in childhood: risk HIV and AIDS behaviours in adulthood. *AIDS Care*, 19, 1313-5.

Hatch, J. P., A. M. de la Peña & J. G. Fisher (1987) Psychometric differentiation of psychogenic and organic erectile disorders. *J Urol*, 138, 781-3.

Hijazi, L., R. Nandwani & P. Kell (2002) Medical management of sexual difficulties in HIV-positive individuals. *Int J STD AIDS*, 13, 587-92.

Hofbauer, L. C. & A. E. Heufelder (1996) Endocrine implications of human immunodeficiency virus infection. *Medicine (Baltimore)*, 75, 262-78.

Kalichman, S. C., K. J. Sikkema, K. DiFonzo, W. Luke & J. Austin (2002) Emotional adjustment in survivors of sexual assault living with HIV-AIDS. *J Trauma Stress*, 15, 289-96.

Lambert, S., A. Keegan & J. Petrak (2005) Sex and relationships for HIV positive women since HAART: a quantitative study. *Sex Transm Infect*, 81, 333-7.

Lawlor, A. & A. Braunack-Mayer (2004) Doctors' views about the importance of shared values in HIV positive patient care: a qualitative study. *J Med Ethics*, 30, 539-43.

Lewis, R. W., K. S. Fugl-Meyer, R. Bosch, A. R. Fugl-Meyer, E. O. Laumann, E. Lizza & A. Martin-Morales (2004) Epidemiology/risk factors of sexual dysfunction. *J Sex Med*, 1, 35-9.

Liebschutz, J. M., G. Feinman, L. Sullivan, M. Stein & J. Samet (2000) Physical and sexual abuse in women infected with the human immunodeficiency virus: increased illness and health care utilization. *Arch Intern Med*, 160, 1659-64.

Lue, T. F. (2000) Erectile dysfunction. *N Engl J Med*, 342, 1802-13.

Luzi, K., G. Guaraldi, R. Murri, M. De Paola, G. Orlando, N. Squillace, R. Esposito, V. Rochira, R. Vincenzo, L. Zirilli & E. Martinez (2009) Body image is a major determinant of sexual dysfunction in stable HIV-infected women. *Antivir Ther*, 14, 85-92.

Merry, C., M. G. Barry, M. Ryan, J. F. Tjia, M. Hennessy, V. A. Eagling, F. Mulcahy & D. J. Back (1999) Interaction of sildenafil and indinavir when co-administered to HIV-positive patients. *AIDS*, 13, F101-7.

Moreira, E. D., C. H. Abdo, E. B. Torres, C. F. Lôbo & J. A. Fittipaldi (2001) Prevalence and correlates of erectile dysfunction: results of the Brazilian study of sexual behavior. *Urology*, 58, 583-8.

Newshan, G., B. Taylor & R. Gold (1998) Sexual functioning in ambulatory men with HIV/AIDS. *Int J STD AIDS*, 9, 672-6.

Nicolosi, A., E. D. Moreira, M. Shirai, M. I. Bin Mohd Tambi & D. B. Glasser (2003) Epidemiology of erectile dysfunction in four countries: cross-national study of the prevalence and correlates of erectile dysfunction. *Urology*, 61, 201-6.

Rabkin, J. G., R. Rabkin & G. J. Wagner (1997) Testosterone treatment of clinical hypogonadism in patients with HIV/AIDS. *Int J STD AIDS*, 8, 537-45.

Rabkin, J. G., G. J. Wagner & R. Rabkin (1999) Testosterone therapy for human immunodeficiency virus-positive men with and without hypogonadism. *J Clin Psychopharmacol*, 19, 19-27.

--- (2000) A double-blind, placebo-controlled trial of testosterone therapy for HIV-positive men with hypogonadal symptoms. *Arch Gen Psychiatry*, 57, 141-7; discussion 155-6.

Richardson, D., D. Goldmeier, G. Frize, H. Lamba, C. De Souza, A. Kocsis & G. Scullard (2007) Letrozole versus testosterone. a single-center pilot study of HIV-infected men who have sex with men on highly active anti-retroviral therapy (HAART) with hypoactive sexual desire disorder and raised estradiol levels. *J Sex Med*, 4, 502-8.

Rogstad, K. E., R. Shah, G. Tesfaladet, M. Abdullah & I. Ahmed-Jushuf (1999) Cardiovascular autonomic neuropathy in HIV infected patients. *Sex Transm Infect*, 75, 264-7.

Rosen, R., C. Brown, J. Heiman, S. Leiblum, C. Meston, R. Shabsigh, D. Ferguson & R. D'Agostino (2000) The Female Sexual Function Index (FSFI): a multidimensional self-report instrument for the assessment of female sexual function. *J Sex Marital Ther*, 26, 191-208.

Rosen, R. C., J. A. Catania, A. A. Ehrhardt, A. L. Burnett, T. F. Lue, K. McKenna, J. R. Heiman, S. Schwarcz, D. G. Ostrow, S. Hirshfield, D. W. Purcell, W. A. Fisher, R. Stall, P. N. Halkitis, D. M. Latini, J. Elford, E. O. Laumann, F. L. Sonenstein, D. J. Greenblatt, R. A. Kloner, J. Lee, D. Malebranche, E. Janssen, R. Diaz, J. D. Klausner, A. L. Caplan, G. Jackson, R. Shabsigh, J. H. Khalsa, D. M. Stoff, D. Goldmeier, H. Lamba, D. Richardson & H. Sadeghi-Nejad (2006) The Bolger conference on PDE-5 inhibition and HIV risk: implications for health policy and prevention. *J Sex Med*, 3, 960-75; discussion 973-5.

Rosen, R. C., A. Riley, G. Wagner, I. H. Osterloh, J. Kirkpatrick & A. Mishra (1997) The international index of erectile function (IIEF): a multidimensional scale for assessment of erectile dysfunction. *Urology*, 49, 822-30.

Rosser, B. R. S., J. M. Gobby & W. P. Carr. 1999. The unsafe sexual behavior of persons. 18-28.

Schiltz, M. A. & T. G. Sandfort (2000) HIV-positive people, risk and sexual behaviour. *Soc Sci Med*, 50, 1571-88.

Schrader, S., A. Mills, M. Scheperle & J. E. Block (2005) Improvement in sexual functioning and satisfaction in nonresponders to testosterone gel: clinical effectiveness in hypogonadal, HIV-positive males. *Clin Cornerstone*, 7 Suppl 4, S26-31.

Seftel, A. D., R. J. Mack, A. R. Secrest & T. M. Smith (2004) Restorative increases in serum testosterone levels are significantly correlated to improvements in sexual functioning. *J Androl*, 25, 963-72.

Segurado, A. C., E. Batistella, V. Nascimento, P. E. Braga, E. Filipe, N. Santos & V. Paiva (2008) Sexual abuse victimisation and perpetration in a cohort of men living with HIV/AIDS who have sex with women from São Paulo, Brazil. *AIDS Care*, 20, 15-20.

Sikkema, K. J., P. A. Wilson, N. B. Hansen, A. Kochman, S. Neufeld, M. S. Ghebremichael & T. Kershaw (2008) Effects of a coping intervention on transmission risk behavior among people living with HIV/AIDS and a history of childhood sexual abuse. *J Acquir Immune Defic Syndr*, 47, 506-13.

Sollima, S., M. Osio, F. Muscia, P. Gambaro, A. Alciati, M. Zucconi, T. Maga, F. Adorni, T. Bini & A. d'Arminio Monforte (2001) Protease inhibitors and erectile dysfunction. *AIDS*, 15, 2331-3.

Speckens, A. E., M. W. Hengeveld, G. A. Lycklama à Nijeholt, A. M. van Hemert & K. E. Hawton (1993) Discrimination between psychogenic and organic erectile dysfunction. *J Psychosom Res*, 37, 135-45.

Srilatha, B. & P. G. Adaikan (2004) Estrogen and phytoestrogen predispose to erectile dysfunction: do ER-alpha and ER-beta in the cavernosum play a role? *Urology*, 63, 382-6.

Srilatha, B., P. G. Adaikan & Y. S. Chong (2007) Relevance of oestradiol-testosterone balance in erectile dysfunction patients' prognosis. *Singapore Med J*, 48, 114-8.

Stein, M., D. S. Herman, E. Trisvan, P. Pirraglia, P. Engler & B. J. Anderson (2005) Alcohol use and sexual risk behavior among human immunodeficiency virus-positive persons. *Alcohol Clin Exp Res*, 29, 837-43.

Trotta, M. P., A. Ammassari, R. Murri, P. Marconi, M. Zaccarelli, A. Cozzi-Lepri, R. Acinapura, N. Abrescia, P. De Longis, V. Tozzi, A. Scalzini, V. Vullo, E. Boumis, P. Nasta, A. Monforte, A. Antinori & A. a. A. S. Group (2008) Self-reported sexual dysfunction is frequent among HIV-infected persons and is associated with suboptimal adherence to antiretrovirals. *AIDS Patient Care STDS*, 22, 291-9.

Trotta, M. P., A. Ammassari, R. Murri, A. Monforte & A. Antinori (2007) Sexual dysfunction in HIV infection. *Lancet*, 369, 905-6.

Wasserman, P., S. Segal-Maurer & D. Rubin (2008) Low sex hormone-binding globulin and testosterone levels in association with erectile dysfunction among human immunodeficiency virus-infected men receiving testosterone and oxandrolone. *J Sex Med*, 5, 241-7.

Whetten, K., J. Leserman, K. Lowe, D. Stangl, N. Thielman, M. Swartz, L. Hanisch & L. Van Scoyoc (2006) Prevalence of childhood sexual abuse and physical trauma in an HIV-positive sample from the deep south. *Am J Public Health*, 96, 1028-30.

Yang, Y., T. Ikezoe, T. Takeuchi, Y. Adachi, Y. Ohtsuki, S. Takeuchi, H. P. Koeffler & H. Taguchi (2005) HIV-1 protease inhibitor induces growth arrest and apoptosis of human prostate cancer LNCaP cells in vitro and in vivo in conjunction with blockade of androgen receptor STAT3 and AKT signaling. *Cancer Sci*, 96, 425-33.

7

Benign and Malignant Lymphoproliferative Disorders in HIV/AIDS

Etienne Mahe and Monalisa Sur
McMaster University, Hamilton, Ontario
Canada

1. Introduction

Owing to the striking lymphotropsism exhibited by the human immunodeficiency virus, HIV/AIDS patients demonstrate a wide breadth of both benign and malignant lymphoproliferative disorders. These disorders span the spectrum from viral lymphadenopathy to lymphocentric opportunistic infections to proliferations of uncertain and frankly malignant potential. This chapter explores a number of the many possible HIV/AIDS associated disorders from the perspective of the lymphoid system. Notably, some of these disorders are themselves AIDS defining illnesses while others are entities known to occur frequently in the HIV/AIDS population but not directly influenced by HIV infection. In most cases, HIV-associated lymphoproliferative disorders are thought to result from an aberrant host immune response in the context of chronic inflammatory stimulation rather than as a direct consequence of HIV infection.

1.1 Pathogenesis

The human immunodeficiency virus is a member of the lentivirus genus (lenti- , *latin* "slow"), a group of viruses in the retrovirus family characterized by tropism for immune cells (Norkin, 2010). HIV demonstrates strong affinity for a specific cohort of human T-cells, the CD4 "Helper" T-cell; this is accomplished by means of the viral gp120 protein's strong affinity for the CD4 molecule (Wain-Hobson, 1996). HIV infects cells with CD4 cell-surface receptor molecules, using them to gain entry into the cell (Verani, et al., 2005). In early infection, HIV is widely disseminated by way of its interaction with antigen presenting cells (e.g. Langerhans and dendritic cells) which direct antigen obtained from mucous membranes toward the tissues of the adaptive immune system (namely the lymph nodes); HIV can accomplish this both by means of CD4 receptor binding but also by exploiting the immune response itself by allowing phagocytosis into these antigen presenting cells through either interations with complement or Fc receptors (Verani, et al., 2005). The result is a systemic dissemination of HIV infection to lymphoid tissues (Pantaleo, et al., 1993). Once gained access to the lymphoid tissues of the body, HIV may engage in a latent infection of T-cells by way of viral integration into resting or memory T-cells; these cells may then serve another reservoir of infection (Sierra, et al., 2005).

A number of studies have explored the biological influences that HIV may have on lymphomagenesis. The primary role of the CD4 T-cell is played out in the adaptive immune response. More specifically, non-infected CD4 T-cells function as immune system modulators through interactions with a multitude of other cells of both the adaptive immune system (i.e. B-cells) as well as the innate immune system (e.g. macrophages and monocytes)(Robbins, et al., 2010). HIV infected CD4 cells cannot execute these normal immunomodulatory functions: HIV replication within CD4 cells is directly cytopathic (Hazenberg, et al., 2000); non-infected CD4 cells will be reduced in number due to activation-induced cell death under the influence of both HIV infection as well as other concomitant infections (McCune, 2001); HIV tropism for CD4 cells will result in colonization and persistent immunostimulation in lymphoid tissues; HIV will also infect immature CD4 positive precursor T-cells thereby further reducing the effective CD4 T-cell pool (Robbins, et al., 2010).

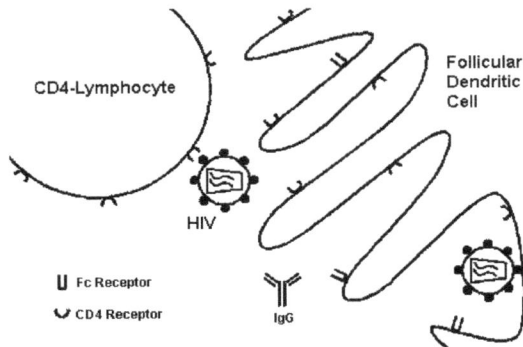

Fig. 1. HIV receptor-specific pathogenesis

In contrast to other viruses associated with neoplasms, HIV is not regarded as a directly transforming virus (i.e. its effect on the host cell genome does not directly initiate neoplastic transformation). This is evidenced by a number of observations regarding HIV-associated lymphomas: there is a wide etiologic range of possible HIV-associated lymphomas; there is frequent association of HIV-associated lymphomas with "super-infecting" known oncogenic pathogens (e.g. Kaposi-sarcoma virus and Epstein-Barr virus); and most HIV-associated lymphomas are lymphomas of B-cells (and not of T-cells, which one would expect if HIV were a uniformly transformative virus). Molecular studies have also noted a propensity for viral genomic integration at random active gene sites; while this may theoretically lead to an insertion at a transformative locus, HIV does not show consistent insertion at a transformative site (Mitchell, et al., 2004).

EBV has been shown to contribute to lymphomagenesis in a number of ways; the latent membrane proteins, in particular, have garnered much research interest in this vein. In the 1980s it was recognized that EBV latent membrane protein-1 gene was able to transform mouse cell models (Wang, et al., 1985). EBV-LMP has also been shown to activate the tumor necrosis factor and p38 mitogenic pathways (Mosialos, et al., 1995; Eliopoulos, et al., 1999); activation of these pathways may contribute to the ability of EBV-infected (and potentially transformed) cells to evade host defense mechanisms. Another EBV encoded protein, latent membrane protein A2 has been shown to stimulate lymphocyte development and proliferation in mouse models outside of the normal immunologic milieu (Caldwell, et al., 1998). Finally, Vockerodt and colleague recently demonstrated that latent membrane protein-1 was capable of inducing a Hodgkin-like state in non-previously transformed germinal centre B-cells (Vockerodt, et al., 2008).

Less commonly, HIV-associated lymphomas demonstrate co-infection with the Kaposi sarcoma herpes virus, HHV-8. A number of HHV-8 viral proteins have been implicated in lymphomagenesis: the HHV-8 latency-associated nuclear antigen has been shown to interfere with normal p53 and Rb gene protein functions; the K13 viral protein interferes with host cell Fas-mediated apoptosis pathways; and the Kaposin B viral protein has been shown to prevent the normal degeneration of stimulatory cytokines (Wen & Damania, 2010). The combined influence of these and other HHV-8 encoded proteins, especially within the context of an already abnormal immunomodulation from HIV infection, places infected B-cells at high risk of malignant transformation.

2. Non-neoplastic lymphoid disorders in HIV/AIDS

2.1 HIV-associated lymphadenopathy

Lymphadenopathy is a characteristic (though certainly not specific) finding in HIV/AIDS patients. Variable definitions of lymphadenopathy exist in the medical literature, typically making reference to enlarged, swollen or painful lymph nodes as definitive. Size cut-offs have been proposed in some definitions and many clinicians will investigate lymph nodes exceeding 1 cm in size. Ioachim notes that lymph nodes larger than 3 cm should raise suspicion of neoplasia (Ioachim & Medeiros, 2009b). Often lymphadenopathy will come to clinical attention as rapidly enlarging lymph nodes; unfortunately, there is little data to suggest how the rapidity of lymph node enlargement pertains to the presence of absence of a neoplastic proliferation. Other features of clinical concern include matting or adherence of multiple nodes to one another, as well as enlargement of several nodes in a given nodal chain (Ioachim & Medeiros, 2009b). Most frequently, due to the frequent clinical concern that an enlarged lymph node may admonish, biopsy and pathological examination of lymph nodes is necessary, especially in the at risk HIV/AIDS community. For our purposes, HIV-associated lymphadenopathy refers to enlarged lymph nodes attributable strictly to a non-neoplastic viral process excluding other opportunistic pathogens (discussed later).

Lymphadenopathy was identified as one of the earliest clinical signs in early epidemiologic studies of patients with AIDS; the closely studied 1982 Vancouver cohort of at risk homosexual men demonstrated a prevalence of 50% of post-seroconversion lymphadenopathy (Boyko, et al., 1987). Similar values were noted in other cohorts, including heterosexual males and females, such as the Zimbabwean cohort of Latif, et al. (Latif, et al., 1989). Lymphadenopathy is also more commonly identified in HIV positive children than in non-HIV infected children (Bakaki, et al., 2001; Nielsen, et al., 1997). HIV-associated lymphadenopathy demonstrates preponderance for the head and neck area, often presenting as cervical lymphadenopathy (Prasad, et al., 2006). Other radiologic studies have also demonstrated frequent (typically occult) intra-abdominal lymphadenopathy in HIV positive patients, most commonly as a result of opportunistic infection but also due to lymphomas (Jasmer, et al., 2002). Concern over the latter not infrequently results in invasive abdominal lymph node biopsies for diagnostic purposes.

HIV-associated lymphadenopathy follows a consistent histological pattern of progression (see Figure 2). Lymphadenopathy typically begins with the onset of HIV viremia; this acute phase of HIV infection (the acute retroviral syndrome) is typically described as a mononucleosis-like cluster of symptoms. Acute retroviral syndrome typically begins 2-6 weeks post-infection and may last for several weeks. Typical symptoms include fever, headache, malaise, pharyngitis and lymphadenopathy (Carpenter, et al., 2004). The lymphadenopathy, however, often persists beyond this acute phase. The histological features of early HIV-associated lymphadenopathy typically demonstrate exuberant hyperplastic changes: large lymphoid follicles with irregular serpiginous shapes are characteristic; irregular enlargement of germinal centres is noted; these large germinal centres typically demonstrate prominent apoptotic bodies and tingible body macrophages; and there may be expansion of the interfollicular zones by numerous transformed B lymphocytes (these have a monocytoid appearance and correspond to antigenically stimulated B-cells). These features are typical of the so-called Grade 1 HIV-associated lymphadenopathy.

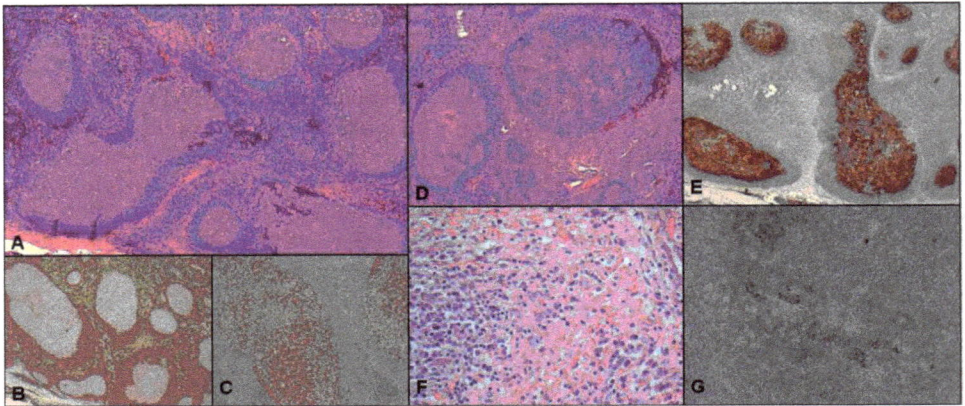

Fig. 2. HIV Lymphadenopathy: A: Early HIV Lymphadenopathy (Grade 1); B: BCL2 stain demonstrating benign follicle staining pattern (negative in follicles and positive in interfollicular zones); C: Ki67 demonstrating benign follicle staining pattern (high index nuclear staining in follicles with low index in interfollicular zones); D: Grade 2 HIV Lymphadenopathy demonstrating early follicular-lysis; E: Corresponding CD21 stain demonstrating hyperplastic moth-eaten follicular dendritic cell meshwork (replaced by fibrosis); F: Grade 3 HIV Lymphadenopathy demonstrating marked fibrosis and loss of follicles; G: Corresponding CD21 stain demonstrating near absence of follicular dendritic meshwork

As HIV infection progresses, the antigenic stimulation within the lymph node begins to wane. This leads to a Grade 2 pattern of HIV-associated lymphadenopathy characterized by a reduction in the number of lymphoid follicles, an increase in the number of plasma cells and a proliferation of perifollicular blood vessels. At the extreme of HIV-associated lymphadenopathy is the Grade 3 pattern in which the residual follicles begin to display sclerosis of their germinal centres.

Although consistent, none of the histologic features noted above are specific to HIV. The Grade 1 pattern, for example, is frequently observed in non-HIV viral lymphadenitides. The Grade 2 and 3 patterns show a significant overlap with those of Castleman's disease (see later). In such cases, a clinical history of known or suspected HIV infection is essential in order that the correct diagnosis be made and that the correct treatment regimen be instituted. The vascular proliferation noted in Grade 2 and 3 may also be misconstrued for Kaposi's sarcoma (see later for the lymph node features of Kaposi's sarcoma); immunohistochemistry for the Kaposi's sarcoma virus is now a commonplace tool to avoid this diagnostic confusion. Other more aggressive lymphoproliferative disorders need to be ruled out in lymph nodes sampled in the context of HIV; the key feature in HIV-associated lymphadenopathy of any Grade is the relative preservation of lymph node architecture which is often lost in lymphoid malignancies.

EBV seropositivity is widespread in HIV positive patients and in the context of lymphadenopathy EBV infection can confuse the histopathologic diagnosis (see Figure 3). More specifically, EBV infection may produce reactive cells demonstrating a striking resemblance to the Reed-Sternberg cells of Hodgkin's lymphoma. In such cases, immunohistochemistry is essential. In order to rule out Hodgkin's lymphoma, the atypical Reed-Sternberg like cells seen in lymphadenitis will typically stain positive for CD20, CD45, and may stain positive for CD30 (an activation marker); these cells, unlike true Reed-Sternberg cells, should not stain for CD15.

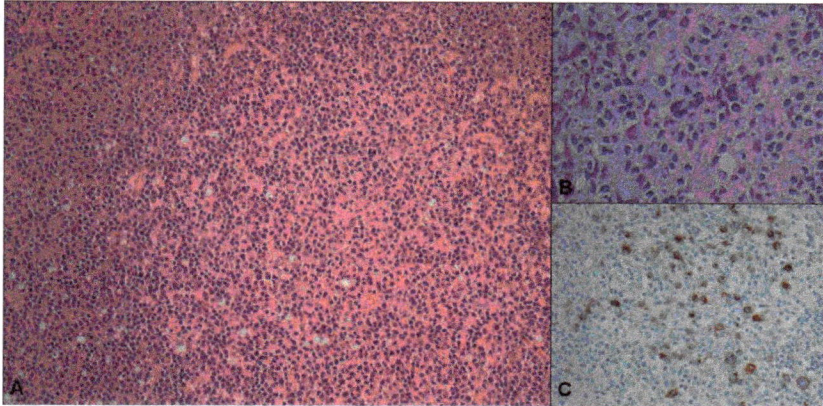

Fig. 3. HIV Lymphadenopathy with EBV related changes: A: Loss of normal lymph node architecture; B: Reed-sternberg-like cells present in EBV-related HIV Lymphadenopathy; C: Corresponding EBV Stain

Treatment for HIV-associated lymphadenopathy is focused around optimizing antiretroviral therapy, treated other concomitant infections as needed and clinical follow-up. The latter point is emphasized in order that lymphoid neoplasia not be missed. Studies have explored the outcomes of patients diagnosed with HIV-associated lymphadenopathy and graded according to the above scheme. In their cohort of HIV patients with lymphadenopathy, Ioachim and colleagues noted that most cases of HIV-associated lymphadenopathy began as Grade 1; many cases subsequently progressed from Grade 1 to 2 and from Grade 2 to 3; most cases with Grade 3 lymphadenopathy subsequently developed AIDS defining illnesses (Ioachim & Medeiros, 2009; Ioachim, et al., 1990). Ioachim et al also noted a distinct survival difference between the various grades of HIV-associated lymphadenopathy (Ioachim & Medeiros, 2009; Ioachim, et al., 1990). Grade 3 HIV-associated lymphadenopathy is also strongly associated with development of Kaposi's sarcoma (Ioachim & Medeiros, 2009c).

2.2 Bacillary angiomatosis

Bacillary Angiomatosis is a lesion of proliferating endothelial cells caused by *Bartonella* species occuring in immunocompromised patients, almost exclusively in patients with AIDS. The first documented case of HIV/AIDS associated bacillary angiomatosis was reported by Stoler and colleagues in 1983 (Cotell & Noskin, 1994; Stoler, et al., 1983); they reported a peculiar case of a young AIDS patient with multiple cutaneous nodules found to consist of proliferating endothelial cells forming lobular networks of small caliber blood vessels. Interspersed within this network were small gram-negative bacillary forms visible only on Warthin-Starry staining. For many years, efforts to speciate the organism observed histologically were unsuccessful; initial attempts at culturing the organism with a range of media produced no results (Cotell & Noskin, 1994; Stoler, et al., 1983). Finally, with the dawning of PCR based techniques, the organism believed to be the causal agent in bacillary angiomatosis was found to be genomically comparable to the species known to cause Cat Scratch Disease, the organism known today as *Bartonella henselae* (Relman, et al., 1990).

It is now known that bacillary angiomatosis may be associated with a number of *Bartonella* species, most common *B. henselae* and *B. quintana* (Maguina, et al., 2009). Interestingly, studies have shown high seroprevalence for *Bartonella* species in the population overall (Lamas, et al., 2010). Furthermore, clinically silent *Bartonella* seroprevalence has been observed in the HIV population, rarely with very high titres (Pape, et al., 2005; Yousif, et al., 1996). These laboratory data mirror the clinically evident divergence of *Bartonella* infection observed in the immunocompromised and immunocompetent populations. In immunocompetent individuals, *Bartonella* infection, if clinically evident, typically manifests as the so-called "cat-scratch disease," characterized by lymphadenopathy demonstrating caseating granuloma formation. In immunocompromised patients, on the other hand, the infection manifests as vascular lesions, sometimes progressing to a potentially fatal systemic infection. This stark contrast has spawned a number of studies demonstrating the importance of an intact adaptive immune system.

Bartonella infection is transmitted either by means of an insect vector (e.g. mites, lice) or by means of trauma by an animal vector (the namesake "cat-scratch" is evident) (Minnick, et al., 2003; Ioachim & Medeiros, 2009a; Wolff, et al., 2005). Studies exploring the comparative genomics of *Bartonella* infections in HIV patients and their pet cats have confirmed this long suspected epidemiologic link (Chang, et al., 2002). After inoculation, *Bartonella* species home to erythrocytes and endothelial cells, thereby allowing it access to multiple sites in the body (Minnick, et al., 2003). *Bartonella* then exploits a number of molecular pathways to evade its host's immune system (Minnick, et al., 2003); this evasion may explain the clinically observed propensity of *Bartonella* to produce granulomatous lymphadenitis. In immunocompromised patients, exploiting an already weakened immune system, *Bartonella* stimulates angiogenesis; *Bartonella* infection stimulates the production of hypoxia-induced factor and other cytokines, thereby upregulating angiogenesis (Minnick, et al., 2003).

Bacillary angiomatosis typically occurs in AIDS patients with low CD4 counts (typically less than $100/mm^3$) (Maguina, et al., 2009). Most patients present with skin lesions, characteristically as multiple violaceous or red papules; these lesions may be painful, typically progress over days to weeks and may resemble cherry hemangiomas or pyogenic granulomas (Wolff, 2005). In most cases a combination of clinical history, known HIV/AIDS status and clinical assessment will result in the correct diagnosis; the differential diagnosis, however, may include Kaposi's sarcoma thereby mandating histopathological assessment

(Maguina, et al., 2009). In a notable number of cases of BA, lymphadenopathy may be identified as the inciting event (Gasquet, et al., 1998). *B. henselae* BA, in particular, tends to demonstrate lymphadenoapthy, both with and without skin lesions (Ioachim & Medeiros, 2009a). Aggressive cases of bacillary angiomatosis may demonstrate splenic or hepatic involvement as bacillary peliosis, often with fatal outcomes.

The histologic features of bacillary angiomatosis in lymph nodes are similar to those seen in skin lesions and elsewhere (see Figure 4). Bacillary angiomatosis typically forms richly vascular nodules. Proliferating endothelial cells are evident, forming variably sized blood-filled vascular spaces into which their nuclei protrude. There may be notable anisonucleosis, multiple nucleoli and numerous mitoses; these features may suggest a malignant entity. Ancillary staining with Warthin-Starry silver stain invariably demonstrates numerous bacilli, 0.2-0.3 μm in size, often noted in clumps (Maguina, et al., 2009; Ioachim & Medeiros, 2009a). Electron microscopy will demonstrate a trilaminar bacillus in association with an obvious proliferation of endothelial cells with characteristic Weibel-Palade bodies (Kostianovsky & Greco, 1994). Modern attempts at developing reliable immunohistochemical markers to aid in the diagnosis of bacillary angiomatosis have been as yet unsuccessful; PCR techniques may be relied upon to confirm the presence of *Bartonella* infection in cases that may be diagnostically equivocal (Caponetti, et al., 2009).

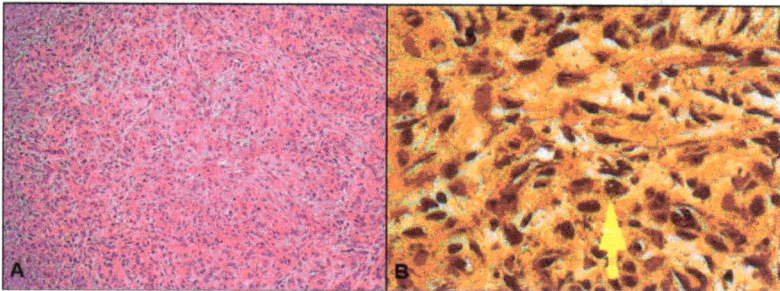

Fig. 4. Bacillary Angiomatosis: A: Low-power view demonstrating proliferating venules; B: Warthin-starry stain demonstrating extracellular clump of bacteria (arrow)

The differential diagnosis of bacillary angiomatosis may include a number of entities, especially if the HIV/AIDS status of the patient is unknown. On hematoxylin & eosin staining alone, bacillary angiomatosis may resemble a hemangioma. Gram staining may help distinguish bacillary angiomatosis from pyogenic granuloma (the former being invariably negative). Bacillary angiomatosis may sometimes be difficult to discern from Kaposi's sarcoma. Histologically, Kaposi's cells are more characteristically spindled and there is a predominance of slit-like vascular spaces. Nonetheless, most authories recommend using an immunohistochemical stain against HHV-8, the causal virus of Kaposi's sarcoma, in order to rule out this more serious condition. Another malignant condition that may be mimicked by bacillary angiomatosis is typical angiosarcoma; this entity is highly aggressive and demonstrates an infiltrative architecture.

Although the clinical course of bacillary angiomatosis is variable, the treatment of choice is antibiotics (typically a course of erythromycin or doxycycline); some cases may also resolve spontaneously even without treatment, however (Wolff, et al., 2005). Care should be taken in HIV/AIDS patients with very low CD4 counts; these patients not only require quick accurate diagnosis to define the appropriate treatment regimen, but further preventative action may also be beneficial, such as prevention of exposure to animals.

2.3 Other common infectious lymphadenitides in HIV/AIDS

While a complete review of the opportunistic and co-infectious agents encountered in HIV/AIDS is beyond the scope of this book, any discussion of the lymph node based disease entities encountered in HIV/AIDS would be remiss if not for a discussion of the commonest node-based co-infections. The following is a brief discussion of the most common opportunistic infections encountered in HIV/AIDS patients from the perspective of lymph node disease.

2.3.1 Pneumocystis

Pneumocystis jiroveci is a ubiquitous organism in nature manifesting as a disease-causing organism only in the immunocompromised. This fungus first came to broad clinical attention in the early 1980s when it was noted in 70-80% of AIDS patients, most commonly manifest as pneumonia. Rarely, however, pneumocystosis does involve the lymph nodes. Anderson and Barrie were probably the first to report pneumocystis in a lymph node, two decades prior to the first identified cases of HIV/AIDS (ANDERSON & BARRIE, 1960). Of the reported extra-pulmonary cases of pneumocystis, the lymphoreticular system is probably the most common (Grimes, et al., 1987; Ioachim & Medeiros, 2009d). When involving lymph nodes, pneumocystis most commonly involves the mediastinum and retroperitoneal lymph nodes (Ioachim & Medeiros, 2009d). The gross features typically reflect the presence of necrotizing granuloma: lymph nodes are typically enlarged with central areas of purulent material. Microscopically, granulomata with central necrotic eosinophilic material will be noted (see Figure 5). The causal microorganisms are generally not overtly evident on routine histologic stains but can be readily identified on fungal silver stains as helmet-shaped organisms within the necrotic foci. Immunohistochemical stains for *Pneumocystis jiroveci* are available, though a combination of clinical history of HIV infection and morphologic features identified on silver staining are often sufficient. The current treatment of choice is trimethoprim-sulfamethoxazole antibiotics; the US centres for disease control also recommend that all HIV-positive patients diagnosed with pneumocystosis be maintained on indefinite prophylactic anti-fungal agents provided that CD4 count remains below 200 cells/μL (Kaplan, et al., 2009).

2.3.2 Mycobacteria

Globally the risk of co-infection with *Mycobacteria tuberculosis* is 20-37 times higher in patients with HIV than those without (WHO Department of HIV/AIDS Stop TB Department, 2010). The WHO also estimates that 25% of HIV-positive patients will die due to concomitant tuberculosis (WHO Department of HIV/AIDS Stop TB Department, 2010). Other non-tuberculous infections are also frequent in (and many are characteristic of) HIV infection. In addition to their primary involvement of the lungs, mycobacteria are also frequently encountered in lymph nodes, especially in the context of HIV infection. Mycobacterial lymphadenitis, regardless of the underlying species, will characteristically produce lymph node enlargement with foci of necrosis. The histologic features are often characteristic, namely central eosinophilic necrosis surrounded by a rim of pallisading histiocytes and giant cells (see Figure 5). In this peripheral rim of histiocytes, mycobacteria may be identified, often few and far between, on acid fast staining (pathologists often use a Ziehl-Neelsen stain for this purpose). Positivity on acid-fast staining does not equate to tuberculosis, however, and in many cases distinguishing between *Mycobacteria tuberculosis*, atypical mycobacteria or the *Mycobacterium avium complex* can be challenging, often requiring molecular testing for speciation (which can fortunately be performed off formalin-fixed and paraffin-embedded tissues). The presence of the so-called Langhans giant cells (with peripherally rimmed nuclei) may hint at the presence of *Mycobacteria tuberculosis* but is by no means specific. Another advantage to molecular testing when acid-fast bacteria are encountered is the ability to test for antimicrobial resistant strains by PCR; this may be an invaluable aid given the burgeoning cohort of multidrug resistant TB cases encountered in HIV/AIDS.

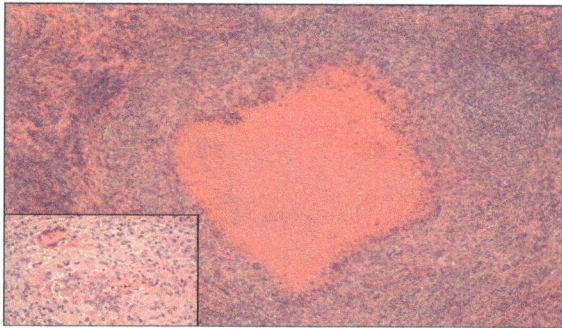

Fig. 5. Tuberculous Lymphadenitis: Granuloma with eosinophilic necrotic centre; inset: characteristics Langhans giant cell (top left) with adjacent necrosis (bottom right)

2.3.3 Toxoplasmosis

Toxoplasma gondii is the causative agent of toxoplasmosis, a parasitic infection believed to be one of the worlds most prevalent. *Toxoplasma gondii* seropositivity in the at-large population has previously been reported as high as 70-90%, though modern estimates in the range of 10-40% seem reasonable (Shin, et al., 2009; Kamani, et al., 2009; Fromont, et al., 2009). Not unexpectedly, the overall seroprevalence of *Toxoplasma gondii* is also high; while the estimates may be lower in North American and Europe, one recent Nigerian cohort demonstrated a seroprevalence of over 50% with active parasitism in the blood detected in over 20% (Lindstrom, et al., 2006). *Toxoplasma gondii* demonstrates parasitism of a number of animal hosts, most commonly of felines (the definitive host). Humans are typically infected by way of consumption of contaminated foods or exposure to contaminated soil or animal droppings. Vertical transmission is also possible, producing a dangerous congenital toxoplasmosis. One of the most frequent presentations of toxoplasmosis in the HIV population is toxoplasma encephalitis (Ioachim & Medeiros, 2009e); a histologically characteristic infection of lymph nodes is also common, however. Toxoplasmosis lymphadenopathy typically affects the lymph nodes of the head and neck; these are typically slightly enlarged and tender to palpation. The most frequently encountered histologic features are nodal follicular hyperplasia with interspersed aggregates and sheets of monocytoid lymphocytes and scattered clusters of epithelioid cells (see Figure 6). The monocytoid cells are immunoglobin producing B-cells (which will stain positive for B-cell markers) and can most typically be found in the subcapsular and paratrabecular locations while the epithelioid cells are histiocytes and are characteristically seen to encroach upon follicles but do not form true granulomas. Many HIV positive cases of toxoplasma lymphadenopathy will demonstrate free or engulfed trophozoites (which may be seen staining hook-like organisms H&E, either free floating or within macrophages); they are rarely observed in immunocompetent patients, however. The giemsa special stain can be used to highlight the organisms and some labs use immunohistochemistry with *Toxoplasma gondii* antibodies; PCR testing is the gold-standard, however. The histologic differential diagnosis is long—as would be expected in most cases with prominent collections of histiocytes. For this reason, it is advisable to use ancillary testing or special stains when examining lymph nodes with prominent collections of histiocytes. In addition to antibiotics for treatment of acute toxoplasmosis (such as pyrimethamine, sulfadiazine or clindamycin), the centres for disease control and prevention also currently recommend antibiotic prophylaxis for HIV patients with low CD4 counts (less than 200 cells/µL) (Kaplan, et al., 2009). Routine serologic testing of HIV positive patients is also recommended (Kaplan, et al., 2009).

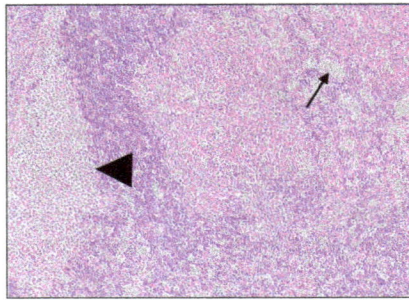

Fig. 6. Toxoplasma Lymphadenitis: Hyperplastic follicle with moth-eaten appearance infiltrated by epithelioid histiocytes (arrow) with adjacent collection of monocytoid B-cells (arrowhead)

2.4 Castleman's disease

Castleman's disease, also known as angiofollicular lymphadenopathy, was first described by Castleman and colleagues in the 1950's. The first studies of Castleman's disease predated the recongnition of HIV and it was not until decades later that its connection to HIV and HHV-8 was recognized. We now recognize two distinct histological forms, the hyaline-vascular and plasma variants. The plasma cell variant may further be categorized into unicentric and multicentric forms, the latter characteristically HIV-associated and of poorer prognosis.

The pathogenetic mechanisms leading to the development of Castleman's disease remain debated. Evidence supports HHV-8 as the etiologic agent in at least some cases; in one study, 50% of the unicentric plasma cell variant cases and nearly all cases of the mulcentric form were noted to be positive for HHV-8 (Soulier, et al., 1995). Further evidence in support of HIV and HHV-8 viral pathogens as etiologic agents stems from studies indicating a response of HIV associated multicentric Castleman's disease to antiviral agents (Casper, et al., 2004). Other studies have identified the lymphokine interleukin-6 (IL-6) as a potential contributor to the development of the plasma cell variant (Oksenhendler, et al., 2002). Interleukin-6 is a chemokine with a number of roles: it acts as an activator of T and B-cells; it also acts to downregulate pro-inflammatory cytokines by inhibiting interleukin-1 and tumour necrosis factor α (Jones, et al., 2001). Another study demonstrated that HHV-8 produces an interleukin-6 homologue (Osborne, et al., 1999). These factors together may account for the pathogenesis of the plasma cell variant, especially the multicentric form. The hyaline vascular variant, however, does not demonstrate as strong an association with HHV-8 and is most common in non-HIV patients, some with no evident immune dysregulation; in these cases, the pathogenesis has yet to be elucidated.

The hyaline vascular variant is the most common variant of the unicentric form, representing 80-90% of cases (Ioachim & Medeiros, 2009f). This variant typically presents as enlargement of a lymph node or lymph node group, often in the mediastinal region. This variant is also is more common than the plasma cell variant to affect younger patients. Few systemic symptoms are present in the hyaline vascular variant and most symptoms are related to mass effect. The classical histological features demonstrate preservation of overall lymph node architecture with an abundance of follicles (see Figure 7). In these follicles are one or two (sometime conjoined) germinal centres demonstrating prominent sclerosis and paucicellularity. The mantle/marginal cells of these follicles can be seen to form concentric layers (termed "onion-skinning") around the sclerosed germinal centres. The classic form also demonstrates a hyalinized penetrating vessel passing into the sclerotic germinal centre from the exterior of the follicle (forming so called "lollipop" lesions). Other interfollicular zone changes may be noted including extensive proliferation of small vascular channels (termed "high endothelial venules"). Sclerosis of the lymph node capsule is also a common finding. As noted previously, similar features may also be noted in cases of high-grade HIV-associated lymphadenopathy. The latter usually lack the classical lollipop lesions and the mantle/marginal zone onion-skinning is usually far less prominent. Ancillary tests for HHV-8 may be helpful but typically the diagnosis is made histologically.

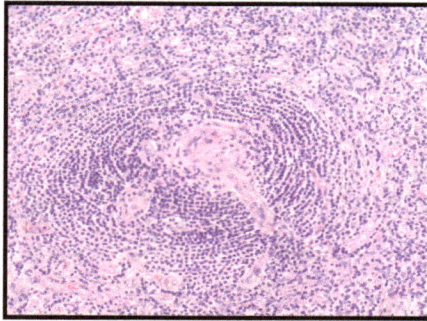

Fig. 7. Hyaline Vascular Variant of Castleman's Disease

The plasma cell variant is the less common of the unicentric forms (Ioachim & Medeiros, 2009f). As in the hyaline vascular variant, the unicentric plasma cell variant may present as an enlarging mass. Patients with this histological variant, however, are more prone to systemic clinical symptoms than those patients with the hyaline vascular variant. Typical symptoms include fevers, night sweats, malaise, and weight loss (these symptoms, in conjunction with enlarged lymph nodes often arouse suspicions of a lymphoproliferative disorder; biopsy for diagnosis is generally recommended). The plasma cell variant demonstrates the similar features of onion skinning and lollipop lesions, though the degree of hyalinization of the germinal centres is markedly reduced relative to the hyaline vascular variant; this may sometimes make the recognition of the lollipop lesions difficult (see Figure 8). Examination of the interfollicular zones is generally very helpful since it demonstrates numerous sheets of mature plasma cells (these generally stand out prominently since prominent plasma cells are rare in lymph nodes). The prominent vascularity noted in the interfollicular zones of the hyaline vascular variant is typically absent. Some cases may have foci demonstrating features of the hyaline vascular variant; when the histologic features of the plasma cell variant dominate, however, the latter diagnosis is appropriate. A number of studies have demonstrated a histological difference between plasma cell variant affected lymph nodes positive and negative for HHV-8 infection. In HHV-8 negative cases, residual hyperplastic follicles are usually notable; in contrast in HHV-8 positive cases, fewer residual follicles are noted and a more prominent interfollicular space vascular proliferation is present. Also, HHV-8 positive immunoblastic cells are also more prominent in the HHV-8 positive cases.

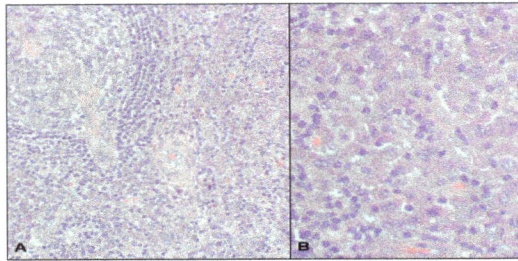

Fig. 8. Plasma Cell Variant of Castleman's Disease: A: Non-hyalinized "lollipop" lesion; B: High-power view demonstrating prominent interfollicular plasma cell infiltrates

Multicentric castleman's disease almost invariably involves multiple lymph nodes most typically demonstrating the histology seen in the unicentric plasma cell variant. The multicentric form has been traditionally under-recognized since its diagnosis requires positive detection of Castleman's disease in multiple locations. This form is also most often present in the context of HIV infection. Patients are nearly always symptomatic, usually presenting with fever, malaise, night sweats and weight loss (the so called B-symptoms) and may also present with hepatosplenomegaly, skin rash, edema and neurologic changes (Ioachim & Medeiros, 2009f). Other laboratory findings include cytopenias, elevated erythrocyte sedimentation rate and elevated C-reactive protein (Ioachim & Medeiros, 2009f). Diagnosis may be confused when a number of the latter clinical signs and symptoms are present, since these are suggestive of the so-called POEMS syndrome (this is a syndrome characterized by the presence of peripheral neuropathy, organomegaly, edema, monoclonal serum paraprotein, and skin changes). POEMS syndrome demonstrates significant diagnostic overlap Castleman's disease, especially the multicentric form. It is felt to be a para-neoplastic syndrome resulting from plasma cell disorders and is felt to have a common pathogenetic link with the plasma cell variant of Castleman's disease via interleukin-6 (Dispenzieri, 2007). The differential diagnosis can be further confused when HIV is considered; the latter, or rather the anti-retroviral drugs used to treat it, can cause peripheral neuropathies, skin changes, edema and other symptoms. In order to avoid diagnostic confusion, specific POEMS criteria have been set forth (Dispenzieri, 2007) and lymphadenopathy should be investigated histopathologically for features of Castleman's disease.

The treatment and prognosis of Castleman's disease depends greatly on both the histologic type as well as the presence of absence of multicentric disease. The hyaline vascular variant is often treated only with excision but adjuvant radiation therapy has been used in cases not amenable to complete resection (Roca, 2009). Some cases of both the hyaline vascular and plasma cell variants may be complicated by recurrence (chiefly the latter more than the former) (Roca, 2009). Cases of unicentric disease with persistent symptoms may also require steroids or chemotherapy (Roca, 2009). The multicentric form often requires aggressive treatment, frequently with chemotherapy (using regimens similar to those used in aggressive lymphomas, often combined with the anti-CD20 antibody rituximab) (Mylona, et al., 2008). There is controversy as to the actual benefit of anti-retroviral therapy; in their systematic review of Multicentric Castleman's disease in HIV, Mylona and colleagues determined that the survival outcomes from Multicentric Castleman's disease with and without antiretroviral therapies were comparable (Mylona, et al., 2008). The caveat to this latter observation is the reduction in incidence of Kaposi's sarcoma in patients on antiretrovirals (Mylona, et al., 2008).

2.5 Polymorphous post-transplant lymphoproliferative disease-like B-cell lymproliferative disorder

With the development of immunosuppressive medications permitting greatly improved successes of allogeneic transplant, it was noted that chronically immunosuppressed patients had a uniquely increased risk of a variety of lymphoproliferative disorders. These proliferations, 80% of B-cell lineage (Jacobson & LaCasce, 2010), were termed post-transplant lymphoproliferative disorders to reflect their unique clinicopathologic characteristics. For our purposes, it is interesting to note that, many decades after the concept of iatrogenic immunosuppression was introduced for the purposes of ameliorating transplant outcomes, the HIV/AIDS epidemic revealed an equally dangerous wave of immunosuppression in which many other cases clinically and histologically similar to post-transplant lymphoproliferative disorder were encountered.

The first series of HIV-associated post-transplant lymphoproliferative disorders was reported in 1987. Four infant autopsy cases from patients with HIV (at that time, the human T-lymphocyte virus-III) and a clinical picture compatible with AIDS were included in the report. At autopsy, splenic and liver infiltrates were noted. These infiltrates, as well as other microscopic infiltrates in the lungs, were noted to consist of a polymorphous collection of inflammatory cells with a preponderance of lymphocytes. These lymphocytes were noted to be polyclonal by kappa and lamda immunohistochemistry. Currently, this entity is known as HIV-associated polymorphous lymphoproliferative disorder (Raphaël, et al., 2008).

Though few cases have been reported, some small series have explored the clinical and pathologic characteristic of this entity. HIV-associated polymorphous lymphoproliferative disorder typically presents in adults with low CD4 counts (typically less than 200 cells/µL) (Nador, et al., 2003). This entity is identified both within and without lymph nodes and tends most often to present unifocally. In contrast to most HIV-associated lymphomas, HIV-associated polymorphous lymphoproliferative disorder tends to lack a monotonous morphology, often demonstrating a mixture of lymphocytes, plasma cells, immunoblasts and histiocytes (see Figure 9). Of particular interest is the tendency for the majority of cells to bear plasmacytoid morphology. A variable degree of cytologic atypia and even necrosis may also be observed.

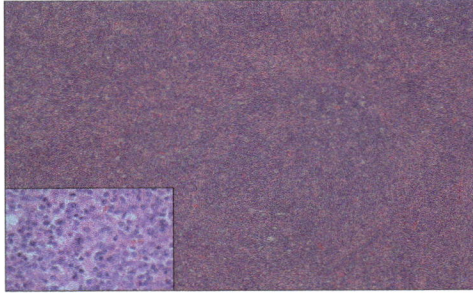

Fig. 9. HIV-associated Polymorphous post-transplant lymphoproliferative disease-like B-cell lymphoproliferative disorder: low-power view demonstrating follicular-lysis; inset: high-power view demonstrating polymorphous infiltrate

The immunophenotypic features of HIV-associated polymorphous lymphoproliferative disorder are also unique. Most cases will demonstrate some form of B-cell phenotype, either in the form of CD20 expression or by prevue of immunoglobulin expression (Nador, et al., 2003). Most, but certainly not all, will demonstrate kappa or lambda light-chain restriction and molecular evidence of clonal immunoglobulin gene rearrangement (Nador, et al., 2003). Some will even demonstrate co-expression of CD20 and CD43, considered an aberrant quality most often observed in B-cell lymphomas (Nador, et al., 2003). The largest series to our knowledge failed to demonstrate any cases demonstrating non-germline T-cell receptor rearrangements (Nador, et al., 2003). Most cases also demonstrate EBV co-infection with few also demonstrating HHV-8 co-infection (Nador, et al., 2003).

HIV-associated polymorphous lymphoproliferative disorders also tend to have a relatively better prognosis than other HIV-associated lymphomas, further reinforcing the debatable malignity of this entity. As noted by Nador and colleagues, many patients will do well, even in the absence of chemotherapy (Nador, et al., 2003). This observation was echoed in one such patient from our institution who responded well by way of optimization of his anti-retroviral therapy. Minimal data is available for the development of optimal treatment regimens, however.

3. HIV-associated lymphomas

HIV patients have a 60-110 fold increased risk of developing a lymphoma relative to the HIV negative population at large (Raphaël, et al., 2008; Lewden, et al., 2005; Whelan & Scadden, 2006). The incidence of HIV-associated lymphomas also increases with duration of disease (Besson, et al., 2001); this is a notable concern in the modern era of antiretrovirals in which the latency period from HIV infection to the development of AIDS is increasing. In recent studies exploring causes of death among HIV/AIDS patients treated with potent antiviral medications, lymphomas were reported as the most common malignancy (Lewden, et al., 2005; Besson, et al., 2001); this is in contrast to the evident predominance of Kaposi's sarcoma in the pre-anti-retroviral era (Carpenter, et al., 2004). Lymphomas in HIV also demonstrate unique preponderances for extra-nodal sites. Characteristic sites of extra-nodal primary involvement include the gastrointestinal tract and the central nervous system (Thirlwell, et al., 2003).

Epidemiological data suggests that the overall incidence of many lymphomas has fallen since the introduction of anti-retroviral treatment. In particular, Besson et al noted a significant reduction in AIDS-related lymphomas in a retrospective review of lymphoma rates before and after the introduction of anti-retroviral treatment (Besson, et al., 2001). The particularly devastating primary central nervous system lymphoma characteristic of AIDS in the pre-antiretroviral era was found to virtually disappear in Besson et al.'s post-antiretroviral cohort (Besson, et al., 2001). Similar observations were made in other studies, noting both improved survival for HIV-associated lymphoma patients and also an overall decrease in incidence (Wolf, et al., 2005; Biggar, et al., 2005; Sacktor, et al., 2001). (One notable exception is Hodgkin's lymphoma in HIV/AIDS patients which, in pre- and post-antiretroviral cohorts has shown an increased incidence; this phenomenon will be explored in the later section "Hodgkin's Lymphoma.")

3.1 Burkitt's lymphoma

Burkitt's lymphoma is a highly aggressive lymphoma eponimized for Denis Burkitt, a British surgeon working in Africa in the 1950s. In his seminal paper, Burkitt described a peculiar "sarcoma" demonstrating a predilection for the jaws of African children. This lesion, Burkitt noted, was first described in 1938 by Christiansen; it was Burkitt's attention to the geographic preponderance of this lesion in Africa, in addition to his detailed clinicopathologic description of 38 cases, which led the disease to be named after him however (BURKITT, 1958). In the 1960s, by way of the work of O'Conor and Wright, the pathologic nature of Burkitt's lymphoma was further detailed: in particular, O'Conor identified the lesion as a lymphoma and Wright demonstrated that the lesion could be accurately histologically distinguished from other lymphomas (O'CONOR & DAVIES, 1960; WRIGHT, 1963). Later, in the 1970s, the association of EBV infection and Burkitt's lymphoma was elucidated with the first publication of EBV viral culture from lymphoblasts obtained from Burkitt's lymphoma samples (EPSTEIN, et al., 1964).

The WHO currently acknowledges three major classes of Burkitt's lymphoma: the endemic form (referring to the entity described by Burkitt with a predilection for the jaws of African children); the sporadic form (more common to adults than children and without a specific geographical or anatomical predilection); and Burkitt's lymphoma arising in the context of immunocompromise (Leoncini, et al., 2008). The latter category was only recently added in order to highlight the unique clinical and pathogenetic features of this entity relative to the other two. Of note, all three entities share the common morphologic, immunophenotypic and molecular features which have come to define Burkitt's lymphoma; they are chiefly distinguished from one another, therefore, on the basis of clinical features.

The first few cases of HIV/AIDS associated Burkitt's lymphoma were reported in the early 1980s; likely the first case was reported by Doll and List (Doll & List, 1982) with a subsequent small case series reported by Ziegler and colleagues (Ziegler, et al., 1982). These cases all presented in homosexual men with AIDS-like clinical features (though these cases were documented prior to the definition of AIDS and before the discovery of HIV) and involved both nodal and extra-nodal sites. Interestingly, these cases were etiologically associated with immunosuppression, despite a lack of awareness of HIV; the immunocompromised in these cases was originally thought to be associated with CMV infection or drug use.

More than two decades later, Burkitt's lymphoma has become one of the most common malignancies in patients with HIV/AIDS. According to the WHO, Burkitt's lymphoma accounts for 30% of all HIV-associated lymphomas (Raphaël, et al., 2008); this number has been noted to reach as high as 40% in some series (Spina, et al., 1998). The WHO also notes that in patients with HIV, Burkitt's lymphoma is 1000 times more likely than in patients without concomitant HIV infection (Raphaël, et al., 2008). An HIV positive patient can furthermore expect a 10-20% lifetime risk of Burkitt's lymphoma (Noy, 2010). In contrast to other HIV/AIDS associated lymphomas, Burkitt's lymphoma often presents relatively early on in the course of infection, often before the severe immunocompromise that precedes most HIV-associated lymphomas (Gaidano, et al., 1998). A recent large study also noted an intriguing decrease in the incidence of Burkitt's lymphoma in cases of profoundly low CD4 counts relative to less immunocompromised AIDS patients (Guech-Ongey, et al., 2010). Despite the distinct classification status afforded to HIV-associated Burkitt's lymphoma relative to other non-immunocompromised Burkitt's cases, controversies persist regarding the need for the distinction. In their cohort of African children with Burkitt's lymphoma, Orem and colleagues noted more similarity than difference between HIV positive and negative patients, with the caveat that HIV-positive Burkitt's patients tended to present with less lymphadenopathy and at higher stage than the others (Orem, et al., 2009). This was in keeping with the previous observations of Spina and colleagues noting similar clinicopathologic features amongst their cohort of HIV-positive and negative Burkitt's patients, including comparable disease free survival rates in HIV patients receiving antiretroviral therapy (Spina, et al., 1998). In contrast, epidemiologic data have suggested that Burkitt's lymphoma age-adjusted incidence may be influenced by HIV status (Mbulaiteye, et al., 2010).

HIV-associated Burkitt's lymphoma demonstrates identical classic histologic features to the other classes of Burkitt's lymphomas (see Figure 10). Whether nodal or extra-nodal, the classic Burkitt's histomorphology is a diffuse effacement of normal tissue architecture by sheets of cohesive intermediately sized (~12 μm) cells with minimal basophilic cytoplasm and central round to oval nuclei usually with multiple distinct nucleoli. These cells are interspersed by larger macrophages (bearing characteristic reniform or kidney-bean shaped nuclei) with enlarged pale cytoplasm often containing engulfed cellular debris; these interspersed "tangible-body" macrophages produced the characteristic "starry-sky" appearance. The macroscopic corollary to this histomorphology is the typical fish-flesh tan white irregular tumour mass. As in most lymphomas, however, there are no macroscopic features characteristic of given specific entity. One unique histopathological feature observed more frequently in HIV-associated Burkitt's lymphomas is Burkitt's lymphoma with a lymphoblastic morphology. In these cases, the tumour cells are notable for their eccentric nuclei, prominent central large nucleoli, and often contain cytoplasmic eosinophilic globules representing immunoglobulin deposits (Leoncini, et al., 2008). These features are observed in up to two-thirds of cases according to the WHO (Leoncini, et al., 2008).

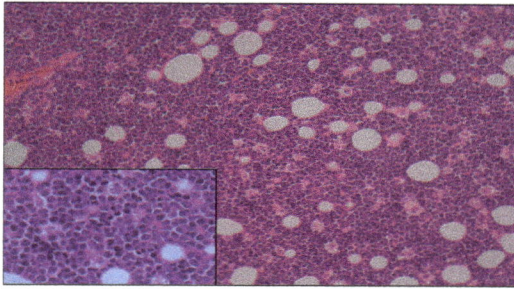

Fig. 10. HIV-associated Burkitt's lymphoma: diffuse "starry-sky" appearance of intermediate-sized cells; inset: high-power of Burkitt cells with scattered macrophages (containing tingible bodies or engulfed debris). The optically clear spaces are fat droplets (this biopsy was taken from a mesenteric lymph node).

Similar immunophenotypic features to the endemic and sporadic Burkitt's forms are observed in HIV-associated Burkitt's lymphoma. The tumour cells are B-cells, demonstrating a variety of possible B-cell antigens including CD19, CD20 and CD22. Burkitt's lymphomas of all types demonstrate characteristic positivity for BCL-6 and CD10 (both immunomarkers of germinal centre phenotype). Unlike diffuse large B-cell lymphomas of germinal centre origin, furthermore, Burkitt's cells are only weakly positive (and often completely negative) for BCL2-. The Ki-67 proliferation immunostain is also characteristically positive nearly in 100%of Burkitt's cells (indicating an extremely high cell proliferation index). To aid in distinguishing Burkitt's lymphomas from precursor B-cell neoplasms (such as pre-B ALL and others, which may have overlapping morphologic features with Burkitt's lymphoma), the TdT stain (a stain indicating a primitive phenotype) is characteristically negative in Burkitt's lymphoma.

The molecular and cytogenetic features in Burkitt's lymphomas (while not entirely specific) are also characteristic. Translocation of the proto-oncogenic MYC region (which encodes a highly conserved cellular transcription factor) to the transcriptionally active IG heavy chain gene, t(8:14), is the most frequently encountered cytogenetic mutation in Burkitt's lymphoma. As previously noted, this translocation is not specific; MYC:IGH translocations have been observed in many diffuse large B-cell lymphomas (often themselves demonstrating high cellular proliferation indices) as well as other malignancies. Using sensitive molecular techniques, EBV virus sequences are observed in 50-70% of HIV-associated Burkitt's lymphomas. This is in contrast to the endemic form, which are virtually all found to contain EBV sequences, as well as the sporadic form which only rarely are found to harbor EBV co-infection.

Chemotherapy for HIV-associated Burkitt's lymphoma is has evolved as the HIV/AIDS epidemic has progressed. Early on, when most HIV-associated Burkitt's patients presented having previously been diagnosed with AIDS, the chemotherapy treatment regimen applied to Burkitt's lymphomas focused on minimizing iatrogenic immunodeficiency. In these cases, the rapid progression characteristic of Burkitt's lymphoma was unfortunately allowed to sway the balance in favor of early mortality from lymphoma (Levine, et al., 2000). Later, with the introduction of anti-retrovirals and the accompanying benefit of improved immunostatus, chemotherapy has evolved toward similar regimens used in the endemic and sporadic Burkitt's lymphomas. Modern HIV-associated Burkitt's lymphomas seem to be treated most commonly with combinations of cyclophosphamide, vincristine, doxorubicin, cytarabine, methotrexate with or without rituximab. Use of the latter anti-CD20 antibody (used frequently to augment the chemotherapeutic response in numerous B-cell lymphomas) remains controversial, in particular relative to the potential immunocompromise that the latter may induce (Levine, et al., 2000); studies exploring optimal treatment regimens in HIV-associated Burkitt's lymphoma are limited given the relative rarity of cases (Noy, 2010).

3.2 Diffuse large B-cell lymphoma

Diffuse large B-cell lymphoma is a heterogeneous category of lymphomas typified by an aggressive clinical aspect, a large cell histomorphology (i.e. neoplastic cells greater than two-times the normal lymphocyte) and B-cell immunophenotype. This category has been the subject of a multitude of classifications over the course of the previous half-century. Currently, the most commonly used WHO classification acknowledges a number of possible "large B-cell" entities, of which diffuse large B-cell lymphoma not otherwise specified is probably the most common. Other diffuse large B-cell lymphoma subtypes (other than the NOS subtype) include rare entities such as primary diffuse large B-cell lymphoma of the central nervous system (an entity characteristically found in HIV/AIDS patients). The current WHO classification schema also allows for molecular and immunohistochemical subgroups in addition to morphologic classes; some of these subgroups have gained notoriety for their distinct therapeutic responses. While a complete description of diffuse large B-cell lymphoma is beyond the scope of this chapter, we will focus heretofore on the specific distinguishing features of HIV/AIDS related diffuse large B-cell lymphomas.

While the most recent edition of the WHO Classification of Hematolymphoid tumours suggests that diffuse large B-cell lymphoma in HIV is second to Burkitt's lymphoma as the most common lymphoma encountered in HIV/AIDS, newer studies have suggested that diffuse large B-cell lymphoma may in fact be more common (Raphaël, et al., 2008; Mantina, et al., 2010; Gucalp & Noy, 2010). There also appear to have been changes in the incidence of diffuse large B-cell lymphoma over the course of the HIV/AIDS epidemic: at the outset in the early to mid 1980s, diffuse large cell lymphoma was very infrequently diagnosed; a marked increase in this diagnosis was seen toward the mid to late 1990s, however (Levine, et al., 2000). These latter results may relate to the observation that diffuse large B-cell lymphoma in HIV/AIDS appears to afflict patients in the setting of long-standing infection with concomitantly low CD4 counts, in contrast to other HIV-associated lymphomas (Raphaël, et al., 2008). As with most HIV-associated lymphomas, diffuse large B-cell lymphoma can often be found in extra-nodal sites; this entity, furthermore, is commonly associated with central nervous system involvement (Agarwal, et al., 2009); furthermore, while overall numbers of central nervous system lymphomas in HIV/AIDS have dropped since the onset of the antiretroviral era, diffuse large-B-cell lymphoma currently seems to be the most frequent offender in the central nervous system (Agarwal, et al., 2009). Important clinical prognostic factors have been noted as pertaining to HIV-associated diffuse large B-cell lymphoma: Vaccher and colleagues noted the importance of CD4 counts, in addition to the other factors incorporated into the international prognostic index (namely age, advanced stage disease, elevated levels of serum lactate dehydrogenase as an indicator of rapid neoplastic cell turnover, extranodal spread and functional performance status) (Vaccher, et al., 1996).

The macroscopic and microscopic features of diffuse large B-cell lymphoma in HIV/AIDS are comparable to those seen in the non-HIV population. Diffuse large B-cell lymphoma generally causes uniform enlargement of a node or group of nodes, often with a characteristic "fish flesh" macroscopic cut surface. On microscopic exam, sheets of large cells typically efface the normal lymph node architecture (these cells are often greater than 12 µm in maximal dimension) (see Figure 11). These neoplastic cells will demonstrate variable cytoplasm, variably sized nuclei, often with clumping or vesciculated chromatin and variable nucleoli. Areas of necrosis may be present, either as individual cells or clusters of cells. Mitotic figures are common and markedly atypical mitoses may be frequent. Often, however, it is difficult to ascribe any specific morphologic features other than diffuse architecture and large cell size to diffuse large B-cell lymphomas. When involving extra-nodal sites, the same diffuse pattern of effaced normal tissue architecture can also be seen, sometimes producing an obvious mass suspicious for a metastatic lesion. The predominant cell type will be the large neoplastic B-cell with variable numbers of intervening fibroblasts and inflammatory cells, sometimes producing a desmoplastic response. In these circumstances, it may be necessary to exclude a malignancy of origin other than the hematolymphoid system such as a carcinoma; these differential diagnoses are usually quickly excluded using a panel of immunohistochemical stains.

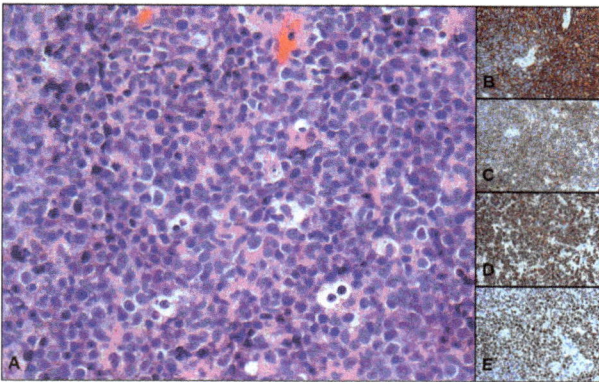

Fig. 11. Diffuse Large B-cell Lymphoma: A: Diffuse pattern of infiltration by pleomorphic large cells; B: CD20 immunostain confirming B-cell lineage; C: CD10 immunostain suggesting germinal centre phenotype; D: BCL2 immunostain strongly and diffusely positive, as is consistent with a B-cell neoplasm; E: BCL6 immunostain suggesting germinal centre phenotype

Immunophenotyping, either by immunohistochemistry or flow cytometry (or ideally both) is required. Diffuse large B-cell lymphomas must, by definition, express one or more of the B-cell markers (e.g. CD19, CD20, CD79a, PAX5, etc.). Diffuse large B-cell lymphomas will frequently be positive for BCL2, though poorly differentiated forms may show only focal or patchy staining. Subsequent stratification of the lesion into "germinal centre" or "non-germinal centre" types is then recommended; the former will generally demonstrate expression of either BCL6 or CD10 (both germinal centre markers) whereas the latter are typically both BCL6 and CD10 negative and may also be MUM-1 positive. This form of stratification can be helpful in directing treatment. More specifically, it has been demonstrated by means of both gene expression profiling (and the surrogate use of immunophenotyping) that diffuse large B-cell lymphomas with a germinal centre phenotype/gene expression profile have a better prognosis (Chang, et al., 2004). Additional staining with Ki67 to demonstrate neoplastic cell proliferation index is also recommended. Diffuse large B-cell lymphomas typically demonstrate a Ki67 proliferation index less than 60-70%; higher indices may suggest a more aggressive entity. High Ki67 index in combination with BCL6 positivity and weak BCL2 staining raises the possibility of a lymphoma intermediate between a diffuse large B-cell and Burkitt's lymphoma. Staining with CD38 or CD138 is also helpful in ruling out a potentially highly aggressive plasmablastic phenotype. Studies have also demonstrated a negative association between HIV-associated diffuse large B-cell lymphoma progression free-survival as well as overall survival and co-infection with EBV (Park, et al., 2007). In our experience however studies exploring the contribution of EBV to the specific pathogenesis of HIV-associated diffuse large B-cell lymphoma are lacking.

The treatment of HIV-associated diffuse large B-cell lymphoma has traditionally been the same as those cases in the HIV-negative population, namely with a combination of cyclophosphamide, doxorubicin, vincristine, and prednisone. This approach has been met with controversy however as a variety of studies using more traditionally "aggressive" chemotherapy regimens, regimens with concomitant rituximab therapy and even regimens incorporating a reduction in antiretroviral therapy have shown promising results in their own rights. Navaro and colleagues demonstrated that patients with HIV-associated diffuse large B-cell lymphoma treated with routine chemotherapy but with additional antiretrovirals demonstrated no significant differences in clinical and laboratory parameters relative to HIV-negative cases of diffuse large B-cell lymphoma (with the caveat that HIV cases were more likely to present with B-symptoms) (Navarro, et al., 2005) Ezzat and colleagues recently indicated that a combination of rituximab with standard chemotherapy and antiretrovirals improved the survival of HIV patients with diffuse large B-cell lymphoma; this study also incorporated epidemiologic data from before and after the antiretroviral era to elucidate a difference in survivability (Ezzat, et al., 2007). In a recent study, Dunleavy and colleagues performed a trial of chemotherapy using short-course etoposide, prednisone, vincristine, cyclophosphamide, doxorubicin and rituximab after having halted antiretroviral therapy for the duration of the chemotherapy (with subsequent restart after completion) (Dunleavy, et al., 2010). In their cohort of 33 authors reported a progression free survival and overall survival of 84% and 68% respectively after a median follow-up of 5 years; 10 deaths were reported with 5 attributed to HIV (3 due to purported previous persistent mycobacterial infection) (Dunleavy, et al., 2010). Head-to-head outcome comparisons, with and without antiretroviral therapy (with particular attention to the long-term effects of short-term iatrogenic HIV-related immunosuppression) have yet to be reported.

3.3 Hodgkin's lymphoma

Thomas Hodgkin, a British physician, first described this strange disease in 1832. Over the course of his work as a pathologist working in Guy's Hospital's anatomical library in London, he noted a number of patients at autopsy with bizarre lymphadenopathy (Mukherhee, 2010). These patients were frequently young and male and died rapidly after a brief fever-stricken illness (Mukherhee, 2010). Having received a less than stellar response to his newly reported disease, he abandoned any further academic exploration of this peculiar lymphadenopathy (and, furthermore, abandoned his life's work soon after) (Mukherhee, 2010). The disease was later further characterized by Samuel Wilks, who coined the eponym "Hodgkin disease" (Stone, 2010). It was not until decades after the first descriptions of Hodgkin's lymphoma that the microscopic feature of the disease — the Reed-Sternberg cell — was discovered by Carl Sternberg of Germany (followed by Dorothy Reed Mendenhall) (Mukherhee, 2010). The current state of the art suggests that the Reed-Sternberg cell is a germinal centre B-cells, as evidenced by the detection of immunoglobulin gene re-arrangements; these cells, it is thought, demonstrate abortive differentiation and therefore do not proceed to produce immunoglobulin (Ioachim & Medeiros, 2009g). Reed-Sternberg cells have also been found to produce a number of pro-inflammatory cytokines; these, it is believed, contribute to the spectrum of "by-stander" non-neoplastic inflammatory cells which make up the majority of the cellular constituents in Hodgkin's lymphomas (Ioachim & Medeiros, 2009g).

One of the earliest series of Hodgkin's lymphomas in a cohort of probable AIDS patients was reported by Ioachim and colleagues (Ioachim, et al., 1985). In this series, only 3 of 21 patients in this study were diagnosed with Hodgkin's lymphoma (Ioachim, et al., 1985). Since these first cases were diagnosed, many more cases of Hodgkin's lymphoma in HIV/AIDS patients have been identified and modern epidemiologic data suggests that HIV-positive patients have at least a 2-10-fold increased risk of developing Hodgkin's lymphoma relative to the HIV-negative population (Carbone, et al., 2009; Sissolak, et al., 2010). Despite this increase, Hodgkin's lymphoma is infrequent relative to diffuse large B-cell lymphoma and Burkitt's lymphoma (the latter two accounting for at least 60% of HIV-associated lymphomas) (Raphaël, et al., 2008).

The pathobiology of HIV-associated Hodgkin's lymphoma serves to demonstrate the unique environment of immunocompromise that HIV infection causes, even in patients with relatively high CD4 counts or on antiretroviral regimens. More specifically, epidemiologists have observed not only an increased incidence of Hodgkin's lymphoma with severe AIDS related immunocompromise but also a paradoxical increased incidence of Hodgkin's lymphoma in HIV-positive patients without AIDS after the introduction of antiretrovirals. In their large cohort study for instance, Biggar and colleagues noted that there was an increased risk of development of Hodgkin's lymphoma in HIV-positive patients with only moderate immunosuppression (Biggar, et al., 2006). Experts have offered hypotheses to explain these unique observations. It is thought that the Reed-Sternberg cell of Hodgkin's lymphoma relies upon intact immunomodulatory signals from T-cells. With T-cell numbers sufficiently stabilized in HIV-infection treated with antiretrovirals — but in an immunologically active environment caused by chronic HIV infection with upregulated inflammatory cytokine production — Reed-Sternberg cells may be inadvertently stimulated and Hodgkin's lymphoma may develop (Sissolak, et al., 2010). Despite the relatively low risk of Hodgkin's lymphoma in HIV-infection, therefore, it is incumbent that HIV patients on anti-retroviral therapy be carefully surveilled for the development of potential Hodgkin's lymphoma.

As noted previously, HIV/AIDS patients are at extremely high risk for lymphadenopathy; when these patients present with symptoms of fever, chills, night sweats and weight loss, furthermore, a long differential must be considered — with lymphomas high on the list. Most HIV-associated Hodgkin's cases will present with lymphadenopathy, typically in a cervical distribution (Sissolak, et al., 2010). Perhaps due to the unique pathobiology of HIV-associated Hodgkin's lymphomas, many HIV-associated Hodgkin patients present at a relatively young age (in addition to possibly presenting earlier on in the course of infection). Many of these patients will also present with advanced stage disease relative to the HIV-negative population (Sissolak, et al., 2010). High clinical suspicion warrants lymph node biopsy, which is required for accurate diagnosis. Most authorities also recommend an initial staging bone marrow biopsy given that 40-60% of cases present with bone marrow involvement (Sissolak, et al., 2010).

While a complete discussion of the possible histological subtypes of Hodgkin's lymphoma is beyond the scope of this chapter, it is warranted to discuss the histopathologic features of the most common form, namely the mixed cellularity subtype of classical Hodgkin's lymphoma. As in all the classical Hodgkin lymphoma subtypes, mixed cellularity subtype is characterized by the presence of scattered Reed-Sternberg cells (see Figure 12). These have a characteristic morphology: the cells are large (~15-40 μm) with abundant lightly basophilic cytoplasm and they have a central bilobed nucleus, each lobe having a central large inclusion-like eosinophilic nucleolus. More importantly relative to the other forms of Hodgkin's lymphoma, the mixed cellularity subtype demonstrates a diffuse effacement of normal lymph node architecture by a mixed population of inflammatory cells consisting of variable number of eosinophils, small lymphocytes, histiocytes, plasma cells and neutrophils. Also, this subtype lacks the characteristic fibrous bands of sclerosis that typify the nodular sclerosing subtype.

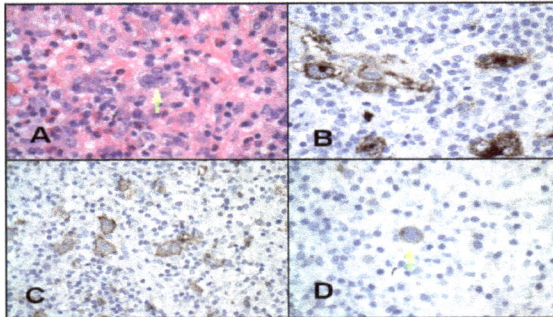

Fig. 12. Hodgkin's lymphoma: A: High-power view demonstrating Reed-Sternberg cell (arrow); B & C: CD15 and CD30 immunostains, respectively; D: EBV stain positive in Reed-Sternberg cell (arrow)

The immunophenotype is also characteristic of mixed cellularity Hodgkin's lymphoma. In particular, the Reed-Sternberg cell is characteristically positive for CD15 (a membrane protein involved in cell adhesion present on a number of hematolymphoid lineage cells) and CD30 (a marker of cell activation). Reed-Sternberg cells seen in Classical Hodgkin's lymphoma are also characteristically negative for the standard B-cell markers CD19 and CD20. Proof of the B-cell nature of Reed-Sternberg cells, however, may be derived from their frequent positive staining for PAX5, a B-cell transcription factor. Most cases of HIV-associated Hodgkin's lymphoma are also positive for EBV co-infection, often identifiable using the immunostain for the EBV-latent membrane protein antigen. This is in contrast to notably fewer cases of EBV positivity outside of HIV-infection (Carbone, et al., 2009).

Treatment approaches for HIV-associated Hodgkin's lymphomas are often similar to those used in non-HIV patients. Limited disease may be treated by a combination of adriamycin, bleomycin, vinblastine and dacarbazine chemotherapy, often with adjuvant radiation therapy to the involved area (if restricted to an amenable nodal region). Advanced cases are not typically amenable to radiation therapy (Sissolak, et al., 2010). Advanced cases may also be considered for bone marrow transplant. The use of rituximab as an adjuvant biological agent may also be considered; those cases demonstrating a large complement of CD20 cells (whether Reed-Sternberg or not) may respond (Sissolak, et al., 2010). Notably, studies looking at the appropriateness of traditional treatments for Hodgkin's disease in the context of HIV-positivity remain ongoing and optimal regimens may yet be discovered. Despite the potential etiologic impact of antiretroviral therapy in cases of HIV-associated Hodgkin's lymphoma, its use is still warranted given the reduction in risk of opportunistic infection (and other HIV-associated malignancies) in order that optimal chemotherapeutic regimens be instituted (Carbone, et al., 2009).

3.4 Plasmablastic lymphoma

Plasmablastic lymphoma is a highly aggressive B-cell lymphoma characterized histologically by a diffuse proliferation of large cells with plasmacytoid features. This entity was only recently recognized and has been shown to occur not only in HIV/AIDS patients but in other immunodeficient individuals, in particular in patients chronically immunosuppressed from solid organ transplants (Rafaniello Raviele, et al., 2009). In its most recent editions, probably owing to its unique clinicopathologic features, plasmablastic lymphoma was classified as an entity unto itself (Raphaël, et al., 2008). Many authors (and other previous classifications) consider plasmablastic lymphoma to be a variant of diffuse large B-cell lymphoma; Chang and colleagues, for example, demonstrated that plasmablastic lymphoma shows a number of overlapping genomic lesions with diffuse large B-cell lymphoma by comparative genomic hybridization techniques (Chang, et al., 2009). Nonetheless, from a treatment and prognostic perspective, plasmablastic lymphoma appears to differ from diffuse large B-cell lymphoma and its classification as a distinct entity is reasonable (Montes-Moreno, et al., 2010).

A number of reports have noted plasmablastic lymphoma arising from transformation from various low-grade lymphomas. Ouansafi and colleagues demonstrated evolution of a follicular lymphoma to plasmablastic lymphoma by means of sequence comparison of the immunoglobulin heavy chain gene rearrangements in both tumours (Ouansafi, et al., 2010). Another report of a plasmablastic lymphoma was described arising in concert with a monoclonal population of plasma cells suggesting potential transformation of the former from the latter (Qing, et al., 2011). Even more intriguing is the case report of concurrent plasmablastic lymphoma and classical Hodgkin's lymphoma arising in a patient with relative immunosuppression from history of chronic lymphocytic leukemia/lymphoma; this case was notably EBV positive (Foo, et al., 2010). The grand majority of cases, however, appear not to represent transformation from a lower grade lesion.

Estimates of the incidence of plasmablastic lymphoma are based on the few reported cases and small series; a recent review of the literature reported approximately 180 cases of plasmablastic lymphoma (Rafaniello Raviele, et al., 2009). While this number is undoubtedly an underestimate (since at least one other unreported case from our own institution in the previous 5 years was encountered), it speaks to the rarity of this entity. The majority of cases are encountered in the HIV/AIDS setting and many, though not all, of the remaining cases are associated with transplant related immunosuppression (Rafaniello Raviele, et al., 2009). The majority of cases, furthermore, were found to be EBV positive (Rafaniello Raviele, et al., 2009). While most cases of plasmablastic lymphoma have demonstrated an odd predilection for the oral cavity, many reports have noted a number of broad ranging almost invariably extranodal sites. A number of reported cases have demonstrated involvement of the central nervous system (Ustun, et al., 2009); involvement of the gastrointestinal tract has also been reported (Rafaniello Raviele, et al., 2009); there are even unique reports of plasmablastic lymphoma involving the penis and vulva (Sun, et al., 2011; Chabay, et al., 2009). Studies have furthermore demonstrated some intriguing clinicopathological factors pertaining to the primary site of plasmablastic lymphomas. Hanra and colleagues for instance, in comparing oral and extraoral cases of plasmablastic lymphoma, demonstrated a distinct survival difference favouring the oral forms (Hansra, et al., 2010).

Plasmablastic lymphoma has also demonstrated different clinicopathologic features in the HIV/AIDS population relative to other immunosuppressed populations. Castillo et al. demonstrated that HIV positive cases of plasmablastic lymphoma tend to occur in younger, typically male patients with a notable preponderance for the oral cavity (Castillo, et al., 2010). Castillo et al. also demonstrated a distinct survival difference between the HIV positive and negative cases of plasmablastic lymphoma, favouring those from HIV positive patients (Castillo, et al., 2010).

Regardless of the primary site or of HIV status, plasmablastic lymphoma demonstrates consistent histological characteristics (see Figure 13). Plasmablastic lymphoma shows a monomorphic morphology comprised of large cells with abundant often-eosinophilic cytoplasm and eccentrically located hyperchromatic nucleus often containing one or more nucleoli. The tumoural cells demonstrate a uniformly diffuse architecture, often with a number of interspersed apoptotic bodies and mitotic figures. Intermingled macrophages or smaller plasma cells may be noted; in some cases in which the latter are particularly abundant, the plasmablastic lymphoma with "plasmacytic differentiation" may be applied.

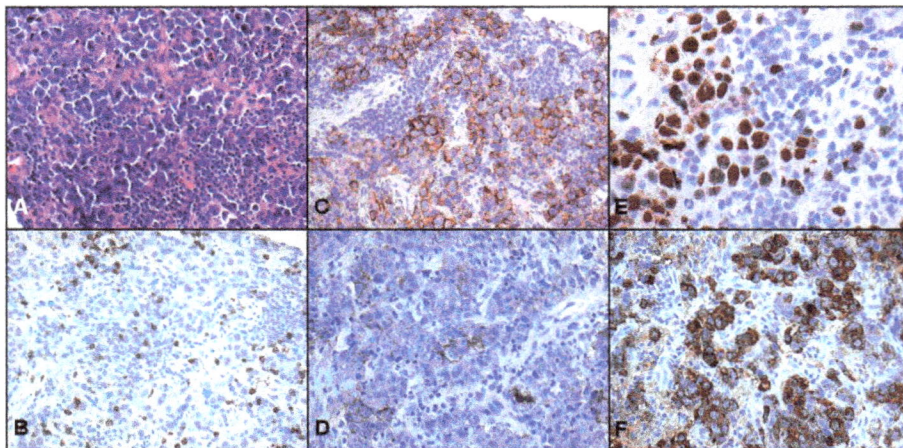

Fig. 13. A: Plasmablastic Lymphoma. B: LCA positive in reactive small T lymphocytes and negative in large neoplastic cells. C: CD138 positive in large neoplastic cells. D: EMA positive in large neoplastic cells. E: MUM-1 positive in large neoplastic cells. F: Lambda light chain positive in large neoplastic cells

In order to distinguish plasmablastic lymphoma for other diffuse lymphomas (and to rule out a simple but more common diffuse large B-cell lymphoma), immunophenotyping is crucial. In plasmablastic lymphoma, in addition to demonstrating minimal positivity for leukocyte common antigen (CD45), CD20 and CD79a, the tumoural cells are invariably positive for CD138; these features are of striking resemblance to the normal immunophenotype of plasma cells. Other post germinal centre markers such as MUM-1 and CD38 are also often positive. Some additional pathologic features that may potentially confuse the diagnosis include positivity for CD3, CD4 and CD56, all of which have been reported to be positive in some cases of plasmablastic lymphoma (Rafaniello Raviele, et al., 2009). Given the primary immunophenotypic differential diagnosis of a plasma cell malignancy (i.e. based on the combination of CD38, CD138, MUM-1 positivity with CD45, CD20 and CD79a negativity), the plasmablastic moniker is assigned given the histomorphology in combination with the absence of clinical features in support of a plasma cell dyscrasia. Plasma cell neoplasms also do not demonstrate positivity for EBV. Other possible differential diagnoses include carcinomas and melanomas, which can be ruled out by the way of an immunohistochemical panel of cytokeratins and melanoma markers. Goedhals et al. explored the electron microscopic features of ten plasmablastic lymphomas and found that 90% of cases demonstrated the consistent plasma cell features of eccentric nuclei with concentric perinuclear endoplasmic reticulum (Goedhals, et al., 2006)

The outcomes in cases of plasmablastic lymphoma are usually poor. In their in depth review, Raviele and colleagues noted disease related deaths in 59.6% of cases of oral-type plasmablastic lymphoma at an average of 10.4 months post-diagnosis as compared to 58.6%at an average of 6.2 months for the extra-oral type (Rafaniello Raviele, et al., 2009). Raviele and colleagues also noted a survival advantage to the use of highly active anti-retrovirals (Rafaniello Raviele, et al., 2009). Given the rarity of plasmablastic lymphoma, there are few studies addressing optimal chemotherapeutics; one large series of published cases noted that the most common chemotherapeutic regimen in plasmablastic lymphoma cases is CHOP (Castillo, et al., 2010). Other more intensive regimens have also been used (e.g. the CODOX-M, often used for HIV-associated Burkitt's lymphoma cases). Two case reports have noted responses to chemotherapy with bortezomib (Bibas, et al., 2010; Bose, et al., 2009); trials looking at optimal treatment regimens are lacking, however.

3.5 Primary effusion/body cavity lymphoma

Primary effusion/body cavity lymphoma is a rare aggressive lymphoma with a peculiar propensity for the serous cavities of the body, namely the peritoneum, pleura and pericardium. These lymphomas are also not primarily associated with a solid component though they may later develop nearby solid tumours and may extend to involve of lymph nodes. Primary effusion lymphoma is characteristically a disease of HIV/AIDS patients, though rare cases have been reported in HIV negative patients. Primary effusion lymphomas are also almost invariably positive for HHV-8 and may show co-infection with EBV.

Knowles and colleagues diagnosed the first cases of primary effusion lymphoma in 1989. Three cases were originally reported, all occurring in homosexual HIV-positive males with clinical features of AIDS. Each case presented with a body cavity effusion containing cytologically malignant cells and quickly died. The effusions were all noted to contain populations of large cells with generous eosinophilic to amphophilic cytoplasm, anisonucleosis and clumped chromatin. Several multinucleated giant cells and abnormal mitotic figures were also noted. The malignant effusion cells were positive for CD45, indicating a hematolymphoid origin, but were negative for B- and T-cell markers as well as a variety of myelomonocytic markers. Subsequent restriction fragment analysis of the DNA obtained from the neoplastic cells revealed immunoglobulin gene rearrangements, suggesting a B-cell origin. The three original cases were also found to be EBV positive; these cases were not tested for HHV-8 positivity in the original publication

Since the first reported cases, several more have been reported; this entity is nonetheless very rare relative to the other HIV/AIDS-associated lymphomas and accounts for approximately 3% (Boulanger, et al., 2005). The WHO notes that this lymphoma is most commonly encountered in HIV patients, but that some cases have been encountered in HIV-seronegative patients and even within the context of immunocompetence (Raphaël, et al., 2008). Primary effusion/body cavity lymphoma cells are almost invariably HHV-8 positive. This is of particular interest in those cases encountered in immunocompetent patients since, as a result of the high prevalence of HHV-8 infection, there is a notably increased risk in peoples (especially males) of the Mediteranean (Said & Cesarman, 2008).

In one of the largest and more recent series of primary effusion/body cavity lymphomas, Boulanger and colleagues reported a wide age range (33-78 years) with only one female of 28 cases (Boulanger, et al., 2005). While the majority of cases were noted to originate in patients from populations with low HHV-8 seroprevalence, Boulanger et al. did note that a substantial number (38%) of patients originated from geographic areas with seroprevalence higher than 5% (Boulanger, et al., 2005). Most cases were noted to present with effusions, predominantly pleural (Boulanger, et al., 2005). Primary effusion/body cavity lymphoma typically remains restricted to the original presenting body cavity (Carbone, et al., 2010). Involved serosal surfaces are often diffusely thickened (Carbone, et al., 2010). Interestingly, 42% of Boulanger et al.'s cases presented with additional extra-cavitary lesions. It has also been documented that many primary effusion/body cavity lymphoma patients have preceding or complicating Kaposi's sarcoma (Boulanger, et al., 2005). Most patients are also profoundly immunosuppressed; in the HIV-positive cohort of Boulanger et al. for example, the average CD4 count was below 200 cells/μL (Boulanger, et al., 2005).

Diagnosis of primary effusion/body cavity lymphoma is typically made on cytologic examination of effusion contents (see Figure 14). As Carbone and colleagues note, the malignant cells of primary effusion/body cavity lymphoma have an appearance resembling a combination of immunoblastic and anaplastic features (Carbone, et al., 2010). A variable degree of plasma cell differentiation may also be noted; a background of pronounced cellular debris and numerous mitoses often accompanies these features. A mixture of reactive inflammatory cells as well as admixed mesothelial cells will also be noted. These morphological features result in a differential diagnosis that may include Burkitt's lymphoma (which may also involve body cavities); as with most lymphomas, however, the immunophenotype will typically indicate the diagnosis. The effusive nature of this lymphoma is highly conducive to flow cytometry. Primary effusion/body cavity lymphoma, as noted previously, demonstrates CD45, CD138 and MUM-1 positivity in the context of dim or negative immunostaining for B-cell markers. This immunohistochemical pattern reflects the plasmablastic phenotype of primary effusion/body cavity lymphoma. Interestingly, a few cases have noted aberrant T-cell antigen expression (Carbone, et al., 2010). The diagnostic clincher, however, is the demonstration of HHV-8 positivity in the tumour cells; this can usually be accomplished reliably with immunohistochemical staining for the HHV-8 latency-associated nuclear antigen.

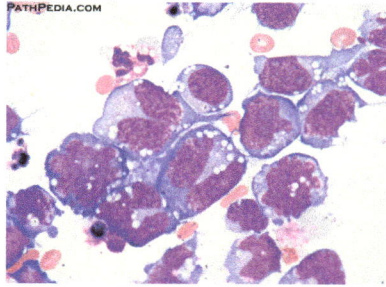

Fig. 14. Primary Effusion Lymphoma: Large cells with clear-coloured cytoplasmic bodies (vescicles containing immunoglobulin); note the eccentrically placed nuclei in a number of the cells, others with large atypical lobated nuclei and prominent nucleoli. Compare the size. difference of the neoplastic cells with the small normally sized (dark stained) round lymphocyte nucleus at the bottom left.

Despite its rarity, a number of studies have explored the molecular pathogenesis of primary effusion/body cavity lymphoma. Gene expression profile studies in primary effusion/body cavity lymphoma have demonstrated a unique profile relative to other aggressive lymphomas; these results tend to substantiate the distinct clinicopathologic distinction of primary effusion/body cavity lymphomas from other lymphomas (Ueda, et al., 2010). Other studies have demonstrated a number of complex cytogenetic abnormalities as well as a reduction in tumour-suppressor gene expression in primary effusion/body cavity lymphoma (Luan, et al., 2010; O'Hara, et al., 2009); these features may further contribute to the aggressiveness of this lesion.

Most published cases appear to be treated with CHOP or derivations thereof. Fewer cases have been treated with a more "aggressive" approach in line with regimens such as doxorubicin, cyclophosphamide, vindesine, bleomycin, prednisone. Some reported cases were also tried on an antiviral regimen (e.g. interferon alpha and cidofovir); the efficacy of these drugs in this context is uncertain, however. Unfortunately, regardless of the chemotherapy regimen, outcomes are poor. In Boulanger and colleagues' cohort, for example, only 14 of 28 patients received clinical remission and only 32% were alive after a median follow-up of 3.2 years (Boulanger, et al., 2005). Most patients who relapse, furthermore, will die of disease (Boulanger, et al., 2005). As in other HIV-associated lymphomas, prognosis appears to be improved with the early incorporation of anti-retroviral medications (Boulanger, et al., 2005; Carbone, et al., 2010).

3.6 T-cell lymphomas

T-cell lymphomas occurring in HIV/AIDS are substantially rarer that B-cell lymphomas. In their large cohort study of 302,834 AIDS patients, Biggar and colleagues noted that only 1.4%of non-hodgkin's lymphomas were of T-cell phenotype (Biggar, et al., 2001). Nonetheless, considering the extreme rarity of T-cell lymphomas in general, Biggar and colleagues estimated a relative risk of 15 of a T-cell lymphoma in the HIV positive population relative to the HIV negative population (Biggar, et al., 2001).

The first documented HIV positive T-cell lymphoma was noted in 1988 by Nasr and colleagues (Nasr, et al., 1988). This case consisted of a large cell lymphoma demonstrating loss of CD3 but with preservation of CD2 and CD4 immunoreactivity. Although CD30 and ALK-1 immunoreactivity were not reported in this case, the reported morphologic features seem most in keeping with anaplastic large cell lymphoma. The earliest reported T-cell lymphoma in a patient with suspected AIDS, however, predated Nasr and colleagues' case by four years; this case was reported in Japan in a patient with AIDS-defining clinical characteristics but co-infected by human t-cell lymphoma/leukemia virus-1 (Kobayashi, et al., 1984).

The most common T-cell lymphoma encountered in HIV-positive patients appears to be peripheral T-cell lymphoma, unspecified (Biggar, et al., 2001; Arzoo, et al., 2004). Several cases of anaplastic large cell lymphoma, NK/T-cell lymphoma and angioimmunoblastic T-cell lymphoma have also been reported, however (Biggar, et al., 2001; Arzoo, et al., 2004; Perez, et al., 2010; Castillo, et al., 2011). A few cases of enteropathy-associated T-cell lymphoma as well as adult T-cell leukemia/lymphoma have also been reported, though little specific information pertaining to the role of HIV in these cases could be gleaned (Arzoo, et al., 2004; Castillo, et al., 2011).

In the largest case series to date, Castilo and colleagues noted that the bulk of HIV-associated T-cell lymphomas occurred in males, typically presenting at high stage (stage III-IV), and often accompanied by B-symptoms (fever, night sweats and weight loss) (Castillo, et al., 2011). Similar clinical characteristics were noted in other smaller cohorts (Arzoo, et al., 2004; Perez, et al., 2010). Many T-cell lymphomas in HIV patients will also present with skin findings, apparently in greater proportions than HIV-associated B-cell lymphomas (Arzoo, et al., 2004).

Peripheral T-cell lymphoma, unspecified, typically occurs in lymph nodes and consists of medium to large-sized lymphocytes with irregular nuclei. The neoplastic T-cells usually show a diffuse pattern of involvement, preferentially involving the paracortical zones, often sparing the lymphoid follicles (see Figure 16). HIV-associated anaplastic large cell lymphoma also demonstrates a range of histological features. A range of cell size may be noted from the typical large anaplastic cell to the so-called small cell variant (see Figure 17). These cells may form loosely cohesive clusters, diffuse sheets and, as is often seen in lymph nodes, may present as subtle subcapsular aggregates. Angioimmunoblastic lymphoma, in contrast, is most common described as a diffuse process often completely obliterating the lymph node architecture; most commonly the lymph node will be replaced by an arborizing network of proliferating endothelial cells interspersed by an infiltrate of atypical lymphocytes, often accompanied by various non-neoplastic inflammatory cells. Mycosis fungoides is characterized by band like superficial dermal infiltrates of atypical lymphocytes (often described as "cerebriform") (see Figure 18). When these atypical cerebriform lymphocytes are noted in the peripheral blood or in lymph nodes, the Sezary syndrome is suspected (sezary syndrome does not always demonstrate the same epidermotropism as mycosis fungoides, however, and the skin changes in this context may be non-specific). NK/T-cell lymphomas occur most often in the aerodigestive tract where they often manifest as mucosal ulceration by atypical lymphocytes. These atypical lymphocytes may have ample cytoplasm and irregular convoluted nuclear membranes. An angioinvasive pattern is also common to NK/T-cell lymphoma, typically with associated areas of necrosis.

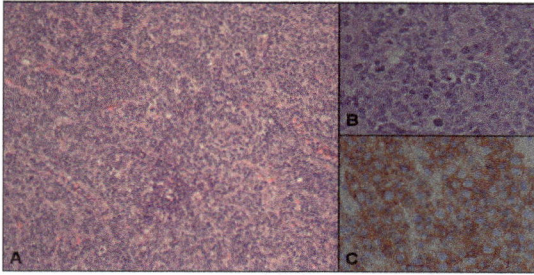

Fig. 15. Peripheral T-cell Lymphoma: A: Atypical cells expanding paracortical interfollicular regions; B: High-power demonstrating atypical cells (larger than normal interfollicular cells) with mitotic figures present; C: Diffuse CD3 positivity confirming T-cell lineage

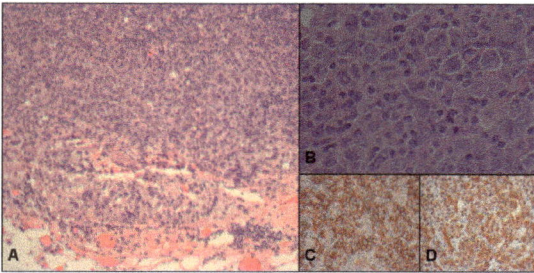

Fig. 16. Anaplastic Large Cell Lymphoma: A: Low-power view of lymph node involved by anaplastic large cell lymphoma showing subcapsular sinus involvement by tumour cells; B: High-power view of tumour cells demonstrating the characteristic hallmark cells (large nuclei with convoluted semi-lunar shapes); C: CD30 immunostain (diffuse positivity in tumour cells); D: ALK-1 immunostain (diffuse positivity in tumour cells)

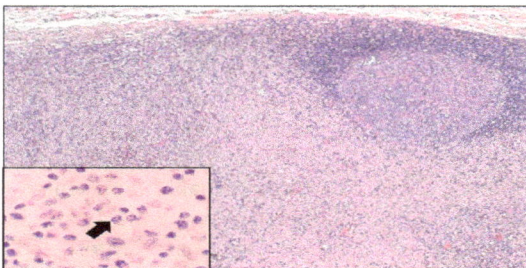

Fig. 17. Mycosis Fungoides: Lymph node demonstrating paracortical expansion by atypical lymphoid infiltrate; inset: large (cerebriform) sezary cells of mycosis fungoides

The typical T-cell lineage markers CD2, CD3, CD5, CD7, CD4, CD8 and CD43 are variably positive in T-cell lymphomas; these markers are useful at demonstrating aberrant phenotype (such as an aberrant CD4:CD8 ratio) or to hint at T-cell lineage neoplasm when the other T-cell markers are negative. The normal progression of T-cell marker ontogenesis proceeds from CD7 to CD2, CD3 and CD5 (in immature T-cells) and then onto CD4 and CD8 (in mature T-cells); the loss of one of the so-called pan-T-Cell markers CD2, CD3, CD5 or CD7 is helpful in the identification of an aberrant (plausibly neoplastic) phenotype. In one of the largest series of HIV-associated anaplastic large cell lymphomas, Perez and colleagues noted that the majority of cases were positive for one or more of CD45, CD2, CD3, CD5, CD4 and CD43 (Perez, et al., 2010); the uniting feature in all cases of ALCL, however, is diffuse strong CD30 positivity. Although the CD30 stain is not entirely specific to anaplastic large cell lymphoma (since this stain is a marker of activated cells), its presence in a diffuse pattern in cells with typically anaplastic morphology is characteristic. Also commonly positive in anaplastic large cell lymphoma is CD45 (also known as leukocyte common antigen, a marker indicating hematolymphoid origin). Interestingly, ALK-1 was noted to be positive in only two of their cases; this is in stark contrast to the non HIV-associated anaplastic large cell lymphomas, which are typically ALK-1 positive (Perez, et al., 2010; Nava, et al., 2008). Although this lack of ALK-1 positivity may represent a distinct molecular feature of HIV-associated anaplastic large cell lymphoma, to our knowledge, no studies have explored this as yet. The neoplastic T-cells in angioimmunoblastic T-cell lymphoma, in addition to staining positive for a number of pan-T-cell markers, are typically positive for CD4 but negative for CD3. These cells also stain positive for a number of markers of follicular centre origin including CD10 and BCL-6. The lymphocytic infiltrates in mycosis fungoides syndrome will often demonstrate a lack of CD3 and CD8 staining often with pronounced CD4 positivity. NK/T-cell lymphoma also demonstrates positivity for one or more pan-T-cell markers, in addition to positivity for CD56 and (unlike most T-cell lymphomas) EBV. These features can easily be demonstrated efficiently, and with only minimal tissue, using flow cytometry.

Most patients with HIV-associated peripheral T-cell lymphomas are treated with a CHOP-based chemotherapy regimen, though a variety of other regimens have also been employed (Castillo, et al., 2011). While most patients seem to demonstrate a complete or partial response to initial therapy, the majority die of progressive disease (Castillo, et al., 2011). A statistically significant improvement in the survival curve of HIV-associated peripheral T-cell lymphomas was also noted in patients treated with anti-retrovirals (Castillo, et al., 2011).

3.7 Lymph node findings in HIV/AIDS related Kaposi's sarcoma

We will limit the discussion of Kaposi's sarcoma in HIV/AIDS to those aspects pertaining to lymph node disease. Whether due to its underlying viral etiology or to the endothelial differentiation of the malignant cell of interest, Kaposi sarcoma often manifests itself in lymph nodes. The disease was first described in 1872 by Moritz Kaposi as a pigmented sarcoma of skin (Mesri, et al., 2010), this form probably represented the modern sporadic subtype seen predominantly in the Mediterranean. In the 1950s, Kaposi's sarcoma was encountered in Africa (Mesri, et al., 2010); this may have represented the first discovery of Kaposi's sarcoma in association with the as yet unknown HIV. When the HIV outbreak was identified, Kaposi's sarcoma was observed to be the most frequent (and AIDS defining) malignancy in this immunocompromised population. It was not until 1996 that a viral pathogen was discovered in association with Kaposi's sarcoma, later named the Kaposi sarcoma herpes virus, or HHV-8 (Mesri, et al., 2010).

Ioachim and colleagues undertook an intriguing study of extra-cutaneous Kaposi's sarcoma in AIDS patients; they noted that lymph nodes were the third most common extra-cutaneous sites of involvement by Kaposi's sarcoma in AIDS cases, next to the gastrointestinal tract and the lungs (Ioachim, et al., 1995). Cases demonstrating primarily nodal involvement may be entirely asymptomatic, with the exception of lymphadenopathy. In these cases the clinical differential diagnosis can be lengthy and histological diagnosis is required.

Lymph nodes involved by Kaposi's sarcoma are typically enlarged and demonstrate preserved architecture in areas not invaded by the tumour, often with follicular hyperplasia (see Figure 18). Involvement of lymph nodes by Kaposi's sarcoma typically begins in the form of triangular nodules with later encroachment into the cortex and medulla; these initial nodules may form wedges with bases parallel to the node capsule. Circular whorled-patterned nodules are also common and can be found throughout the nodal parenchyma. The cells within Kaposi's nodules are spindled with intervening slit-like vascular spaces. The neoplastic cells are usually fairly uniform with plump nuclei; mitoses may be present but are usually not numerous. Characteristic hyaline globules may be seen within Kaposi cells and in nearby histiocytes. Infiltration of tumour foci by lymphocytes, plasma cells and hemosiderin-laden macrophages is also frequent.

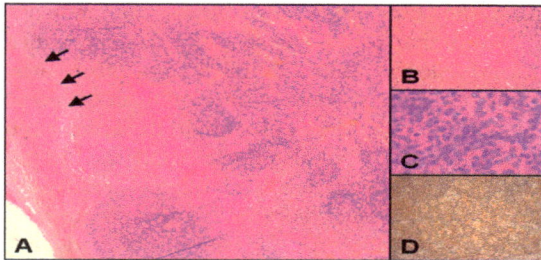

Fig. 18. Kaposi's Sarcoma: A: Low-power view of a lymph node involved by subcapsular nodules of Kaposi's sarcoma; B: Focus of neoplastic endothelial cells encroaching upon a follicle; C: High-power view of neoplastic endothelial cells with notable tumour cell cytoplasmic hyaline globules; D: HHV-8 immunostain demonstrating diffuse positivity

The morphologic differential diagnosis includes many vascular lesions, though the morphologic features are usually characteristic in Kaposi's sarcoma. Bacillary angiomatosis may show nodule formation but typically does not contain the uniformly plump monotonous spindle cells with intervening slit-like spaces seen in Kaposi's sarcoma. The vascular proliferation and hyalinization that may be seen in HIV-associated lymphadenopathy or Castleman's disease may be confused with Kaposi's sarcoma. Angiosarcomas should also be included in the differential diagnosis, though this typically demonstrates are much more sarcomatoid appearance with more marked atypia, necrosis and numerous mitoses. Confusion is avoided by using an immunohistochemical panel including markers for endothelial cells (such as CD31, CD34 or Factor VIII) in combination with a stain for HHV-8.

Antiretroviral therapy is used both to prevent Kaposi's sarcoma but also to treat it. Nonetheless, HIV patients with Kaposi's sarcoma may not respond curatively to antiretroviral optimization and some cases treated with antiretrovirals de novo have been known to develop more severe disease due to the so-called immune reconstitution inflammatory syndrome (in which the presumed increased in inflammatory mediators results in unintentional cytokinetic stimulation of the sarcoma) (Mesri, et al., 2010; Di Lorenzo, et al., 2007). Localized disease may respond to surgery or radiation therapy (though lymph node disease is frequently not localized) and more widespread disease is treated with chemotherapeutic regimens, typically including liposomal anthracyclines and taxanes (Di Lorenzo, et al., 2007). Newer biological therapies including the vascular endothelial growth factor receptor and tyrosine kinase inhibitors are currently being investigated (Di Lorenzo, et al., 2007). Some early studies exploring the use of antivirals (such as gancyclovir and foscarnet) have noted encouraging results though more definitive studies are ongoing (Di Lorenzo, et al., 2007).

4. Conclusion

In the three decades since the beginning of the modern HIV/AIDS epidemic, a great deal of advancement has been made in the understanding of retrovirology, immunology and hematolymphoid pathology. In these 30 years, the recognition of a unique and fastidious retrovirus causing AIDS has occurred, its biologic interaction with human cells has been detailed, and the variety of possible resulting illnesses following infection have been documented. In particular, the range of malignant disease that may occur in HIV/AIDS has been widely enumerated and, thankfully, has shown a distinct reduction in incidence and prevalence since the introduction of antiretroviral therapy, truly a modern medical elixir able to prolong life in a medical context once tantamount to a death sentence.
The above discussion should not only serve to highlight the unique clinical features of HIV-associated hematolymphoid disorders but also demonstrate the unique pathologic work-up necessary to ensure accurate classification and clinical follow-up. In particular, we emphasized the need to obtain tissue biopsies in any scenario in which a potential malignancy is considered. Furthermore, for the pathologist readership, it is imperative to properly handle and work-up a lymph node biopsy from any case in which there is a suspicion of lymphoma; we especially encourage the use of flow cytometry which is an invaluable tool in the diagnosis of lymphoid neoplasms and is extremely helpful in proper classification. Also, in addition to the standard H&E evaluation, a panel of immunohistochemical stains is usually needed to properly identify the lineage, malignant potential and classification of a lymphoid lesion. Many hematolymphoid malignancies require further molecular or cytogenetic work-up as well, the latter requiring fresh tissue.

5. References

Agarwal, P. A., Menon, S., Smruti, B. K. & Singhal, B. S.(2009).Primary central nervous system lymphoma: a profile of 26 cases from Western India.*Neurol.India,*Vol.57, No.6,(Nov-Dec),pp.756-763,0028-3886

Anderson, C. D. & Barrie, H. J.(1960).Fatal pneumocystis pneumonia in an adult. Report of a case. *Am.J.Clin.Pathol.,* Vol.34, (Oct), pp.365-370, 0002-9173

Arzoo, K. K., Bu, X., Espina, B. M., Seneviratne, L., Nathwani, B. & Levine, A. M.(2004).T-cell lymphoma in HIV-infected patients.*J.Acquir.Immune Defic.Syndr.,*Vol.36,No.5,(Aug 15),pp.1020-1027,1525-4135

Bakaki, P., Kayita, J., Moura Machado, J. E., et al.(2001).Epidemiologic and clinical features of HIV-infected and HIV-uninfected Ugandan children younger than 18 months.*J.Acquir.Immune Defic.Syndr.,*Vol.28,No.1,(Sep 1),pp.35-42,1525-4135

Besson, C., Goubar, A., Gabarre, J., et al.(2001).Changes in AIDS-related lymphoma since the era of highly active antiretroviral therapy.*Blood,*Vol.98,No.8,(Oct 15),pp.2339-2344,0006-4971

Bibas, M., Grisetti, S., Alba, L., Picchi, G., Del Nonno, F. & Antinori, A.(2010).Patient with HIV-associated plasmablastic lymphoma responding to bortezomib alone and in combination with dexamethasone, gemcitabine, oxaliplatin, cytarabine, and pegfilgrastim chemotherapy and lenalidomide alone.*J.Clin.Oncol.,*Vol.28,No.34,(Dec 1),pp.e704-8,1527-7755; 0732-183X

Biggar, R. J., Engels, E. A., Frisch, M., Goedert, J. J. & AIDS Cancer Match Registry Study Group(2001).Risk of T-cell lymphomas in persons with AIDS.*J.Acquir.Immune Defic.Syndr.,*Vol.26,No.4,(Apr 1),pp.371-376,1525-4135

Biggar, R. J., Engels, E. A., Ly, S., et al.(2005).Survival after cancer diagnosis in persons with AIDS.*J.Acquir.Immune Defic.Syndr.,*Vol.39,No.3,(Jul 1),pp.293-299,1525-4135

Biggar, R. J., Jaffe, E. S., Goedert, J. J., Chaturvedi, A., Pfeiffer, R. & Engels, E. A.(2006).Hodgkin lymphoma and immunodeficiency in persons with HIV/AIDS.*Blood,*Vol.108,No.12,(Dec 1),pp.3786-3791,0006-4971

Bose, P., Thompson, C., Gandhi, D., Ghabach, B. & Ozer, H.(2009).AIDS-related plasmablastic lymphoma with dramatic, early response to bortezomib.*Eur.J.Haematol.,*Vol.82,No.6,(Jun),pp.490-492,1600-0609; 0902-4441

Boulanger, E., Gerard, L., Gabarre, J., et al.(2005).Prognostic factors and outcome of human herpesvirus 8-associated primary effusion lymphoma in patients with AIDS.*J.Clin.Oncol.,*Vol.23,No.19,(Jul 1),pp.4372-4380,0732-183X

Boyko, W. J., Schechter, M. T., Craib, K. J., et al.(1987).The Vancouver Lymphadenopathy-AIDS Study: 7. Clinical and laboratory features of 87 cases of primary HIV infection.*CMAJ,*Vol.137,No.2,(Jul 15),pp.109-113,0820-3946

BURKITT, D.(1958).A sarcoma involving the jaws in African children.*Br.J.Surg.,*Vol.46,No.197,(Nov),pp.218-223,0007-1323; 0007-1323

Caldwell, R. G., Wilson, J. B., Anderson, S. J. & Longnecker, R.(1998).Epstein-Barr virus LMP2A drives B cell development and survival in the absence of normal B cell receptor signals.*Immunity,*Vol.9,No.3,(Sep),pp.405-411,1074-7613

Caponetti, G. C., Pantanowitz, L., Marconi, S., Havens, J. M., Lamps, L. W. & Otis, C. N.(2009).Evaluation of immunohistochemistry in identifying Bartonella henselae in cat-scratch disease.*Am.J.Clin.Pathol.,*Vol.131,No.2,(Feb), pp.250-256,1943-7722; 0002-9173

Carbone, A., Cesarman, E., Gloghini, A. & Drexler, H. G.(2010).Understanding pathogenetic aspects and clinical presentation of primary effusion lymphoma through its derived cell lines.*AIDS,*Vol.24,No.4,(Feb 20),pp.479-490,1473-5571; 0269-9370

Carbone, A., Gloghini, A., Serraino, D. & Spina, M.(2009).HIV-associated Hodgkin lymphoma.*Curr.Opin.HIV.AIDS.,*Vol.4,No.1,(Jan),pp.3-10,1746-6318; 1746-630X

Carpenter, C. C., Flanigan, T. P. & Lederman, M. M.(2004).Chapter 107: HIV Infection and the Acquired Immunodeficiency Syndrome, In:*Cecil essentials of medicine,*Andreoli, T. E. and Cecil, R. L., pp.917-935,W.B. Saunders,0721601472,Philadelphia, Pa.

Casper, C., Nichols, W. G., Huang, M. L., Corey, L. & Wald, A.(2004).Remission of HHV-8 and HIV-associated multicentric Castleman disease with ganciclovir treatment.*Blood,*Vol.103,No.5,(Mar 1),pp.1632-1634,0006-4971; 0006-4971

Castillo, J. J., Beltran, B. E., Bibas, M., et al.(2011).Prognostic factors in patients with HIV-associated peripheral T-cell lymphoma: a multicenter study.*Am.J.Hematol.,*Vol.86,No.3,(Mar),pp.256-261,1096-8652; 0361-8609

Castillo, J. J., Winer, E. S., Stachurski, D., et al.(2010).Clinical and pathological differences between human immunodeficiency virus-positive and human immunodeficiency virus-negative patients with plasmablastic lymphoma.*Leuk.Lymphoma*,Vol.51,No.11,(Nov),pp.2047-2053,1029-2403; 1026-8022

Chabay, P., De Matteo, E., Lorenzetti, M., et al.(2009).Vulvar plasmablastic lymphoma in a HIV-positive child: a novel extraoral localisation.*J.Clin.Pathol.*,Vol.62,No.7,(Jul),pp.644-646,1472-4146; 0021-9746

Chang, C. C., Chomel, B. B., Kasten, R. W., Tappero, J. W., Sanchez, M. A. & Koehler, J. E.(2002).Molecular epidemiology of Bartonella henselae infection in human immunodeficiency virus-infected patients and their cat contacts, using pulsed-field gel electrophoresis and genotyping.*J.Infect.Dis.*,Vol.186,No.12,(Dec 15),pp.1733-1739,0022-1899

Chang, C. C., McClintock, S., Cleveland, R. P., et al.(2004).Immunohistochemical expression patterns of germinal center and activation B-cell markers correlate with prognosis in diffuse large B-cell lymphoma.*Am.J.Surg.Pathol.*,Vol.28,No.4,(Apr),pp.464-470,0147-5185

Chang, C. C., Zhou, X., Taylor, J. J., et al.(2009).Genomic profiling of plasmablastic lymphoma using array comparative genomic hybridization (aCGH): revealing significant overlapping genomic lesions with diffuse large B-cell lymphoma.*J.Hematol.Oncol.*,Vol.2,(Nov 12),pp.47,1756-8722

Cotell, S. L. & Noskin, G. A.(1994).Bacillary angiomatosis. Clinical and histologic features, diagnosis, and treatment.*Arch.Intern.Med.*,Vol.154,No.5,(Mar 14),pp.524-528,0003-9926

Di Lorenzo, G., Konstantinopoulos, P. A., Pantanowitz, L., Di Trolio, R., De Placido, S. & Dezube, B. J.(2007).Management of AIDS-related Kaposi's sarcoma.*Lancet Oncol.*,Vol.8,No.2,(Feb),pp.167-176,1470-2045

Dispenzieri, A.(2007).POEMS syndrome.*Blood Rev.*,Vol.21,No.6,(Nov),pp.285-299,0268-960X

Doll, D. C. & List, A. F.(1982).Burkitt's lymphoma in a homosexual. *Lancet,* Vol.1, No.8279, (May 1), pp.1026-1027,0140-6736

Dunleavy, K., Little, R. F., Pittaluga, S., et al.(2010).The role of tumor histogenesis, FDG-PET, and short-course EPOCH with dose-dense rituximab (SC-EPOCH-RR) in HIV-associated diffuse large B-cell lymphoma.*Blood,*Vol.115,No.15,(Apr 15),pp.3017-3024,1528-0020; 0006-4971

Eliopoulos, A. G., Gallagher, N. J., Blake, S. M., Dawson, C. W. & Young, L. S.(1999).Activation of the p38 mitogen-activated protein kinase pathway by Epstein-Barr virus-encoded latent membrane protein 1 coregulates interleukin-6 and interleukin-8 production.*J.Biol.Chem.*,Vol.274,No.23,(Jun 4), pp.16085-16096, 0021-9258

EPSTEIN, M. A., ACHONG, B. G. & BARR, Y. M.(1964).Virus Particles in Cultured Lymphoblasts from Burkitt's Lymphoma.*Lancet,*Vol.1,No.7335,(Mar 28),pp.702-703,0140-6736

Ezzat, H., Filipenko, D., Vickars, L., et al.(2007).Improved survival in HIV-associated diffuse large B-cell lymphoma with the addition of rituximab to chemotherapy in patients receiving highly active antiretroviral therapy.*HIV.Clin.Trials,*Vol.8,No.3,(May-Jun),pp.132-144,1528-4336

Foo, W. C., Huang, Q., Sebastian, S., Hutchinson, C. B., Burchette, J. & Wang, E.(2010).Concurrent classical Hodgkin lymphoma and plasmablastic lymphoma in a patient with chronic lymphocytic leukemia/small lymphocytic lymphoma treated with fludarabine: a dimorphic presentation of iatrogenic immunodeficiency-associated lymphoproliferative disorder with evidence suggestive of multiclonal transformability of B cells by Epstein-Barr virus. *Hum.Pathol.*, Vol.41, No.12, (Dec), pp.1802-1808,1532-8392; 0046-8177

Fromont, E. G., Riche, B. & Rabilloud, M.(2009).Toxoplasma seroprevalence in a rural population in France: detection of a household effect.*BMC Infect.Dis.*,Vol.9,(May 28),pp.76,1471-2334

Gaidano, G., Carbone, A. & Dalla-Favera, R.(1998).Pathogenesis of AIDS-related lymphomas: molecular and histogenetic heterogeneity .*Am. J. Pathol.*, Vol.152, No.3, (Mar), pp.623-630, 0002-9440

Gasquet, S., Maurin, M., Brouqui, P., Lepidi, H. & Raoult, D.(1998).Bacillary angiomatosis in immunocompromised patients.*AIDS*,Vol.12,No.14,(Oct 1),pp.1793-1803,0269-9370

Goedhals, J., Beukes, C. A. & Cooper, S.(2006).The ultrastructural features of plasmablastic lymphoma.*Ultrastruct.Pathol.*,Vol.30,No.6,(Nov-Dec),pp.427-433,1521-0758; 0191-3123

Grimes, M. M., LaPook, J. D., Bar, M. H., Wasserman, H. S. & Dwork, A.(1987).Disseminated Pneumocystis carinii infection in a patient with acquired immunodeficiency syndrome.*Hum.Pathol.*,Vol.18,No.3,(Mar),pp.307-308,0046-8177

Gucalp, A. & Noy, A.(2010).Spectrum of HIV lymphoma 2009. *Curr. Opin. Hematol.*, Vol.17,No.4,(Jul),pp.362-367,1531-7048; 1065-6251

Guech-Ongey, M., Simard, E. P., Anderson, W. F., et al.(2010).AIDS-related Burkitt lymphoma in the United States: what do age and CD4 lymphocyte patterns tell us about etiology and/or biology?*Blood*,Vol.116,No.25,(Dec 16),pp.5600-5604,1528-0020; 0006-4971

Hansra, D., Montague, N., Stefanovic, A., et al.(2010).Oral and extraoral plasmablastic lymphoma: similarities and differences in clinicopathologic characteristics. *Am. J. Clin. Pathol.*, Vol.134,No.5,(Nov),pp.710-719,1943-7722; 0002-9173

Hazenberg, M. D., Hamann, D., Schuitemaker, H. & Miedema, F.(2000).T cell depletion in HIV-1 infection: how CD4+ T cells go out of stock. *Nat. Immunol.*, Vol.1, No.4,(Oct), pp.285-289,1529-2908

Ioachim, H. L., Adsay, V., Giancotti, F. R., Dorsett, B. & Melamed, J.(1995).Kaposi's sarcoma of internal organs. A multiparameter study of 86 cases.*Cancer*,Vol.75,No.6,(Mar 15),pp.1376-1385,0008-543X

Ioachim, H. L., Cooper, M. C. & Hellman, G. C.(1985).Lymphomas in men at high risk for acquired immune deficiency syndrome (AIDS). A study of 21 cases.*Cancer*,Vol.56,No.12,(Dec 15),pp.2831-2842,0008-543X

Ioachim, H. L., Cronin, W., Roy, M. & Maya, M.(1990).Persistent lymphadenopathies in people at high risk for HIV infection. Clinicopathologic correlations and long-term follow-up in 79 cases.*Am.J.Clin.Pathol.*,Vol.93,No.2,(Feb),pp.208-218,0002-9173

Ioachim, H., L. & Medeiros, J., L.(2009a).Chapter 18: Bacillary Angiomatosis of Lymph Nodes, In:*Ioachim's Lymph Node Pathology*,Ioachim, H., L. and Medeiros, J., L., pp.115-118,Wolters Kluwer, Lippincott Williams & Wilkins,0-7817-7596-5,Philadelphia, PA

Ioachim, H., L. & Medeiros, J., L.(2009b).Chapter 1: The Normal Lymph Node, In:*Ioachim's Lymph Node Pathology*,Ioachim, H., L. and Medeiros, J., L., pp.2-14,Wolters Kluwer, Lippincott Williams & Wilkins,0-7817-7596-5,Philadelphia, PA

Ioachim, H., L. & Medeiros, J., L.(2009c).Chapter 15: Human Immunodeficiency Virus Lymphadenitis, In:*Ioachim's Lymph Node Pathology*,Ioachim, H., L. and Medeiros, J., L., pp.99-105,Wolters Kluwer, Lippincott Williams & Wilkins,0-7817-7596-5,Philadelphia, PA

Ioachim, H., L. & Medeiros, J., L.(2009d).Chapter 28: Pneumocystis Lymphadenitis, In:*Ioachim's Lymph Node Pathology*,Ioachim, H., L. and Medeiros, J., L., pp.156-158,Wolters Kluwer, Lippincott Williams & Wilkins,0-7817-7596-5,Philadelphia, PA

Ioachim, H., L. & Medeiros, J., L.(2009e).Chapter 29: Toxoplasma Lymphadenitis, In:*Ioachim's Lymph Node Pathology*,Ioachim, H., L. and Medeiros, J., L., pp.159-164,Wolters Kluwer, Lippincott Williams & Wilkins,0-7817-7596-5,Philadelphia, PA

Ioachim, H., L. & Medeiros, J., L.(2009f).Chapter 42: Castleman Lymphadenopathy, In:*Ioachim's Lymph Node Pathology*,Ioachim, H., L. and Medeiros, J., L., pp.227-237,Wolters Kluwer, Lippincott Williams & Wilkins,0-7817-7596-5,Philadelphia, PA

Ioachim, H., L. & Medeiros, J., L.(2009g).Chapter 57: Hodgkin Lymphoma: Classical, In:*Ioachim's Lymph Node Pathology*,Ioachim, H., L. and Medeiros, J., L., pp.306-324,Wolters Kluwer, Lippincott Williams & Wilkins,0-7817-7596-5,Philadelphia, PA

Jacobson, C. A. & LaCasce, A. S.(2010).Lymphoma: risk and response after solid organ transplant.*Oncology (Williston Park)*,Vol.24,No.10,(Sep),pp.936-944,0890-9091; 0890-9091

Jasmer, R. M., Gotway, M. B., Creasman, J. M., Webb, W. R., Edinburgh, K. J. & Huang, L.(2002).Clinical and radiographic predictors of the etiology of computed tomography-diagnosed intrathoracic lymphadenopathy in HIV-infected patients.*J.Acquir.Immune Defic.Syndr.*,Vol.31,No.3,(Nov 1),pp.291-298,1525-4135

Jones, S. A., Horiuchi, S., Topley, N., Yamamoto, N. & Fuller, G. M.(2001).The soluble interleukin 6 receptor: mechanisms of production and implications in disease.*FASEB J.*,Vol.15,No.1,(Jan),pp.43-58,0892-6638

Kamani, J., Mani, A. U., Egwu, G. O. & Kumshe, H. A.(2009).Seroprevalence of human infection with Toxoplasma gondii and the associated risk factors, in Maiduguri, Borno state, Nigeria.*Ann.Trop.Med.Parasitol.*,Vol.103,No.4,(Jun),pp.317-321,0003-4983

Kaplan, J. E., Benson, C., Holmes, K. H., et al.(2009).Guidelines for prevention and treatment of opportunistic infections in HIV-infected adults and adolescents: recommendations from CDC, the National Institutes of Health, and the HIV Medicine Association of the Infectious Diseases Society of America.*MMWR Recomm Rep.*,Vol.58,No.RR-4,(Apr 10),pp.1-207; quiz CE1-4,1545-8601; 1057-5987

Kobayashi, M., Yoshimoto, S., Fujishita, M., et al.(1984).HTLV-positive T-cell lymphoma/leukaemia in an AIDS patient.*Lancet*,Vol.1,No.8390,(Jun 16),pp.1361-1362,0140-6736

Kostianovsky, M. & Greco, M. A.(1994).Angiogenic process in bacillary angiomatosis.*Ultrastruct.Pathol.*,Vol.18,No.3,(May-Jun),pp.349-355,0191-3123

Lamas, C. C., Mares-Guia, M. A., Rozental, T., et al.(2010).Bartonella spp. infection in HIV positive individuals, their pets and ectoparasites in Rio de Janeiro, Brazil: serological and molecular study.*Acta Trop.*,Vol.115,No.1-2,(Jul-Aug),pp.137-141,1873-6254; 0001-706X

Latif, A. S., Katzenstein, D. A., Bassett, M. T., Houston, S., Emmanuel, J. C. & Marowa, E.(1989).Genital ulcers and transmission of HIV among couples in Zimbabwe.*AIDS*,Vol.3,No.8,(Aug),pp.519-523,0269-9370

Leoncini, L., Raphaël, M., Stein, H., Harris, N., L., Jaffe, E., S. & Kluin, P. M.(2008).Burkitt Lymphoma, In:*WHO Classification of Tumours of Haematopoietic and Lymphoid Tissues*,Swerdlow, S., H., Campo, E., Harris, N., L., et al, pp.262-264,IARC,9283224310,Lyon, France

Levine, A. M., Seneviratne, L., Espina, B. M., et al.(2000).Evolving characteristics of AIDS-related lymphoma.*Blood*,Vol.96,No.13,(Dec 15),pp.4084-4090,0006-4971

Lewden, C., Salmon, D., Morlat, P., et al.(2005).Causes of death among human immunodeficiency virus (HIV)-infected adults in the era of potent antiretroviral therapy: emerging role of hepatitis and cancers, persistent role of AIDS.*Int.J.Epidemiol.*,Vol.34,No.1,(Feb),pp.121-130,0300-5771

Lindstrom, I., Kaddu-Mulindwa, D. H., Kironde, F. & Lindh, J.(2006).Prevalence of latent and reactivated Toxoplasma gondii parasites in HIV-patients from Uganda.*Acta Trop.*,Vol.100,No.3,(Dec),pp.218-222,0001-706X

Luan, S. L., Boulanger, E., Ye, H., et al.(2010).Primary effusion lymphoma: genomic profiling revealed amplification of SELPLG and CORO1C encoding for proteins important for cell migration.*J.Pathol.*,Vol.222,No.2,(Oct),pp.166-179,1096-9896; 0022-3417

Maguina, C., Guerra, H. & Ventosilla, P.(2009). Bartonellosis. *Clin.Dermatol.*, Vol.27, No.3, (May-Jun), pp.271-280,1879-1131; 0738-081X

Mantina, H., Wiggill, T. M., Carmona, S., Perner, Y. & Stevens, W. S.(2010).Characterization of Lymphomas in a high prevalence HIV setting.*J.Acquir.Immune Defic.Syndr.*,Vol.53,No.5,(Apr),pp.656-660,1944-7884; 1525-4135

Mbulaiteye, S. M., Anderson, W. F., Bhatia, K., Rosenberg, P. S., Linet, M. S. & Devesa, S. S.(2010).Trimodal age-specific incidence patterns for Burkitt lymphoma in the United States, 1973-2005.*Int.J.Cancer*,Vol.126,No.7,(Apr 1),pp.1732-1739,1097-0215; 0020-7136

McCune, J. M.(2001).The dynamics of CD4+ T-cell depletion in HIV disease. *Nature,* Vol.410, No.6831,(Apr 19),pp.974-979,0028-0836; 0028-0836

Mesri, E. A., Cesarman, E. & Boshoff, C.(2010).Kaposi's sarcoma and its associated herpesvirus.*Nat.Rev.Cancer.*,Vol.10,No.10,(Oct),pp.707-719,1474-1768; 1474-175X

Minnick, M. F., Smitherman, L. S. & Samuels, D. S.(2003).Mitogenic effect of Bartonella bacilliformis on human vascular endothelial cells and involvement of GroEL.*Infect.Immun.*,Vol.71,No.12,(Dec),pp.6933-6942,0019-9567

Mitchell, R. S., Beitzel, B. F., Schroder, A. R., et al.(2004).Retroviral DNA integration: ASLV, HIV, and MLV show distinct target site preferences. *PLoS Biol.,* Vol.2, No.8, (Aug), pp.E234,1545-7885; 1544-9173

Montes-Moreno, S., Gonzalez-Medina, A. R., Rodriguez-Pinilla, S. M., et al.(2010).Aggressive large B-cell lymphoma with plasma cell differentiation: immunohistochemical characterization of plasmablastic lymphoma and diffuse large B-cell lymphoma with partial plasmablastic phenotype. *Haematologica,* Vol.95, No.8, (Aug), pp.1342-1349,1592-8721; 0390-6078

Mosialos, G., Birkenbach, M., Yalamanchili, R., VanArsdale, T., Ware, C. & Kieff, E.(1995).The Epstein-Barr virus transforming protein LMP1 engages signaling proteins for the tumor necrosis factor receptor family.*Cell,*Vol.80,No.3,(Feb 10),pp.389-399,0092-8674

Mukherhee, S.(2010).Part 2: An Impatient War An Anatomist's Tumor, In:Anonymous pp.151-161,Scribner, A division of Simon & Schuster, Inc.,978-1-4391-0795-9,New York, NY

Mylona, E. E., Baraboutis, I. G., Lekakis, L. J., Georgiou, O., Papastamopoulos, V. & Skoutelis, A.(2008).Multicentric Castleman's disease in HIV infection: a systematic review of the literature.*AIDS.Rev.*,Vol.10,No.1,(Jan-Mar),pp.25-35,1139-6121

Nador, R. G., Chadburn, A., Gundappa, G., Cesarman, E., Said, J. W. & Knowles, D. M.(2003).Human immunodeficiency virus (HIV)-associated polymorphic lymphoproliferative disorders.*Am.J.Surg.Pathol.*,Vol.27,No.3,(Mar),pp.293-302,0147-5185

Nasr, S. A., Brynes, R. K., Garrison, C. P. & Chan, W. C.(1988).Peripheral T-cell lymphoma in a patient with acquired immune deficiency syndrome.*Cancer,*Vol.61,No.5,(Mar 1),pp.947-951,0008-543X

Nava, V. E., Cohen, P., Kalan, M. & Ozdemirli, M.(2008).HIV-associated anaplastic large cell lymphoma: a report of three cases.*AIDS,*Vol.22,No.14,(Sep 12),pp.1892-1894,1473-5571; 0269-9370

Navarro, J. T., Lloveras, N., Ribera, J. M., Oriol, A., Mate, J. L. & Feliu, E.(2005).The prognosis of HIV-infected patients with diffuse large B-cell lymphoma treated with chemotherapy and highly active antiretroviral therapy is similar to that of HIV-negative patients receiving chemotherapy.*Haematologica,*Vol.90,No.5,(May),pp.704-706,1592-8721; 0390-6078

Nielsen, K., McSherry, G., Petru, A., et al.(1997).A descriptive survey of pediatric human immunodeficiency   virus-infected   long-term survivors.*Pediatrics,*Vol.99,No.4,(Apr),pp.E4,1098-4275; 0031-4005

Norkin, L.(2010).The Retroviruses: Lentiviruses, Human Immunodeficiency Virus, and AIDS, In:*Virology Molecular Biology and Pathogenesis,*Norkin, L., pp.597-671,ASM Press,9781555814533,Washington, DC

Noy,   A.(2010).Controversies   in   the   treatment   of   Burkitt   lymphoma   in AIDS.*Curr.Opin.Oncol.,*Vol.22,No.5,(Sep),pp.443-448,1531-703X; 1040-8746

O'CONOR, G. T. & DAVIES, J. N.(1960).Malignant tumors in African children. With special reference to malignant lymphoma.*J.Pediatr.,*Vol.56,(Apr),pp.526-535,0022-3476

O'Hara, A. J., Wang, L., Dezube, B. J., Harrington, W. J.,Jr, Damania, B. & Dittmer, D. P.(2009).Tumor suppressor microRNAs are underrepresented in primary effusion lymphoma and Kaposi sarcoma.*Blood,*Vol.113,No.23,(Jun 4),pp.5938-5941,1528-0020; 0006-4971

Oksenhendler, E., Boulanger, E., Galicier, L., et al.(2002).High incidence of Kaposi sarcoma-associated herpesvirus-related non-Hodgkin lymphoma in patients with HIV infection and multicentric Castleman disease.*Blood,*Vol.99,No.7,(Apr 1),pp.2331-2336,0006-4971

Orem, J., Maganda, A., Mbidde, E. K. & Weiderpass, E.(2009).Clinical characteristics and outcome of children with Burkitt lymphoma in Uganda according to HIV infection.*Pediatr.Blood Cancer.,*Vol.52,No.4,(Apr),pp.455-458,1545-5017; 1545-5009

Osborne, J., Moore, P. S. & Chang, Y.(1999).KSHV-encoded viral IL-6 activates multiple human IL-6 signaling pathways.*Hum.Immunol.,*Vol.60,No.10,(Oct),pp.921-927,0198-8859

Ouansafi, I., He, B., Fraser, C., et al.(2010).Transformation of follicular lymphoma to plasmablastic lymphoma with c-myc gene rearrangement. *Am. J. Clin. Pathol.,*Vol.134,No.6,(Dec), pp.972-981,1943-7722; 0002-9173

Pantaleo, G., Graziosi, C., Demarest, J. F., et al.(1993).HIV infection is active and progressive in   lymphoid   tissue   during   the   clinically   latent   stage   of disease.*Nature,*Vol.362,No.6418,(Mar 25),pp.355-358,0028-0836; 0028-0836

Pape, M., Kollaras, P., Mandraveli, K., et al.(2005).Occurrence of Bartonella henselae and Bartonella   quintana   among   human   immunodeficiency   virus-infected patients.*Ann.N.Y.Acad.Sci.,*Vol.1063,(Dec),pp.299-301,0077-8923

Park, S., Lee, J., Ko, Y. H., et al.(2007).The impact of Epstein-Barr virus status on clinical outcome in diffuse large B-cell lymphoma.*Blood,*Vol.110,No.3,(Aug 1),pp.972-978,0006-4971

Perez, K., Castillo, J., Dezube, B. J. & Pantanowitz, L.(2010).Human Immunodeficiency Virus-associated anaplastic large cell lymphoma.*Leuk.Lymphoma,*Vol.51,No.3,(Mar), pp.430-438,1029-2403; 1026-8022

Prasad, H. K., Bhojwani, K. M., Shenoy, V. & Prasad, S. C.(2006).HIV manifestations in otolaryngology.*Am.J.Otolaryngol.,*Vol.27,No.3,(May-Jun),pp.179-185,0196-0709

Qing, X., Sun, N., Chang, E., French, S., Ji, P. & Yue, C.(2011).Plasmablastic lymphoma may occur as a high-grade transformation from plasmacytoma. *Exp. Mol. Pathol.,* Vol.90, No.1, (Feb),pp.85-90,1096-0945; 0014-4800

Rafaniello Raviele, P., Pruneri, G. & Maiorano, E.(2009).Plasmablastic lymphoma: a review.*Oral Dis.,*Vol.15,No.1,(Jan),pp.38-45,1601-0825; 1354-523X

Raphaël, M., Said, J., Borisch, B., Cesarman, E. & Harris, N., L.(2008).Lymphomas associated with HIV infection, In:*WHO Classification of Tumours of Haematopoietic and Lymphoid Tissues,*Swerdlow, S., H., Campo, E., Harris, N., L., et al, pp.340-342, IARC, 9283224310, Lyon, France

Relman, D. A., Loutit, J. S., Schmidt, T. M., Falkow, S. & Tompkins, L. S.(1990).The agent of bacillary angiomatosis. An approach to the identification of uncultured pathogens.*N.Engl.J.Med.,*Vol.323,No.23,(Dec 6),pp.1573-1580,0028-4793

Robbins, S. L., Kumar, V. & Cotran, R. S.(2010).Chapter 6: Disease of the Immune System, In:*Robbins and Cotran Pathologic Basis of Disease,*Robbins, S. L., Kumar, V. and Cotran, R. S., Saunders/Elsevier,9781416031215,Philadelphia, PA

Roca, B.(2009).Castleman's Disease. A Review.*AIDS.Rev.,*Vol.11,No.1,(Jan-Mar),pp.3-7,1139-6121

Sacktor, N., Lyles, R. H., Skolasky, R., et al.(2001).HIV-associated neurologic disease incidence changes:: Multicenter AIDS Cohort Study, 1990-1998.*Neurology,*Vol.56,No.2,(Jan 23),pp.257-260,0028-3878

Said, J. & Cesarman, E.(2008).Primary effusion lymphoma, In:*WHO Classification of Tumours of Haematopoietic and Lymphoid Tissues,*Swerdlow, S., H., Campo, E., Harris, N., L., et al, pp.260-261,IARC,9283224310,Lyon, France

Shin, D. W., Cha, D. Y., Hua, Q. J., Cha, G. H. & Lee, Y. H.(2009).Seroprevalence of Toxoplasma gondii infection and characteristics of seropositive patients in general hospitals in Daejeon, Korea.*Korean J.Parasitol.,*Vol.47,No.2,(Jun),pp.125-130,1738-0006; 0023-4001

Sierra, S., Kupfer, B. & Kaiser, R.(2005).Basics of the virology of HIV-1 and its replication.*J.Clin.Virol.,*Vol.34,No.4,(Dec),pp.233-244,1386-6532

Sissolak, G., Sissolak, D. & Jacobs, P.(2010).Human immunodeficiency and Hodgkin lymphoma.*Transfus.Apher.Sci.,*Vol.42,No.2,(Apr),pp.131-139,1473-0502

Soulier, J., Grollet, L., Oksenhendler, E., et al.(1995).Kaposi's sarcoma-associated herpesvirus-like DNA sequences in multicentric Castleman's disease.*Blood,*Vol.86,No.4,(Aug 15),pp.1276-1280,0006-4971

Spina, M., Tirelli, U., Zagonel, V., et al.(1998).Burkitt's lymphoma in adults with and without human immunodeficiency virus infection: a single-institution clinicopathologic study of 75 patients.*Cancer,*Vol.82,No.4,(Feb 15),pp.766-774,0008-543X

Stoler, M. H., Bonfiglio, T. A., Steigbigel, R. T. & Pereira, M.(1983).An atypical subcutaneous infection associated with acquired immune deficiency syndrome.*Am.J.Clin.Pathol.,*Vol.80,No.5,(Nov),pp.714-718,0002-9173

Stone, M. J.(2010).Samuel Wilks: the "grand old man" of British medicine.*Proc.(Bayl Univ.Med.Cent),*Vol.23,No.3,(Jul),pp.263-265,0899-8280; 0899-8280

Sun, J., Medeiros, L. J., Lin, P., Lu, G., Bueso-Ramos, C. E. & You, M. J.(2011).Plasmablastic lymphoma involving the penis: a previously unreported location of a case with aberrant CD3 expression.*Pathology,*Vol.43,No.1,(Jan),pp.54-57,1465-3931; 0031-3025

Thirlwell, C., Sarker, D., Stebbing, J. & Bower, M.(2003).Acquired immunodeficiency syndrome-related lymphoma in the era of highly active antiretroviral therapy.*Clin.Lymphoma,*Vol.4,No.2,(Sep),pp.86-92,1526-9655

Ueda, K., Ito, E., Karayama, M., Ohsaki, E., Nakano, K. & Watanabe, S.(2010).KSHV-infected PEL cell lines exhibit a distinct gene expression profile.*Biochem.Biophys.Res.Commun.,*Vol.394,No.3,(Apr 9),pp.482-487,1090-2104; 0006-291X

Ustun, C., Reid-Nicholson, M., Nayak-Kapoor, A., et al.(2009).Plasmablastic lymphoma: CNS involvement, coexistence of other malignancies, possible viral etiology, and dismal outcome.*Ann.Hematol.,*Vol.88,No.4,(Apr),pp.351-358,1432-0584; 0939-5555

Vaccher, E., Tirelli, U., Spina, M., et al.(1996).Age and serum lactate dehydrogenase level are independent prognostic factors in human immunodeficiency virus-related non-Hodgkin's lymphomas: a single-institute study of 96 patients. *J.Clin.Oncol.,*Vol.14,No.8,(Aug), pp.2217-2223,0732-183X

Verani, A., Gras, G. & Pancino, G.(2005).Macrophages and HIV-1: dangerous liaisons.*Mol.Immunol.,*Vol.42,No.2,(Feb),pp.195-212,0161-5890; 0161-5890

Vockerodt, M., Morgan, S. L., Kuo, M., et al.(2008).The Epstein-Barr virus oncoprotein, latent membrane protein-1, reprograms germinal centre B cells towards a Hodgkin's Reed-Sternberg-like phenotype.*J.Pathol.,*Vol.216,No.1,(Sep),pp.83-92,0022-3417

Wain-Hobson, S.(1996).HIV. One on one meets two.*Nature,*Vol.384,No.6605,(Nov 14),pp.117-118,0028-0836

Wang, D., Liebowitz, D. & Kieff, E.(1985).An EBV membrane protein expressed in immortalized lymphocytes transforms established rodent cells.*Cell,*Vol.43,No.3 Pt 2,(Dec),pp.831-840,0092-8674

Wen, K. W. & Damania, B.(2010).Kaposi sarcoma-associated herpesvirus (KSHV): molecular biology and oncogenesis.*Cancer Lett.,*Vol.289,No.2,(Mar 28),pp.140-150,1872-7980; 0304-3835

Whelan, P. & Scadden, D. T.(2006).Cancer in the Immunosuppressed Patient, In:*Oncology,*Anonymous pp.1689-1716,Springer,978-0-387-31056-5,New York, NY

WHO Department of HIV/AIDS Stop TB Department(2010).Guidelines for intensified tuberculosis case-finding and isoniazid preventive therapy for people living with HIV in resource-constrained settings.Vol.1,No.1,(December 2010),pp.1-50,978 92 4 150070 8

Wolf, T., Brodt, H. R., Fichtlscherer, S., et al.(2005).Changing incidence and prognostic factors of survival in AIDS-related non-Hodgkin's lymphoma in the era of highly active antiretroviral therapy (HAART).*Leuk.Lymphoma,*Vol.46,No.2,(Feb),pp.207-215,1042-8194; 1026-8022

Wolff, K., Johnson, R. & Suurmond, D.(2005).Bacillary Angiomatosis, In:*Fitzpatrick's Color Atlas & Synopsis of Clinical Dermatology,*Wolff, K., Johnson, R. and Suurmond, D., pp.648-650,McGraw-Hill,0071440194,New York, NY

WRIGHT, D. H.(1963).Cytology and histochemistry of the Burkitt lymphoma. *Br. J. Cancer,* Vol.17,(Mar),pp.50-55,0007-0920

Yousif, A., Farid, I., Baig, B., Creek, J., Olson, P. & Wallace, M.(1996).Prevalence of Bartonella henselae antibodies among human immunodeficiency virus-infected patients from Bahrain.*Clin.Infect.Dis.,*Vol.23,No.2,(Aug),pp.398-399,1058-4838

Ziegler, J. L., Drew, W. L., Miner, R. C., et al.(1982).Outbreak of Burkitt's-like lymphoma in homosexual men.*Lancet,*Vol.2,No.8299,(Sep 18),pp.631-633,0140-6736

8

AIDS Changed America with the Twin Breast Cancer Epidemic: Exploring the Consequences of Condomization

Arne N. Gjorgov
Retired Lecturer Epidemiologist, Skopje,
Republic of Macedonia

1. Introduction

Breast cancer as an epidemic disease which suddenly emerged along with the AIDS in the United States at the beginning of the 1980s, continued its unabated rise ever since and steadily continued its unprecedented epidemic advance worldwide. Initially affecting mainly the advanced, developed and 'rich' countries of the West, the breast cancer epidemic is now increasingly affecting the developing, less-advanced and 'poor' countries of all parts of the world. The 'latent period' of transition from the 'West" to the East and South, took less than a decade to extend. The epidemic of breast cancer along with the other accompanying, widespread diseases in women of all ages became better apparent now and is increasingly attracting more attention and concern

More than 34 years ago, a case-control study was initiated and completed in the U.S. in order to test an *a priori* hypothesis that a reduced or eliminated exposure to human seminal factors during the reproductive life-spans of women is an etiologic risk factor of developing breast cancer in American married women (Gjorgov, 1978a,b; Gjorgov, 1979; 1980, 1990, 1991, 1994a,b,c, 1996, 1998b). The hypothesis-testing study was jointly carried out at the University of North Carolina, School of Public Health (Epidemiology), at Chapel Hill, NC, and at the University of Pennsylvania School of Medicine and Hospital, in Philadelphia, PA, between 1974 and 1978, more than eight years before mutual epidemics of AIDS and breast cancer ever emerged. The results of the study corroborated the evidence of a significant association between exposure to barrier contraception (condom use and withdrawal practice) and the development of breast cancer in American and other women. In addition, the results provided evidence of a potential for primary (non-chemical) prevention/protection against breast cancer at individual, familial and community levels. Quantifying the risk, the results of the study indicated that women who used condoms and/or practiced withdrawal had a risk of developing breast cancer of 5.2 times greater (95%CI 3.1 – 8.7) than women who used non-barrier methods for fertility-control and family-planning purposes (diaphragm, IUDs, rhythm, oral-contraceptive pills, cream-jellies, and tubal ligation). By using Bayes' conditional theorem, it was estimated that 17% of women in the mainstream population using condoms / withdrawal were likely to develop breast cancer, versus 3.9% of women using non-barrier contraceptive methods. The evidence challenged head on the widespread misperception that all women are at an 'equal risk of breast cancer' and that the disease is a 'random' event in the lives of women (Gjorgov, 1980; 2009b). The newly revealed carcinogenic and other devastating effects and consequences of condomization of female sexuality showed to be operative even at a frequency of use of 50% of condom use. The quantification in the study of the latent period of development of breast cancer was shown to be between 2½ and 5 years, rather than the prevailing arbitrary assumptions of 15-20 years. Almost 80 percent of the etiologic fraction of the putative risk factor, which could indicate a potential preventive gain, was attributed in the study to the condomized and coitus interruptus birth control. One of the most favored inferences of the study was that the marriage is a profoundly biological woman-man union, with physiologic impact on spouses/couples, particularly on woman, along with the customary definition of marriage is a social, economic, psychological, traditional, and legal man-woman unit. Anticipation turned postulate has been that condomization could adversely affect this oldest human institution, the marriage.

The major unforeseen development in the epidemiology of breast cancer, lingering during the past three decades, beginning from the early 1980s, and continuing through the 1990s and 2000s, is the introduced policy of condomization of women's sexuality, as a supposed 'safe' prophylaxis against the HIV/AIDS transmission in the populations. As postulated, the newly introduced mechanical device, the condom, in the intimate (sexual) reproductive ecosystem, has substantially changed (corrupted) the primordial inter-human microenvironment, by eliminating the postulated putative protective factors (the prostaglandins?), that is, by introducing on an unprecedented scale technical effects of absolute male sterility in intimate (sexual) woman-man communication and other marital relations. The new development seem almost for certain to have had substantially supported / confirmed both an indirect causality of the tested evidence of the condom to breast cancer link, and the potential of primary (non-chemical, natural) prevention of the current, excess and unabated breast cancer epidemic.

There is a variety of gender- (sex-) specific diseases or dysfunction in women of all ages, related or not to the perpetual changes of the physiology of the reproductive system and changes of functions and events during the women's the child-bearing life-span. The definition of female-specific diseases is a pragmatic one and consists of specific female organs and systems (the internal and external reproductive organs), and mutual organs in both genders (breast, thyroid, bones) which are preponderantly and 'specifically' present in female. The central postulate is that the condomization is deleterious to all of the normal life functions of women and their reproductive events.

By entering the New Millennium, the beginning of the 21st Century in particular, the twin epidemics and burden of the HIV/AIDS transmission and breast cancer epidemic are likely to remain a major medical problem and great public health burden. The objective of this study was to try to explore the magnitude of the unknown impact and "unintended consequences" of a social action (Fox, 2004), such as the mass condomization, upon the health and lives of women. Accordingly, the study will attempt to provide answer(s) to what is the problem and what has to be done about the worsening morbidity and mortality of women in the changing world, what has been done--or not done--in the past, and especially what seems to be needed to investigate and to be done in the future, in terms of prevention and protection of reproductive health, life processes, truthful birth control, and (un)happiness of women in today's contemporary societies. The methods of the study are assessments of the trends, postulated etiology (root causes), epidemiology and the potential of primary prevention of the most frequent diseases of women of all ages, the cancer of the breast as an epidemic diseases, especially in the industrialized and affluent world of the West, in the last three decades, since the early 1980s, and ever since.

Cancer of the breast is the truly a major marker of the condomization impact upon the health and lives of women in urgent need for solution. Other manifestations of the ill-effect of condomization of women's sexuality are also taken into considerations. All-inclusive data of female specific diseases and phenomena were collected from epidemiologic and clinical studies as well as from psychological and social investigations of female predominance, higher incidence, prevalence and mortality rates, and female to male ration (F:M) of various conditions and diseases **(Table 1).** Because of data limitations, only some of the most frequent afflictions of women and girls were subject to review in the study.

Exclusively female diseases and dysfunctions:
Ovarian cancer, (incidence and death rates), cysts, polycystic syndrome (PCOS), and dysfunctions,
Endometrial cancer (incidence and death rates), other pelvic tumors-fibroids
Cervical cancer (incidence and death rates), and lesions
Vulvodynia, Pain during sex
Endometriosis,
Female sexual dysfunctions (FSD),
Dysmerrhea, menstrual irregularities, cessation, breast pain, hot flashes, craps
Abortion: Spontaneous, habitual, artificial, and 'missed abortion'; Pseudocyesis
Chronic pelvic pain, Pelvic congestion syndrome, Bloating
Specific, predominantly female diseases: Ratio female : male
Breast cancer, incidence cases and rates is 100 : 1 in males;
Thyroid cancer, incidence cases and rates is 3.5 - 7 : 1 in females to males;
Osteoporosis, fractures, prevalence, more than 80 : 20 in female to males;
Anorexia-bulimia ('eating') disorders, prevalence, in 90 : 10 girls / young women to boys / young men.
Other female predominant diseases: Ratio female : male (referred)
Thyroid disease (Hashimoto), prevalence 10 : 1
Graves disease, prevalence 7 : 1
Sjogren's syndrome, prevalence 9 : 1
Lupus erythematosus, prevalence 8 : 1
Rheumatoid arthritis, prevalence 2.5 : 1
Scleroderma, prevalence 3 : 1
Multiple sclerosis, prevalence 3 : 1   (National Academy of Sciences,.2011)

Table 1. Comprehensive woman's health: specific sex- (gender-) diseases in women, and female-to-male ratios

It should be mentioned here that some of the gender specific morbidly is also observed in domestic female animals, such as the **BSE**, *bovine spongiform encephalopathy,* and created in laboratory animals' mammary carcinomas and other tumors as well. It has been assumed, perhaps with some justification, that the persistent disproportion of higher female prevalence rates and aggregates of the specific gender diseases in females is also related to their specific, reproductive and natural functions. (Gjorgov, 1996b)

2. Evidence-based and theoretical etiology of the breast cancer epidemic

The provided evidence and inferences of the initial, hypothesis-testing study of etiology and prevention of breast cancer showed to be new and different from the widely and routinely accepted conceptions about the women's ill-health. The etiological link between the use of condom and breast cancer development in American and other married women, corroborated in a field study, was subsequently confirmed in a dramatic way by the explicitly predicted, natural experiment of the breast cancer outbreak/epidemic and the perplexing, rapid rise (Dinse et al. 1999), related to condomization campaigns and rumors for prophylaxis against the emergent mysterious infections.

The biological plausibility off the purported causal link of the carcinogenic effects between the of use of barrier methods of contraception, that is, use of condoms and/or withdrawal (*coitus interruptus*) and breast cancer in American and other women has been also corroborated elsewhere (Lê et al., 1989 in France, and Pikhut et al, 1991 in the former USSR). The indirect causality of breast cancer exposure to condom use was defined as an inverse ecological risk factor due to the absence, elimination or reduction of certain protective biological factors in the seminal fluid (the prostaglandins?), thus inducing technical effects of absolute male sterility in the prime biological woman-man communications. It has also been observed that the dichotomy of sexuality and procreative functions of female is much more complex, moving through incrementally deteriorating phases, than it has been presumed. Although intertwined, the distinct sexuality and reproduction capacities in women might offer a 'window of opportunity' to act coherently in achieving the imperatives of both control of the individual fertility and control of the global population growth.

Population-growth control could hardly proceed successfully by applying incorrect, deadly, and deceptive values of the technological method. The carcinogenic effects and life-threatening consequences of the barrier contraceptive methods, such as the new/old, high-tech condom device, along with the ancient technique of withdrawal, are cases in point: they cannot be assumed to be appropriate methods upon which a mass application of a proper population-growth control policy could be maintained. The contemporary social life and norms are practically incompatible with the bygone tradition of large families and multi-parity households. It has been calculated and observed that a woman has to have at least eight or more full term normal pregnancies (FTNPs), i.e., children, in order to be virtually protected against breast cancer. The Nature has not changed and made no adjustments to facilitate the modern human tendency for reduced reproduction. The modern medical history, not yet written, has already shown that any misconception and even inadvertent error in the sphere of human reproduction is bound to inflict tremendous harm on women and society, such as the mass condomization of female sexuality in the mainstream population. It is the purpose of this study to try to clarify the damage of the condom-related "reproductive freedom" fallacy and the scientific and individual ignorance and errors in condomized control of fertility, without passing judgment.

Although the main attention and concern has been focused on the 'hormonal,' oral contraceptive pills, the condom use and the uncritical campaigns for its use in any situation resulted in grave consequences on health and lives of women and girls, in terms of the on-going breast cancer epidemic and rampant 'eating' disorders. Even though the use of condoms dates for more than one century (in England at least), the condoms have been overlooked as the possible cause of the widespread ill-effects and grave consequences in women. The introduction of mass condomization of female sexuality has completely corrupted and destroyed the micro-environment of intimate (sexual) human ecosystem, by creating technical effects of sterile mating and un-physiological primordial woman-man communication and other relations. The unspoken ideas and intuitive popular knowledge of sex as a necessary part of life, health and survival of woman in marriage, and perhaps her beauty, was replaced by a conceptual vacuum in research, attitude and mindsets of sex and sexuality as a trivial, only 'recreational' gender activity.

3. Sources, population and methods

3.1 Sources
Global breast cancer data are updated in five-year reports published by the World Health Organization International Agency on Cancer Research (IARC), in Lyon, France, titled: "Cancer Incidence in Five Continents" (CI5s), volumes III-IX. (Waterhouse et al, 1977, 1982; Muir et al., 1987; Parkin et al, 1992; Parkin et al., 1997, 2002; Cirado et al., 2007). For achieving the objectives volumes III to IX, 1968 to 2002, inclusive, in duration of 35 years for most centers.

3.2 Population
Population under study consists of contingencies of women affected by breast cancer and other malignant diseases, collected by the national or regional Cancer Registries in 180 to 300 countries and population situations globally, with data quantified in average incidence rates (crude and age-standardized), collected in five-year periods, and reported by the regular editions of the WHO-IARC CI5 volumes.

3.3 Methods
For appraisal of existing, reliable and controlled data, collected internationally by the World Health Organization throughout several decades. Common statistical procedures [means, standard deviations, 95% CI (confidence intervals) of the risks, correlation coefficients, two-way statistical significances at P<.01 and P<.05 levels] were used for testing the differences, the temporal and spacial changes of the epidemic disease. Correlation and regression analyses, in order to test the statistical significance of the trends and rates of the diseases, and possible extrapolations. The necessary graphical figures and tables of the results and trends are also presented. The analysis of the multitude of data was done by using the SPSS (Statistical Package for Social Sciences), Version 16, 2008.

4. Epidemiological and clinical results and consequences

4.1 Perplexing breast cancer incidence rise worldwide
The rapid rise of breast cancer in the U.S. was first noted by the media, perplexed over the "highest breast cancer incidence rate (of 92.1) ever seen" in the U.S., in 1984. The type of tidal wave ('tsunami') onslaught of breast cancer heralded an emerging, unprecedented epidemic of a malignant (not contagious) disease in the medical history. Thus reaching for a first time in human medical history an unprecedented epidemic of malignant disease. Starting by 1987, the crude incidence rate (based on the number of new cases) was almost entirely replaced by age-adjusted incidence rates (computed on out of sight number of new cases). Correlation between the breast cancer incidence rates and prevalence rates of condom use were invariably positive at statistically significant levels, as presented in **Table 2** (Gjorgov, 1998; Gjorgov, 2000; UN Secretariat, 1994):

Region and number of countries/centres	Breast cancer age-adjusted incidence rates,[+] 1983-1987 (Lowest and highest rates)	Condom-use prevalence, estimates, in %[++] 1987	Correlation coefficient (Spearman r)
• WORLDWIDE (166)	6.4 - 104.2	1 - 15	.860**
• NORTH AMERICA (46) (USA and Canada)	52.2 - 104.2	10 - 15	.748**
• SOUTH AMERICA (12) (Columbia, Costa Rica, Cuba, Equador, Paraguay, Puerto Rico, Martinique, Brazil and other)	26.2 - 40.5	2 - 3	.548*
• WEST EUROPE (42) (Portugal, Spain, Italy, France, Norway, Finland, Denmark, Sweden, Holland, Iceland, West Germany, Switzerland and other)	35.7 - 73.5	5 – 13	.777**
• EAST EUROPE (17) (Czechoslovakia, GDR, Poland, Estonia, Latvia, Slovenia, Romania, Russia, and other)	31.1 - 43.7	3 - 5	.438
• UK, AUSTRALIA, NEW ZEALAND (22)	56.1 - 64.3	10 – 14	.564**
• AFRICA and ASIA (27) (Algeria, Gambia, Mali; China, India, Japan & other)	6.4 - 24.6	1 - 3	.558**
• DEVELOPMENTAL STAGE			
Developed regions (140)	35.7 - 104.2	5 - 15	.834**
Developing countries/regions (25)	6.4 - 43.7	1 - 3	.594**
• RACE			
White women (131)	31.1 - 104.2	2 - 15	.855**
Africans & Afro-Americans (12)	10.2 - 71.6	1 – 12	.541*
Orientals (23)	16.9 - 64.0	2 - 3	.821**
• URBANIZATION			
Urban populations (21)	31.1 - 104.2	3 - 15	.907**
Rural populations (26)	6.4 - 58.8	1 - 10	.932**

SOURCES: Parkin DM et al. 1992; United Nations Secretariat,.1994; Gjorgov AN., 1998, 2000 *p < .05 (significance level); **p < .01 and/or **p < .0001 (significance levels)

Table 2. Breast Cancer: Age-adjusted Rates (per 100,000) and Condom-Use Prevalence (percentages), 1983-1987, and Correlation coefficients, by Global Regions, Developmental Stage, Race, and Rural-Urban Places,

Quantifying the impact of condomization on breast cancer epidemic, it was estimated that an increase of condom use by 1 (one) percentage point, the gradient of increase of the breast cancer incidence will correspond to rate of 3.85 per 100,000 female population, globally. For North America, the increase of breast cancer incidence would correspond to a rate of 4.4/100,000 per one percent condom-use prevalence increase, and increase between 2.1 and 3.6 breast cancer incidence rates for various European countries. (Gjorgov, 1998a).

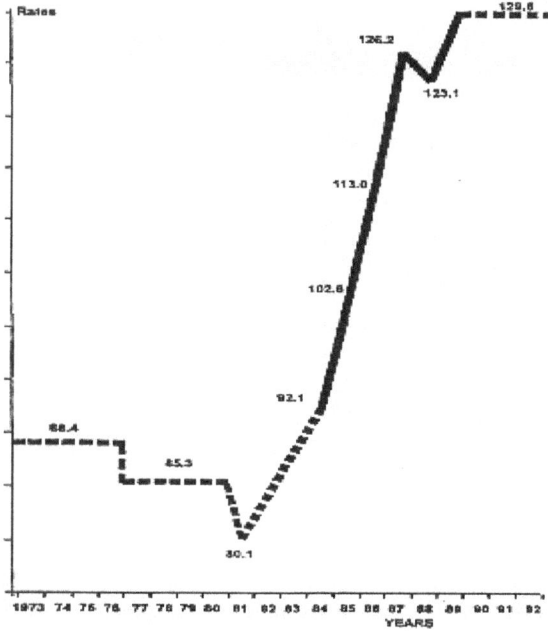

Fig. 1. Breast cancer rise in the United States, 1973-1987. Crude incidence rates, per 100,000 (female) population

Whether the condomization was intended for the feminist's allure only and latter adjusted for prophylaxis of the newly discovered HIV virus, is hard to come by. In one of available sources, the assertion about 'political decision' for condom-use promotion remained ambivalent: Ehrchardt "For the male condom, no controlled trials were demanded before it gained approval as an HIV prophylactic" (Ehrchardt, 1992).

Globally, the average number of breast cancer cases rose by 22% in the last two periods, between 1993-1997 and 1998-2002 (between CI2 VIII and IX Editions), showing difference in the medians of cases 1893.0 and 2735.5, and mode between 595 and 1840, respectively. The upsurge of breast cancer as an epidemic disease emerged rapidly in the United States after 1981, the first and 'the highest ever recorded' reported by the mass media incidence rates, foreboding the trends during the time period 1981 and 1986 and later. The escalation of breast cancer of 57.7 percent increase was recorded in a short period of six years between 1981 and 1986, with 80.1 incidence rate (per 100.000 female population) and 126.2 incidence rate, respectively (**Figure 1**).

4.2 Breast cancer epidemic changes in time, places and populations

The force of the rising incidence of breast cancer has been seen all over the world, the attempts of denigrating its surprise emergence and astonishing effect and magnitude notwithstanding. The new development of breast cancer as an epidemic disease could be best seen in **Figure 2**, as recorded for **Connecticut**, in the last 35 years.

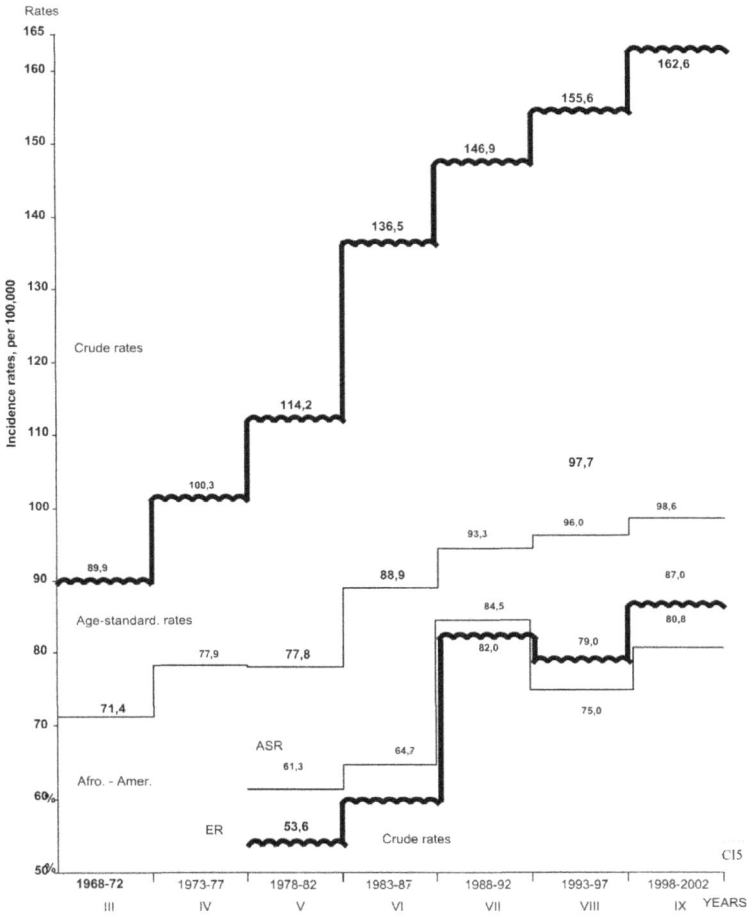

Fig. 2. Breast cancer trends in Connecticut, 1968-2002. Crude and age-adjusted incidence rates, per 100,000

The **Figure 2** reliably confirms the fact of a steep and steady increase of the breast cancer epidemic, for both races, since the Cancer Registry of Connecticut in New Haven, was first cancer registry in the world, established in 1936. (It may be of interest to note that there was a fluctuation of the breast cancer incidence rates for the Afro-Americans, an event rarely observed before.)

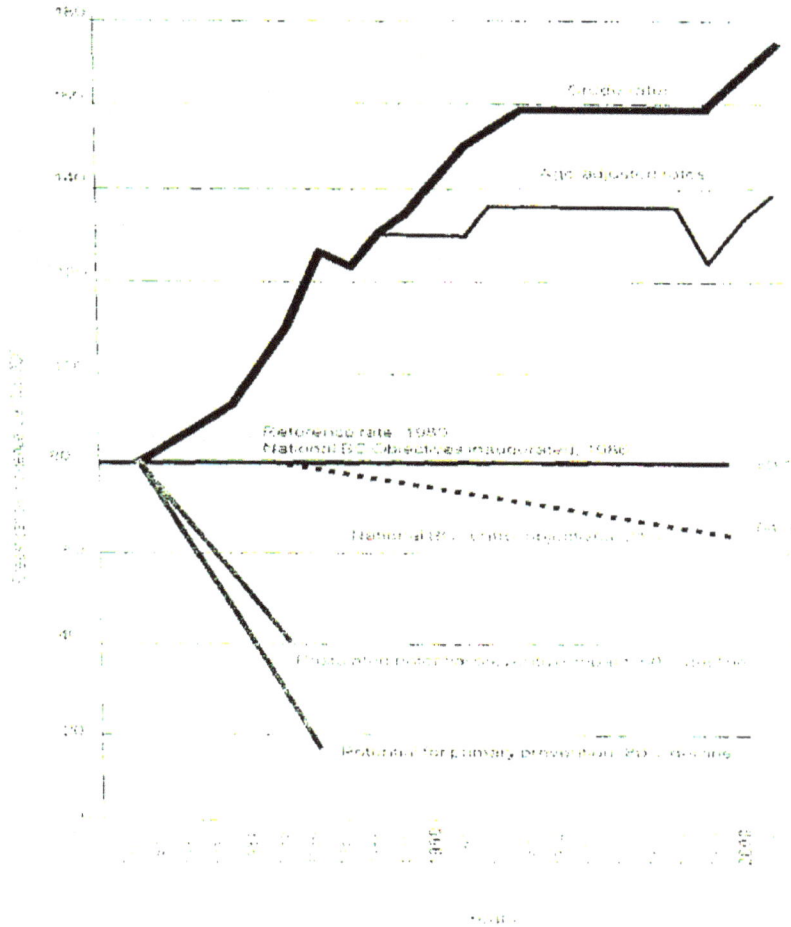

Fig. 3. Breast cancer trends in the U.S., 1980-2002. Observed crude and age-adjusted incidence rates: Projected 21% decline 1986-2000, and Postulated preventive impact, in percentages tested.

The overall epidemiology of the breast cancer epidemic in the **United States** is presented in the **Figure 3**. There is a dual presentation of the trends of the breast cancer progression in the past two-and-a-half decades, from 1980 to 2002. The breast cancer rising trends are presented in crude and age-adjusted incidence rates. The two incidence rates differ considerably, mainly because the age-adjusted rates, showing lower rates, were derived according to moving U.S. census populations, instead to the conventional World Standard Population 1960 (WSP). In the same **Figure 3** is presented the official, wrong prediction (in 1986) of 'declining' breast cancer trend until 2000, and also are presented two personal predictions of the future, postulated downward trends of 50 to 80 percent of breast cancer in the U.S.

Additional data support the analogous development of breast cancer rise in other parts of the country, such as the **San Francisco Bay Area** (**Figure 4**), which was subsequently and perhaps justifiably called "the Breast Cancer Capital of the World," for the highest incidence in America in the 1983-1987 period, reaching the excess incidence rate.

The first, the NCI confident forecast of decline of breast cancer incidence rates between 1986 until 2000, by 21 percent, was patently wrong from the outset. The predicted decline of breast cancer, published in 1986 proved to be quite off center: the incidence rates of the disease almost doubled by the end of the 20th Century. The wrongly computed forecast of decline probably reflected the same percentage of decline of the disease during the 1970s, and was computed maybe before the statistical data were in following the 1981unexpected breast cancer jump; The second prediction of decline of the breast cancer incidence rates between 50 to 80 percent, as related to the 1980 situation, remained theoretical estimates, based on etiological fraction percent, contingent on implementation of primary prevention and elimination of the corroborated etiological risk factor of semi-official policy of condomization of the mainstream population(s) against the HIV/AIDS transmissions, along with the application of Bayes' probability theorem computation, and yet to be

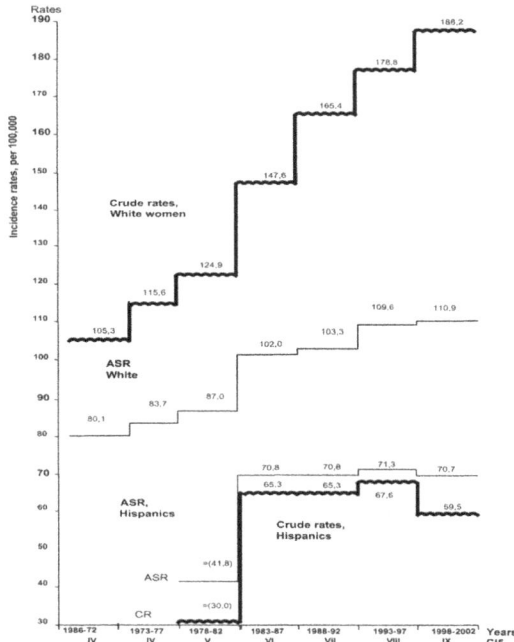

Fig. 4. Breast cancer in San Francisco Bay Area, CA, 1986-2002, by race. Crude and age-adjusted incidence rates, per 100,000

The same pattern of rapid rise of breast cancer was recorded in **Seattle, WA**, with an extraordinary jump of 27.8 percent of crude incidence rate (from 95.8 to 121.8) within one period of 1978-82 (before AIDS epidemic) to 1983-87 (the initial tide of the AIDS outbreak in the U.S.). (Figure not presented.) According to the data in the latest (IX) volume of the CI5, it seems that the infamous title of "Breast cancer capital of the world" has shifted from the San Francisco Bay Area to the Ferrara Region, Italy, with a crude incidence rate of 201.8 in the 1998-2002 period, and an increase of 263 percent in the number of breast cancer cases (from 527 to 1833) since 1998-1992.

In other parts of the Western world, the **Oxford** Region, the UK experienced immediate high increase of breast cancer and without apparent delay after the U.S. (**Figure 5**). The steady rise of the breast cancer incidence has been happening continuously and all 5-year time periods after 1980. In the mid-1990s, the Cancer Research UK organized, in cooperation with other European countries and North-American regions, so-called population-based, chemo-preventive community trials against epidemic breast cancer, by giving the drug *tamoxifen* to great number healthy women, in duration of five years, The enthusiastic chemo-preventive trials ended prematurely, with impractical results for breast prevention. No other idea or projects were envisioned or proposed for testing a potential primary (non-chemical) prevention of breast cancer. Circumstantial and fragmentary evidence seems to suggest that the idea of global condomization has originated at the 'R. Doll' Institute of Epidemiology in Oxford, probably thought of during the decade 1960s.

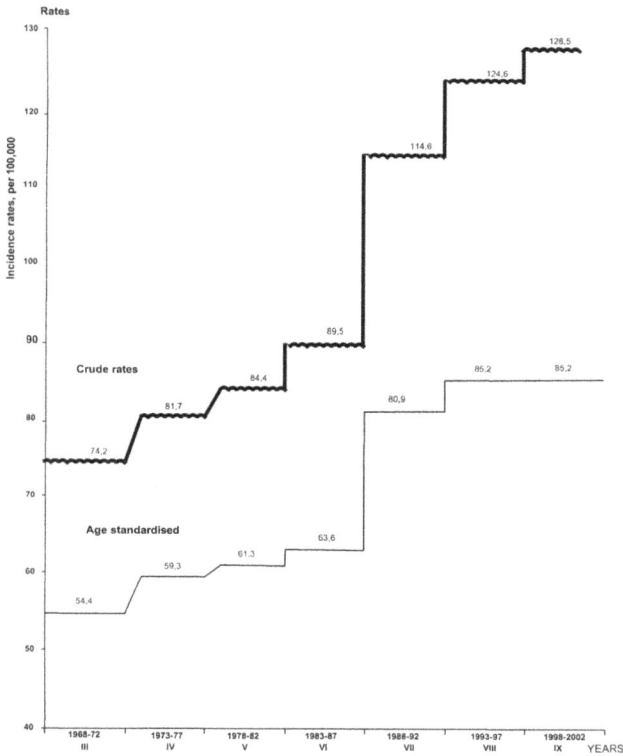

Fig. 5. Breast cancer in Oxford, UK, 1968-2002. Crude and age-adjusted incidence rates, per 100,000

At least two more high-risk regions of breast cancer epidemic in Europe deserve mention, in France and Sweden. The breast cancer epidemic in **France** (**Figure 6**) may prove of interest because of the fact that the North-Rhine Region is both one of the best developed regions, and one with the highest incidence rates in EU. The City of Strasbourg, where the multinational European Parliament is located, is also an important place where much of the debates and policies about breast cancer control, mainly for rectifying the early-detection screening policy, has been and is expected to continue to eventually consider primary prevention of the breast cancer epidemic soon.

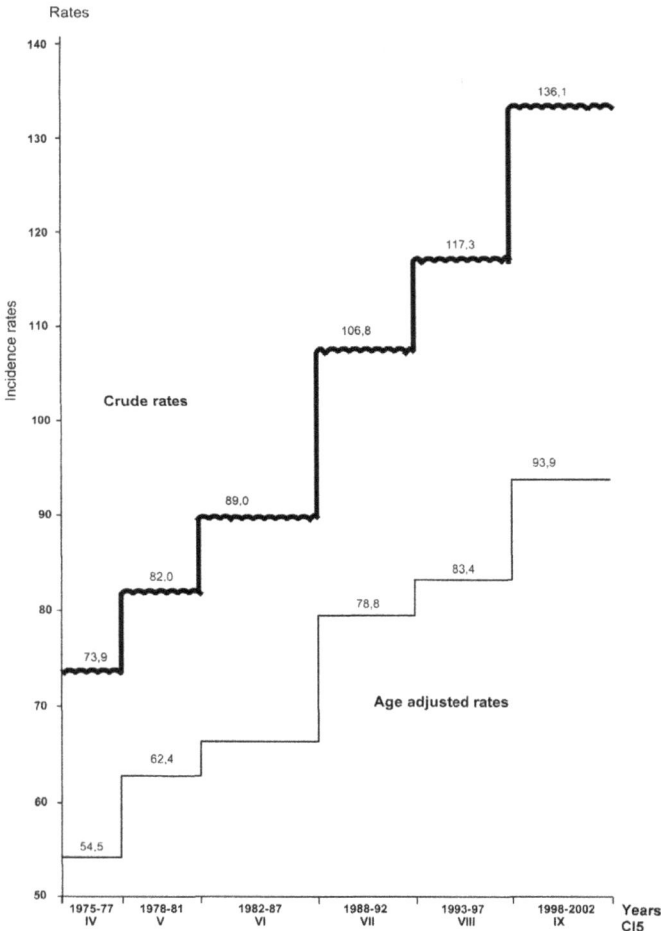

Fig. 6. Breast cancer in Bas-Rhin, France, 1975-2002. Crude and age-adjusted incidence rates, per 100,000

Sweden has always been a lead-country of high breast cancer incidence (**Figure 7**). The country has an interesting epidemiology of the disease, since the current, global breast cancer epidemic seems to have started much earlier there, during the decade of the 1970s, ten years before the epidemic was first recorded in the U.S. in the 1980s. Part of the puzzle lies in the information that condomization ("for non-contraceptive use") was first introduced in Sweden (Hinman, 1978; Valdiserri, 1988), in the 1970s decade, before campaigns of condomization were carried out in the rest of the world.

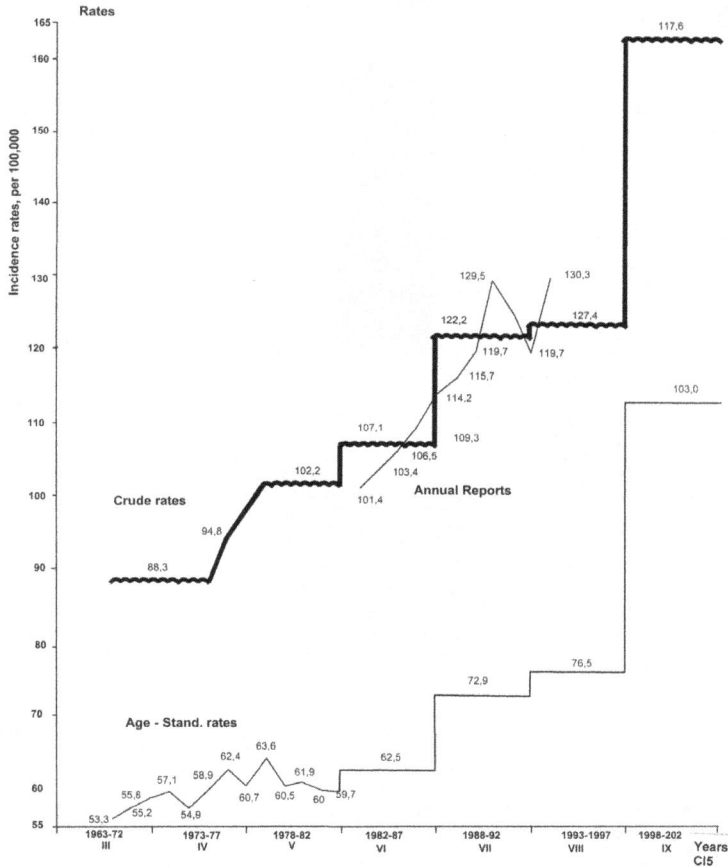

Fig. 7. Breast cancer in Sweden, 1971-2002. Crude and age-adjusted incidence rates, per 100,000

On the other side of the globe, in Australia, the rise of the breast cancer epidemic in the **New South Wales** showed the familiar European model of advent (**Figure 8**). According to the separate Annual Reports of the Cancer Registry of the Province NSW, the rise of breast cancer was apparently steeper than presented by the presentation in 5-year periods of the WHO-IARC CI5 reports.

Rates

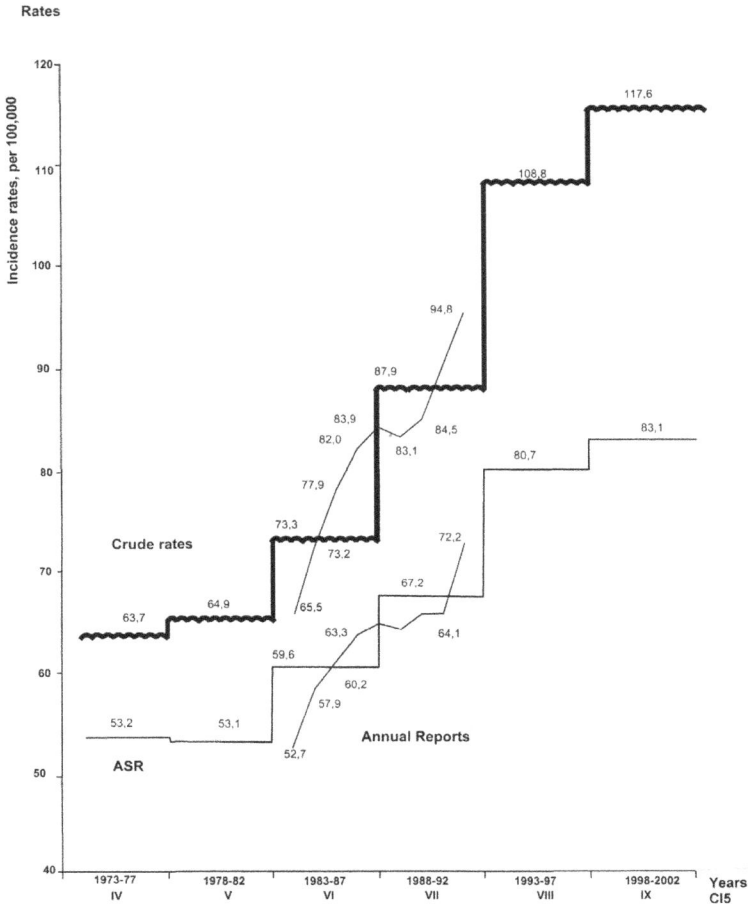

Fig. 8. Breast cancer in New South Wales, Australia, 1973-2002. Crude and age-adjusted incidence rates, per 100,000

In Asia, the experience of **Kuwait** (**Figure 9**) of the breast cancer epidemic rise was somewhat peculiar. First, Kuwait long enjoyed the distinction to be listed as a country with the lowest rate of breast cancer in the world. I worked and as Director of the National Cancer Registry at the Kuwait Cancer Control Centre for a long while, was able to observe the situation and the ensuing profound changes with regard breast cancer. (Gjorgov, 1986). Second, the breast cancer onslaught happened fast and affected very young, married multipara-women (not less than 4 pregnancies), between 23 to 35 years of age. The surgeons from Europe, worked in the local hospitals, were the first to voice alarm of the unusual in their practice pattern of performing mastectomies to such a young-age group of patients. Third, contrary to the American and European experience, the Non-Kuwaiti, immigrant women, had persistently had a higher incidence rate of breast cancer than the Kuwaiti women. During the past three decades, the increase of breast cancer in Kuwaiti women did not reach the higher incidence of the immigrant, Non-Kuwaiti women in the country.

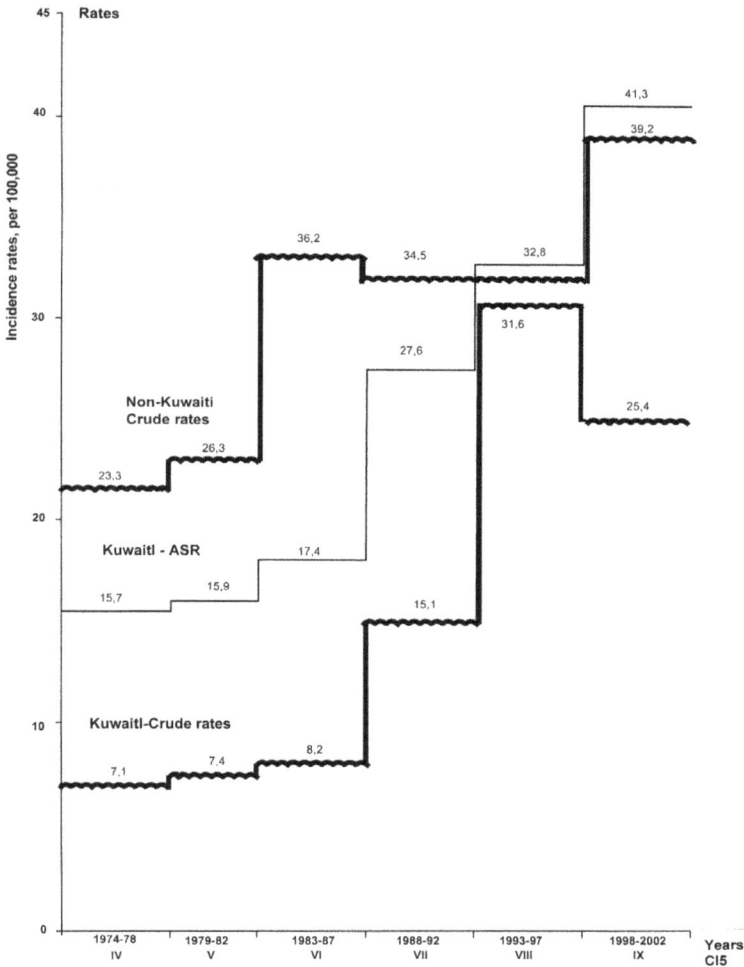

Fig. 9. Breast cancer in Kuwait, 1974-2002, by Kuwaiti and Non-Kuwaiti women. Crude and age-adjusted incidence rates, per 100,000

The other regions and countries of the world followed suit. In **Miyagi, Japan**, the **Figure 10** shows a steadily but moderately increasing breast cancer incidence rates. Nevertheless, the slow-moving breast cancer epidemic revealed an extraordinary evidence / proof of the peculiar characteristics of the breast cancer epidemic, the increase of the incidence in the younger women, most notably in the reproductive age-span of women **(Figure 11)**.

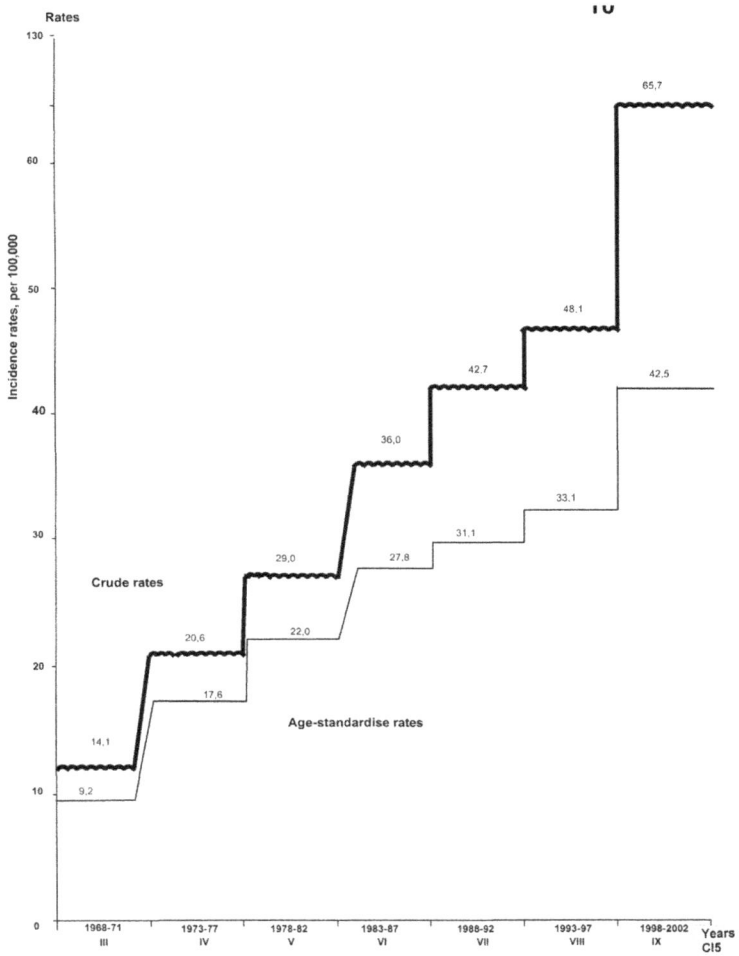

Fig. 10. Breast cancer in Miyagi, Japan, 1968-2002. Crude and age-adjusted incidence rates, per 100,000

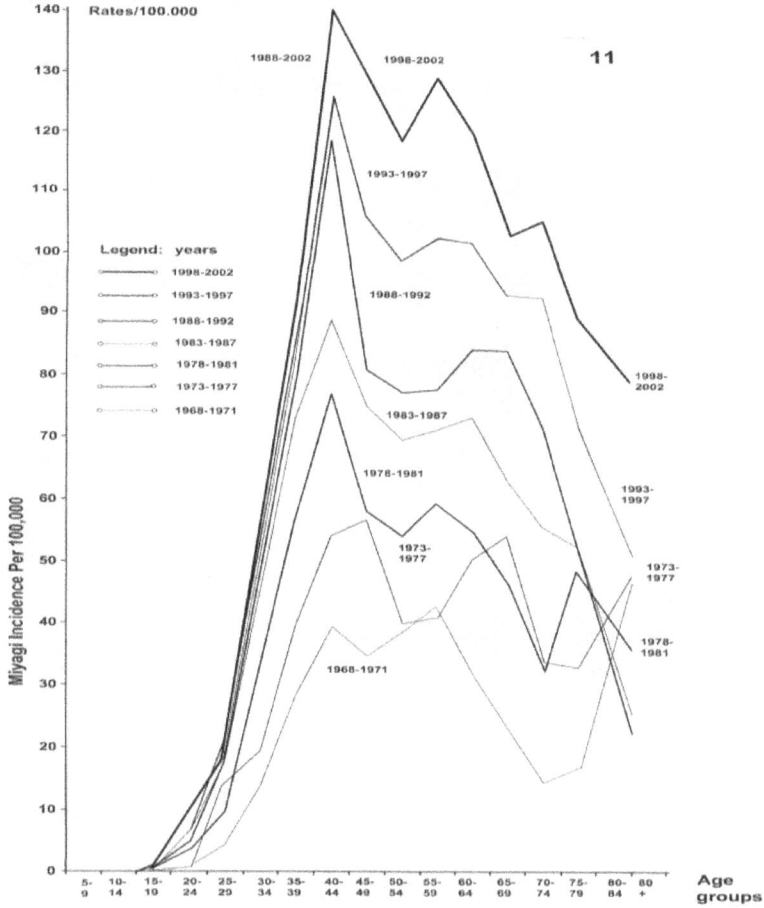

Fig. 11. Breast cancer Age-specific incidence rates in Miyagi, Japan, 1968-2002, by five-year periods, per 100,000

The conventional view that breast cancer is a "disease of affluence" had to be changed in the meantime by the epidemiology and empirical research of the disease in Afro-American women in the U.S., as well as in less industrialized (Krieger, 2002) and other "poor" countries. Three more situations could demonstrate the sudden changes in the trends of breast cancer developments (in %) in a number of centers in the **United States (Figure 12)** and in **Europe (Figure 13)**, from negative-decreasing to positive-increasing breast cancer trends.

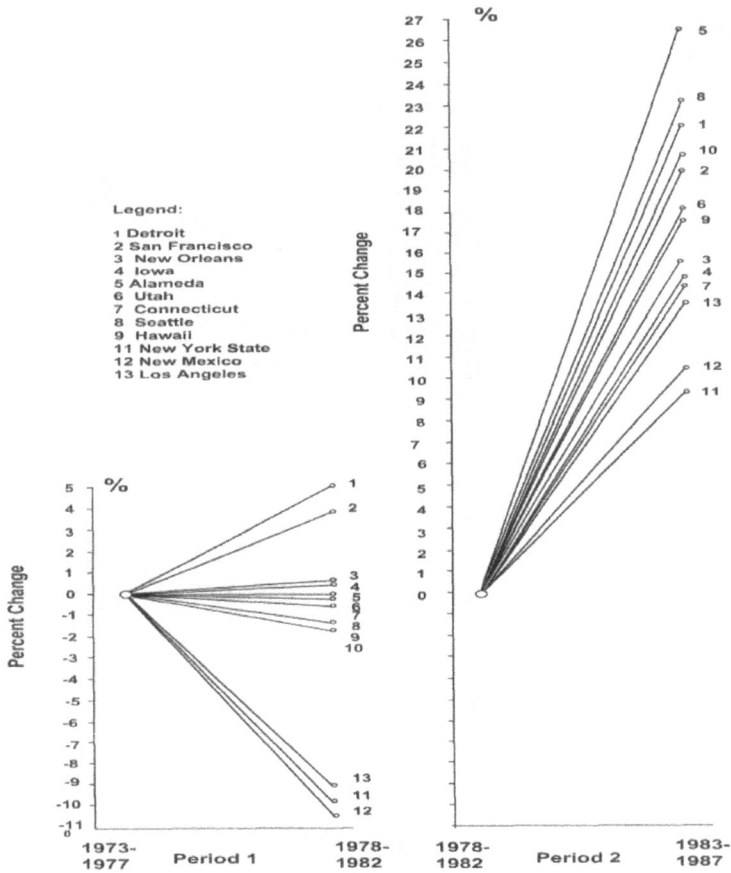

Fig. 12. Shift of breast cancer trends in the United States, 1983-1987, by time periods and regions. Changes of age-adjusted incidence rates, in percentages.

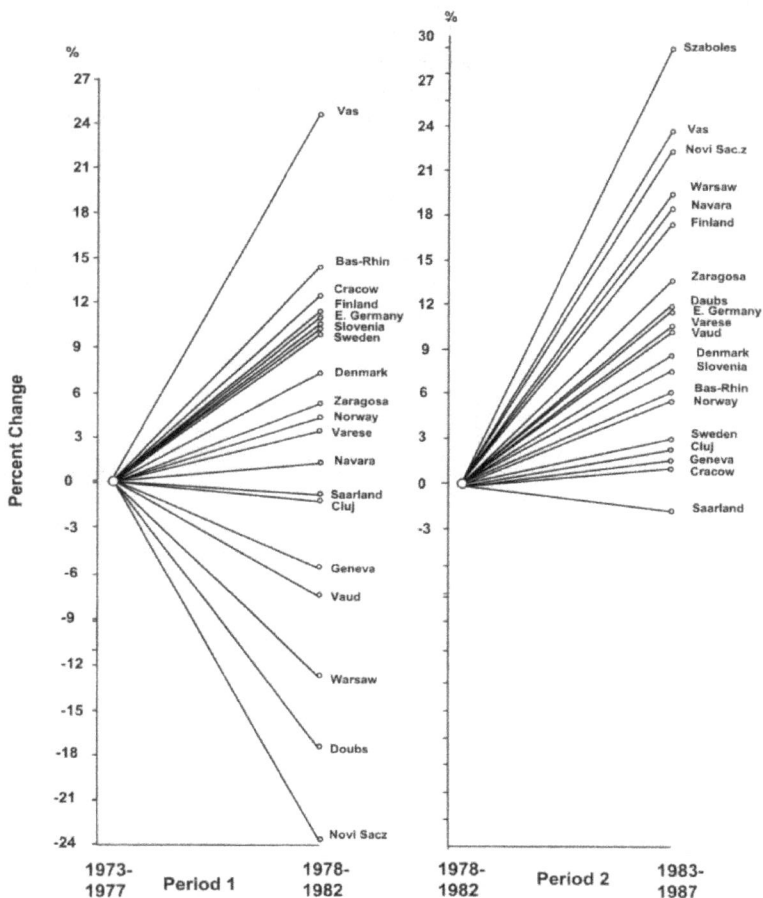

Fig. 13. Shift of breast cancer trends in Europe, 1983-1987, by time periods and countries. Changes of age-adjusted incidence rates, in percentages.

4.3 Inner developments of the breast cancer epidemic

The distribution of the age-specific incidence rates among young women, bellow 45 years of age, during the seven period of five-year intervals (35 years duration), between 1968 and 2002, clearly demonstrates the shift of the breast cancer epidemic towards younger, reproductive-age groups, ostensibly most frequently exposed to the purported risk factor of condomization. In addition to the situation in **Miyagi** (**Figure 11**), an extraordinary evidence of breast cancer descending in young women is evident in **Shanghai,** China (**Figure 14**). Perhaps a foreboding development of the disease in the country, the extraordinary shift of breast cancer incidence towards younger women was recorded in Shanghai in just a single five-year period, 1973-1978. In 2008, an alarming among many other studies appeared that rightly claimed that "China is on the point end of a breast cancer epidemic" (Linos et al. 2008). However, the solution in averting the predicted, impending breast cancer epidemic was seen and recommended in reductions of "modifiable risk factors," such as, alcohol intake, parity, hormone use, and adult weight gain... Condomization as a means for the restrictive reproductive policy was neither investigated nor mentioned in the study.

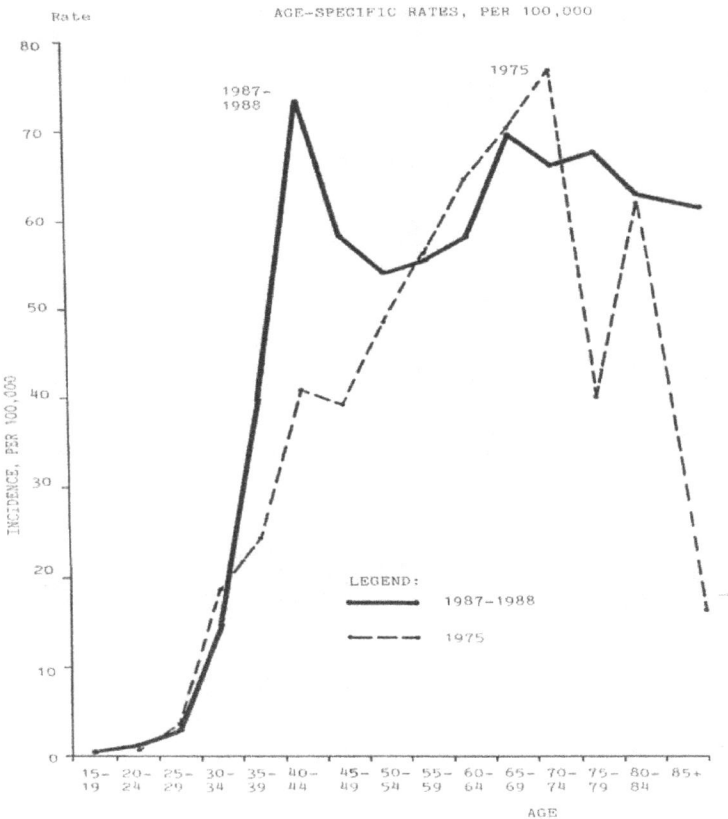

Fig. 14. Breast Cancer in Shanghai, China, 1975 and 1987-1988: "Debut" peak. Age-specific incidence rates, per 100,000

The unexpected shift towards young women was manifested in a remarkable peak of the disease in the of 35-39 year age-group, as a "debut" phenomenon, assuming that condomization was the first and perhaps the main mode of fertility control and family planning. Almost exactly the same situation was observed in Warsaw City (Poland), with the "debut" peak in 1987, compared with the age-specific distribution before the condom-use campaigns, in the period 1968-1972. (Figure not shown.) In the Volume VII of the CI5 (Parkin et al., 1997), and to a lesser degree in the Volumes VIII (Parkin, 2002) and IX (Cirado, 2007), there were more than 60 cases of age-specific distribution in which the first highest incidence of breast cancer was located in younger age groups, bellow 50, and even below 40 years of age. The "debut" phenomenon was mainly seen in countries with low baseline breast cancer incidence and where the breast cancer epidemic has been developing at a faster pace afterwards, such as, for instance, Italy.

The debut peaks showed that they are not static phenomena and not a rare situation. Data from the Malta National Cancer Registry (2010) showed that "debut" peaks popped up in the past decades in almost every year in a ten-year decade, and continued to be still present in subsequent cohorts of women **(Table 3).** Not less than 50-60 breast cancer age-specific distributions in the 1988-1992 period (CI5-VII) showed the highest peaks in younger women. The pattern of "debut" peaks is reminiscent to the epidemiological pattern of breast cancer age-specific incidence in Europe before and immediately after the WWII, with the so-called 'Clemmesen's hook' (Storm, 2011), similar but not equal with the "debut" phenomenon, because it happens to young women, in the prime of their reproductive sexuality, rather than at the end of the reproduction life time of menopause.

Age groups	1998	1999	2000	2001	2002	2003	2004	2005	2006	2007
15-19	0	0	0.07	0	0	0	0	0	0	0
20-24	0	0	0.07	0	0	0	0	0	0	0
25-29	0	0.08	0	0	0	0	0	0	0	0
30-34	0.17	0.18	0.09	0.60	0.33	0.24	0.08	0.07	0.15	0.35
35-39	0.36	0.29	0.37	030	0.79	0.40	0.41	0.58	0.33	0.41
40-44	1.13	1.68	0.75	0.60	0.87	1.09	1.39	1.44	1.27	1.48
45-49	1.76	1.43	1.57	1.68	0.97	1.02	0.80	2.05	1.32	1.40
50-54	2.47	1.60	1.91	2.22	2.19	1.77	2.14	1.53	1.80	1.92
55-59	2.29	2.26	2.29	2.18	2.07	2.68	2.33	2.00	2.52	2.04
60-64	1.50	2.56	2.62	1.59	2.89	3.59	2.61	3.76	3.20	3.00
65-69	3.23	3.27	3.09	2.34	1.64	2.28	2.13	3.50	3.30	3.65
70-74	4.12	2.28	3.21	2.56	3.15	1.27	3.58	2.19	3.62	3.44
75-79	2.09	4.71	3.83	3.07	2.50	4.26	2.95	4.53	4.41	3.82
80-84	4.12	3.75	6.34	3.43	2.36	3.48	2.86	4.39	2.87	3.85
85+	3.60	3.95	1.55	4.10	3.02	3.72	4.63	3.65	2.90	4.22
Crude rates	106.75	110.34	110.44	100.75	99.57	108.40	109.67	128.81	127.50	131.74
Age-adj. rates	72.61	72.30	70.55	64.35	64.99	67.70	66.84	79.56	75.82	77.78

Table 3. Cancer of the breast: Maltese Islands-Trends in Incidence 1998-2007. Incidence rates, by age and year of cancer registration (February 2010)

Most likely, the "debut" phenomenon is closely related with another puzzling issue of the breast cancer epidemic, the growing cases of ductal carcinoma in-situ (DCIS), or simply in-situ breast cancer, whose incidence, has gone up exponentially, up to 30 percent of the annual number of registered breast cancer cases, since the 1980s (National Cancer Institute, 2001). The in-situ (DCIS) cases in fact, testify of the evolving nature and lack of understanding of the global breast cancer epidemic. The in-situ breast cancer epitomizes also the conceptual vacuum in professional dealing with the breast cancer epidemic, because of misconception of DCIS as a random event in lives of women; not reporting of DCIS in the annual reports of incidence rate of breast cancer; exaggerated and not true claims of excellent ("nearly 100%") survival rate; unduly and unreasonably defined in-situ cases as non-breast cancer (0-zero stage); the systemic background of the in-situ cases is ignored and treatment is as a local disease. The early-detection screening, for finding most and more of the DCIS cases, has always been mired with uncertainty of further course of the in-situ finding into aggressive and metastatic breast cancer, the extent of treatment, and the dilemma about the usefulness of the early detection as the basic tenet of the breast cancer strategy.

4.4 Reproductive age and breast cancer
Age of women as such has almost invariably been defined among the strongest risk factor of breast cancer. The assertion of randomness has frequently accompanied the age factor. The international experience, however, points out to the long held observation that this assessment is not universally correct and that is in principle wrong. **Figure 15** shows that breast cancer in **Korea** is confined to middle-aged women, to the reproductive-age span women, with declining incidence after the peri-menopausal age of 50. In most of Asian populations (Japan, Malaysia, India), the breast cancer profiles exhibit the same pattern.

The pattern of breast cancer age distribution in Korea was similar to those in many European countries, which could still be seen in Porto, Portugal, evocative to the old rather than new European models. (Figure not presented)

Hidden behind the common reference of "cancer incidence increase" lies the fact that the increase is created to a high extent by the rise of breast cancer, while the category of "the rest of cancers" is actually decreasing. [The categories of breast cancer and "all cancers without skin cancer (C44)" are given as such and, for the purposes of this study, is computed a new category of "rest of cancers," meaning 'all cancers' minus breast cancer)]. The data of the **SEER** (Surveillance, Epidemiology, and End Results) program, containing nine registration centers in the U.S. and, since it stands for about 10 percent of the U.S. population, considered representative sample of the country, showed that the number of breast cancer rose by 11.6 percent, while the "rest" of cancers increased by 8.7 percent, between the two consecutive periods of 1993-97 and 1998-2002. The **Figure 16** presents data of increasing breast cancer age-adjusted incidence rates (16.8%) compared to the decreasing "rest" of cancer (-7.5%) in Afro-American women during the aforementioned two 5-year periods. There was exactly the same reciprocal increase of breast cancer (7.7%) and decrease (-4.3%) of the 'rest of cancers' in Afro-American women in Connecticut, and unexpected decrease (of -4.9%) of the 'rest' of cancers (age-adjusted incidence rates), and increase (1.2%) in white women in the San Francisco Bay Area, CA.

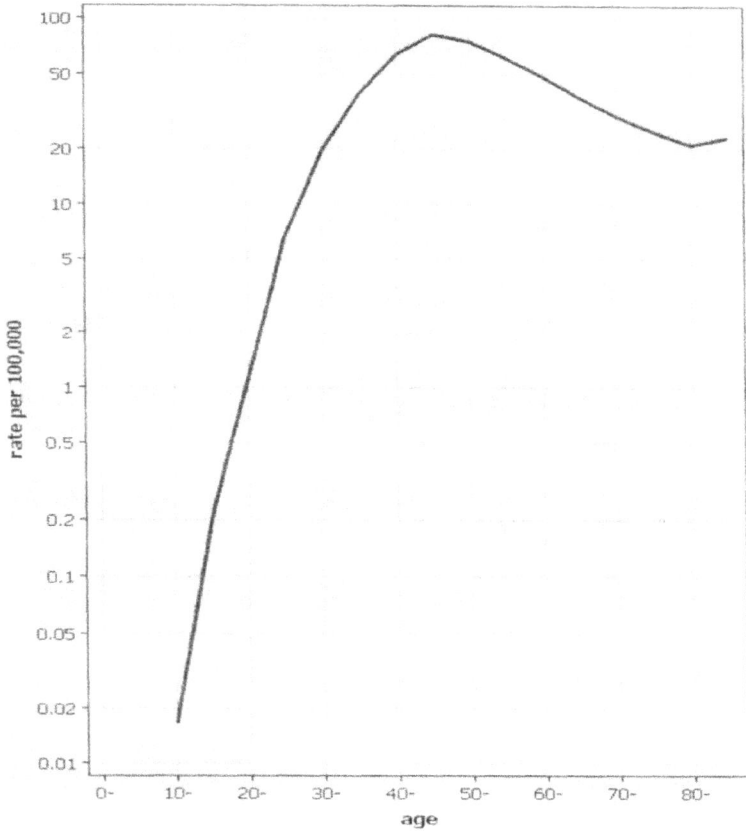

Fig. 15. Breast Cancer in Korea, 1988-2002. Age-specific incidence rates, per 100,000

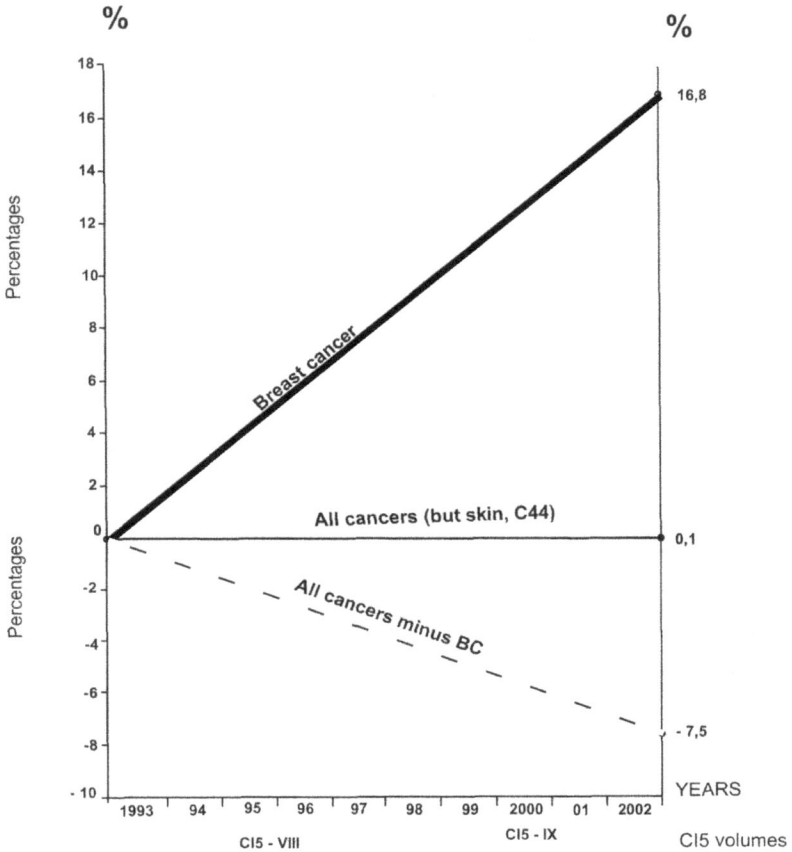

Fig. 16. Diverging trends of increase of breast cancer, and decrease of the 'rest' of all cancers in Afro-American women, 1993-2002, SEER - 9 regions. Age-standardized incidence rates, per 100,000

The differences in incidence rates and the diverging, comparative trends of increase and decrease of breast cancer and the 'rest' of cancers in women of both races (white and Afro-American), living in a reasonably same environment, gives credence to the evidence that the environmental chemicals/toxins, and of the women's nature culprit estrogen theory, are not the likely risk factors of the disease. The root cause of the modern-time women's suffering (breast cancer), is in certain other areas, such as, the "inverse" etiological risk factor at play at personal, intimate (sexual) and familial levels, as postulated.

Exactly the same pattern of diverging trends of rising breast cancer incidence rates as contrasted to decreasing incidence all other forms of cancer ('rest" of cancers) has been determined in Sweden in the past, Poland (Warsaw City) at the recent past and other centers in the world, according to the latest CI5 data (1998-2002). The same source shows that breast cancer incidence rates increased for 14.1% in Hong Kong, while the "rest" of cancer declined for minus 6.7% between decades 1993-97 and 1998-2002. The Shanghai City, a fast developing urban conglomerate, and similar to Hong Kong in population and number of breast cancer cases, showed the same trends of increase, of 29.8%, of breast cancer (age-adjusted incidence rates), and increase of 9.7% of the "rest" of cancers. Once again, the differing end-results of breast cancer between the two Chinese metropolises may corroborate the evidence that increase of the disease in Hong Kong, along with the decrease of the "rest" of cancers, is more related to other than poisonous risk factors in the environment, than the (fast) increase of breast cancer in Shanghai (together with the "rest" of cancers), which might be related to ecological pollution of presumed exposures to noxious workplace environments. The notion of better controlled environment-related cancers, defined as "rest" of cancers and excluding breast cancer, might be seen in the following examples for the two periods between 1993-97 and 1998-2002: Higher breast cancer rise and trailing rise of the "rest" of cancers is observed in Sweden, at country level again, with 3.3% breast cancer rise and -1.6% decline of the "rest" of cancers), Geneva (Switzerland, with a 6.2% breast cancer rise and -3.0% decline of the "rest" of cancers), Tyrol (Austria, with 4.9% breast cancer rise, and a practically stalled rise of "rest" of cancers, of 0.3%). Virtually, almost all centers of cancer registration in the world, for the two aforementioned periods, showed much higher percentages of breast cancer rises as compared with the increase of the "rest" of cancers.

The intermediate figures and other tabulated data which are to be presented, will try to corroborate once again the underlying tested theory (hypothesis) of the exposure forces of the misconceived barrier contraception as the main risk factor, attributed as the root cause of the epidemic of the gender-specific diseases. Almost no other known alteration in the inter-human environment or corruption of the intimate (sexual) woman-man ecosystem has taken place in the population(s), but the misconceived ubiquitous mass condomization, making this overlooked fallacy an exceedingly hazardous "minefield" to the health, lives and happiness of women and girls in the modern world. In contemporary dictionary of profit-driven healthcare system, the biological risk factors and exposure to ever-rising breast cancer and other epidemic diseases in women are considered as "keeping the healthy people in the risk pool" and "death spiral." From the deliberately maintaining the "risk pool" leading to scare, anxiety and "death spiral" of cost and uncertainties, new health-care dynamics are created, by which the insurance companies recruit eternal number of cases of breast-cancer affected women for "downstream" clinical activities, deceptively defined and disguised as "preventive health care for women," and which include "preventive screening," "preventive mammography programs" for "early detection," and clinical treatments (surgery and chemotherapy). (The failed, previously carried out community "chemo-prevention" trials on healthy women with *tamoxifen* against breast cancer, in a number of European and North American regions, in the 1990s, is not an active option anymore.)

Most of the results and data evaluated in the study would stay open-ended, to monitor the further developments of the increasing trends of the breast cancer epidemic, until after the decision and public option for intervention is implemented for practical elimination of the breast cancer epidemic and the accompanied diseases-tumors of female reproductive system. (Practical elimination of the excess breast cancer epidemic worldwide might be defined as is a virtual 'eradication' of the disease(s) to low incidence rates of sporadic cases the disease(s) at individual, familial and community levels.)

4.5 Ovarian cancer
Besides breast cancer, an integral part of the comprehensive research of the reproductive health of women is the ovarian and endometrial cancers. In this regard, observations and results in joint breast-ovarian cancer research experience are presented. The following commentary to highly publicized results in prevention of ovarian cancer by oral contraceptive pills is presented: Adjacent to cancer of the ovary are considered the polycystic syndrome, menstrual irregularities, endometriosis, female sexual dysfunction, low pelvic pain, craps, bloating.

The following critical comment was communicated to Prof. Valerie Beral, the Director of the **Cancer Research UK** and the lead author of the "Study: the Pill Protects against Ovarian Cancer," as reported by Washington Post Online, January 25, 2008 (Fragments):

"The Oxford study reported only a partial truth about the prevention / protection against ovarian cancer in the United Kingdom and elsewhere. Yet, the research of the root cause of the epidemic extent of ovarian cancer has NOT been done.

Despite the brief, but interrupted, heated exchange with the author and other presiding colleagues 14 years ago, at the 'Lancet International Breast Cancer Challenge Conference' (Brugge, Belgium, April 1994), about the tested evidence... that the CONDOMIZATION of women's sexuality, as the main root cause of the rising epidemics of epidemic breast cancer and other malignancies (ovarian and endometrial cancers), has been ignored and circumvented time and again, and not investigated to date...

It is a real wonder that there were such women who used oral contraceptive pills during the long era of indiscriminate promotion of 'condom culture;' a minority of 'non-politically correct' women and couples who rejected, even periodically the use of condoms, perhaps by listening to their inner sense of impaired sexuality and health consequences. For, many millions of women suffered and died mainly in the Western world, including the UK, during the twin breast and ovarian epidemics. The deadly, false belief of the exposure to (use of) condoms as a "safe" device for fertility-control and family-planning purposes has apparently taken a heavy human toll, and puts many more lives in jeopardy.

Despite the controversial assertion (that OC pills 'increase' breast cancer while decreasing ovarian cancer), the fact remains that the OC pills (with prevalent use during the 1970s), did not create the breast cancer epidemic, but the condomization of female sexuality (since the beginning of the 1980s), has predictably precipitated the unprecedented natural experiment of rapid breast cancer rise as an epidemic disease, or has 'coincided' with the emergence of the current, unabated breast / ovarian / gynecological cancer epidemics. According to previous evidence, the preventive effect is recognized not because of the OC-pill chemical content, i.e., "the first medication...(which) cuts ovarian cancer," as claimed by the authors of the aforementioned statistical study, but rather because of the non-use or abandoned barriers contraceptive methods (mainly condoms), associated with the observed protection of ovarian / breast cancer.

The OC-pill claim as protective factor also contradicted the added statement by the authors of 'other protective measures' against ovarian cancer which included 'advice' for "having children or getting tubes tied." Those two human conditions (pregnancies or tubal ligation) oppose the presumed OC-pill preventive effects, for they contain neither exogenous, OC pill's estrogens nor any other medication. Consequently, the role of the

OC pills as a presumed preventive measure against cancer in women should be questioned and rejected as an interpretation of its effects, as highlighted previously in a discussion about 'Tubal ligation and risk of ovarian cancer" in the same journal, Lancet 2001; 358: 1467-70 (pp. 843-44).

Women may change the contraceptive methods during their reproductive lifetimes, and may frequently, even sporadically still use condoms, because of planned ignorance of its carcinogenic effects. It is anticipated that the termination of the main and perhaps the sole risk factor of breast / ovarian cancers, the universal condomization of women's sexuality, will bring about immediate health gain in the community. A practical 'eradication' of the diseases to levels of sporadic cases, is expected to reached in a speedy decline of the current, excess epidemics of breast and ovarian cancers, in a mirror image of the rapid rise of the sex- (gender-) specific malignant epidemics as they entered the human race more than two-and-a-half decades ago. What might help in defining and providing primary prevention of ovarian and breast cancer epidemics in the advanced courtiers of the West, including the UK, is the empowerment of the British and other women with the "Right to Know" legislation about life and death matters."

4.6 Thyroid cancer

An initial hypothesis-testing study, in the mid-1970s, showed evidence of a significant association between the exposure to condom use and the breast cancer development in American and other married women. During the mid-1980s, another field study corroborated the evidence of a postulated association between condom use and thyroid cancer in women as well. The study also confirmed the close relationship between these two female "sex- (gender-) specific" diseases of the breast and thyroid glands along with other accompanying diseases, tumors and cancers of female reproductive tract (Gjorgov, 1999).

A feedback was communicated to the New York Times, entitled: "Pseudo Answers to the Thyroid Cancer Contingency: Times Essentials" - "The Rising Incidence of Thyroid cancer," by **Carolyn Sayre** (NY Times, Oct. 15, 2010), as follows:

"The thyroid disorders and tumors, along with the other epidemic diseases that afflict women, such as breast cancer, showed to have the same etiologic root cause: the CONDOMIZATION of women's sexuality. I have investigated in the field of thyroid cancer and I strongly believe that the aforementioned Times essentials of thyroid cancer are incomplete and out of reality.

Firstly, the information in the article should have provided separate data of women (i.e., for the so-named in the article "certain groups"?) and should not referred to "people" rather than women throughout the article. The existing evidence suggests that the female thyroid cancer may etiologically differ from that in males. Besides the assumed environmental causes, the reproductive causes apparently play a major, additional causative role in the development of thyroid cancer in women. The female-male difference of the root causes of thyroid cancer in the past three decades (since the beginning of 1980s) may confirm or provide further evidence of the potential of primary (non-chemical) prevention of the disease in women to a great extent. The existing epidemiological evidence points out to a situation that thyroid cancer falls into the same category of the female sex- (gender-) specific diseases, along with breast cancer. While the ratio of breast cancer is about 100 in women to 1 in men, the ratio of thyroid cancer in women is unanimously around or greater than three times of that of men.

Perhaps no one should be so mystified about the emerging, epidemic thyroid diseases nowadays, including the erratic thyroid cancer. Along with the other epidemic diseases which afflict women, such as breast cancer and the thyroid disorders have, almost certainly, the same etiologic root cause: the condomization of women's sexuality.

Inferring from the NYT article, it could be assumed that out the 45,000 thyroid cancer cases in the U.S. there were at least 1,125,000 thyroid-nodule biopsies, out of which about 843,750 thyroid-nodule biopsies were performed to about 33,750 women a year. It may confirm the assessment that the magnitude of the number of biopsies and other diagnostic procedures equal the scale of clinical diagnostic activities conducted to the epidemic of breast cancer.

It is anticipated that both widespread, epidemic diseases in women, breast cancer and thyroid disorders / nodules, could practically be eliminated ('eradicated' to sporadic cases), by a still pending, primary (non-chemical) prevention of the current breast cancer epidemic.."

(The comment was first communicated to the 'mystifying emergence' of Oprah's Thyroid Club almost three years earlier, on October 25, 2007),

The idea of similarity of risk factors of breast and thyroid cancers along with other female specific cancers, diseases and other phenomena was not widely known. The availability of the exceptionally rich cancer data in the WHO-IARC editions of the 'Cancer Incidence in Five Continents' (in last six editions) offered an opportunity to test the association, on global as well as regional scale (North America, South America, Europe, Asia, Australia, Africa), in addition to race (white, Afro-American), and developmental stage (developed and developing countries). The following **Table 4** presents the correlation coefficients and significance levels, of world data.

Country / Population	Vol. III: 1968-1972	Vol. IV: 1973-1977	Vol. V: 1878-1982	Vol. VI: 1983-1987	Vol. VII: 1988-1992	Vol. VIII: 1993-1997	Vol. IX: 1998-2002
# of places	80	104	159	166	183	211	300
Breast Ca.	.212*	.265*	.205*	.323*	.166*	.284**	.225**
Cervix Ca.	-.027	-.142	.041	-.060	-.118	-.208**	-.084
Uterus Ca.	.400**	.232**	.274**	.205**	,230**	..322**	.271**
Ovary Ca.	.078*	.080	.294**	.158*	.029	.224**	.538**

Legend:
⁺Age-adjusted according to World Standard Population (WSP), *Statistical significance p<.05
**Statistical significance p<.01 or p<.001

Table 4. Thyroid Cancer: Correlation coefficients with Breast cancer and other Cancers of reproductive system in women, World data: 1968-2002. Age-adjusted incidence rates, per 100,000.female population.

The results showed positive associations for breast, ovarian and endometrial cancer on global scale, and negative association with the cancer of the cervix uteri. The results are in accord with the postulated condomization exposure of women. The correlations coefficients

controlling for regional, especially on American and European variables and other developmental and racial variables reiterated the conclusion of a common root cause of breast and thyroid cancers. A series of dietary factors investigated in the study showed no significant results. The study was published in the journal
"Libri Oncologici" in Zagreb, Croatia. A brief summary of the "(Gjorgov, 1998a), is presented below:

Risk Factors Of Female Thyroid Cancer In Kuwait: A Retrospective Study (Summary)
Background. A case-control study was conducted in Kuwait during 1984-1985, in order to ascertain the reproductive characteristics, contraceptive practice, and dietary habits of 101 women with primary thyroid cancer (TC), aged 19-65 years, and a comparative group of 98 control women, free of the disease, and matched by age and nationality status. Information was obtained by personal interview with a questionnaire. **Objectives.** The study investigated the relationship between the risk factors in the domain of fertility control, known or postulated to be related to breast cancer, and the risk of TC in women. **Results.** The study showed that both groups of cases and controls were homogeneous and comparable in almost all studied factors. Differences at statistically significant levels were observed, however, in two contraceptive exposures: the TC patients reported more frequent and more extended use of condoms than the controls (P<.05), whereas the controls reported more extended exposure to oral contraceptives than the TC cases (P<.01). The highest relative risk (odds ratio) to the disease, OR = 4.3 (95%CI: 0.5--39.2), and adjusted OR = 7.1 (95%CI: 0.6--78.9), was observed for women with condom use of more than two years. In regard to the dietary factors, no appreciative differences were found for most of the investigated food items, except a difference of borderline significance of higher consumption of sugared products among the TC cases, and a significant difference of a higher consumption of sugared drinks among the controls. **Conclusions.** The findings of barrier contraceptive risk factors (condoms) in this study may help explain the similarity and analogy of the epidemiology of these predominantly female sex-specific neoplasms, cancer of the thyroid and cancer of the breast.
Key words: Reproduction, Contraception, Barrier methods, Condom, Non-barrier methods, Oral contraceptive, Diet

---

4.7 Other reproductive-health adverse effects
4.7.1 Adverse effects of condomization on female sexual dysfunction
Besides the new investigations into some new phenomena falling under a diagnosis of "FSDs" (female sexual dysfunctions), as further collateral, potential side effects of changed inter-human (woman-man) micro-environment could also come under consideration for investigation both the increased frequencies of divorce, and the more frequent reports of women's unhappiness. The assumption of condomization being associated with allegedly newly defined condition 'FSD' – Female sexual dysfunction – and the ensuing discussion in the **British Medical Journal**-Online, 2003, is presented in the following rapid response (Gjorgov, 2003):

Condomization of female sexuality - the cause of the FSD (Female Sexual Dysfunction) (Gjorgov, 2003)
"In the recent article about the female sexual dysfunction (FSD) (Moynihan, 2003) and in the ensuing rapid reactions and debate about the subject matter, the keystone factor of the

female sexuality is amazingly missing across the board: the factor MAN. This background of culturally conditioned deficit convinced me that the research on FSD is being taken out of context. In addition, it seems that the FSD is not a static condition, developing by random choice and aimless. As emphasized in the article and the comments, the FSD has certainly a poorly understood etiology, but it might be evolving into some realms of unknown end-result(s).

More than 25 years ago, a hypothesis-testing study[2] on primary breast cancer prevention and etiology was completed jointly at the University of North Carolina School of Public Health, at Chapel Hill, NC, and at the University of Pennsylvania School of Medicine and Hospital, in Philadelphia, PA, USA, during the mid-1970s. The study has tested and corroborated an a priori hypothesis on "semen factors" (deficiency) that an extended exposure to (use of) barrier contraception, specifically, the long-term condom use, and/or withdrawal practice, is significantly associated with the development of breast cancer in married American and other women, including the British women. Besides defining a new approach to the etiology of and the potential for a primary (non-chemical) prevention of breast cancer, another main contribution, I believe, of my cancer research has been the evidence-based inference that SEX along with marriage and love is a fundamental PHYSIOLOGICAL unit, above and beyond the psychological, social, economic, reproductive and legal linkage. The final report of the study, entitled, "BARRIER CONTRACEPTION AND BREAST CANCER" (Gjorgov, 1980) was published as a monograph by S. Karger Med. Publ., Basel-New York, in the distant 1980. (Since the book has been effectively banned from the public view and professional information, the breast cancer research was first published in the dissertation format, in 1979, by the University of Michigan Dissertation International, Ann Arbor, MI 48106; UMI publication # 79-14352.)

It was further indicated in the study that breast cancer is a systemic disease and not a random event, and that the breast carcinogenesis is most likely passing through nonspecific and unrecognized phases, manifesting itself in a number of trivial or undistinguishable symptoms in women's lives (Gjorgov, 1995), presumably such as the FSD, and eventually reaching a definite stage of overt breast cancer and other accompanying disease end-results, as predicted (Gjorgov, 1993, 1994a; Gjorgov, 1994b). An experimental trial (Gjorgov, 1999) of sterile mating on a colony of small laboratory animals corroborated the preventive efficacy of the semen factors (the prostaglandins) on mammary neoplastic tumors, and on the general impact on animal-female lives and health. The condom use introduces technical effects of absolute male sterility in marriages, placing an impregnable wall between the protective biology of man and woman, and converting their marriages into infertile male partners. It is quite conceivable that many a woman may feel the ill- effects ("female sex problems") because of the persistent and un-physiological condom use, and that the woman is reflexively trying to protect herself by escape, distancing, separation or reluctance against the unwittingly afflicting insults (!) upon her done by her technically sterile husband. It seems quite evident and certain that during the long evolution, Nature has not adjusted the species to sterile mating, including the humans.

Within the framework of the tested "semen-factor" (condom) hypothesis in breast cancer, partial comments, opinion and paraphrases on the FSD debate: - Perhaps "Body-mind" rather than "Mind-body" relationships is a better model than the psychiatric and social understanding of the FSD; - Contrary to what was mentioned, sex is NOT "Like Dancing": Sex is a physiological impact; - There is evidence that the continuing promotion of condoms use as a "normal sexual behavior" and/or (PC) contraceptive practice is lethal (breast cancer); - "Sexual functioning is an integral part of our lives" and perhaps of (gender) physical survival; - The feminist nonsense as a recipe for producing FSD: "masturbation" in females; - The "Conspiracy of Silence" for FSD is even more so for the unabated breast cancer epidemic; - The FSD, "as potentially epidemic condition" could and should be better handled in the services and domain of the Gynecologists-Obstetricians rather than the Urologists. - The "environmental intervention" in FSD, like in the breast cancer epidemic: Eradication of the "INVERSE" environmental factor, the barrier of the condom use that is eliminating, reducing or making absence the protective biological mechanisms in the intimate and subtle, inter-human (sexual) environment and ecosystem.

No wonder that the FSD is so prevalent in British and American women (reportedly, about 43%), for both are "high-risk" populations of breast cancer and are among the leading breast-cancer epidemic countries, with the highest breast cancer incidence and death rates in the world. Since the CONDOMIZATION of human sexuality seems to be the singular most important factor in the women's sexual dysfunction, my humble and evidence-based suggestion is simple and brief:

ABOLISH THE USE OF CONDOMS FOR CONTRACEPTIVE, FERTILITY-CONTROL AND FAMILY-PLANNING PURPOSES in the British marriages and couples, and make an urgent shift to the "non-barrier" methods of contraception (Gjorgov & Narod, 2001a). It is long overdue to make the British and other women happy."

4.7.2 Condomization, abortions, 'missed abortions,' and pseudopregnancy

The following letter to the **Editor of the New York Times**, referring to the editorial "Abortion, Condoms and Bush," by **Nicholas D. Kristof**, NYT November 5, 2006, tackles the issue of condoms, "missed abortion," and breast cancer:

Condoms, Condoms, Condoms…and Abortions. A critical reply
"Mr. Kristof seems biased and medically ill-informed by discussing a biological issue like abortions and condoms. What kind of abortion "rise" and "fall" throughout the past (three) decades and during (six) presidential periods? Discussion of temporal changes of all (i) the artificial, (ii) spontaneous, and (iii) so-called "missed" abortions? And, on top of this professional mix-up and mystery of abortions, a cause-and-effect link is added to the (predominant) use of condoms?

The (i) artificial abortions are carried out by demands, and reflect a fertility capacity of at least the woman. The artificial abortions burden the soul of the women in tremendous psychological pain, are reluctantly performed, and socially have always been quite controversial.

The (ii) spontaneous abortions reflect an infertility / sub-fertility status of both partners, usually married, and may indicate a hidden plight in building the family. The infertility condition is an acknowledged risk factor of development of breast cancer and other women's ill health.

The (iii) "missed abortion" is an utterance of professional, clinical perplexity. As a pastime term it could only be found in older editions of gynecology textbooks. The contemporary professionals try hard to avoid diagnosis of "missed abortion," for its occurrence is not understood, and indicates a situation of false pregnancy. The condition is connected with the use of condoms. The 'failure-rate' of the use of condoms as contraceptive device is (uncritically) estimated to be around 9 percent. In fact, the use of condoms is induction of technical effects of absolute male sterility in the intimate (sexual) relations. (The prolonged or repetitious condition of false pregnancy is presumed as the initial, still reversible stage of breast cancer and other sex- (gender-) specific diseases in women of all ages.)

In my informed view, the reported, intermittent phrasing of "sharp rise," "tiny increase" and/or "tiny fall" of abortions throughout time are misleading, inaccurate and incomplete. Actually, who knows whether the reports of abortions could ever be better exact?

On the other hand, the sharp rise and spiraling advent of the breast cancer epidemic in the country, in the last two-and-a-half decades (since the beginning of 1980s), the unending epidemic of malignant disease associated with the persistent condom use, is strangely overlooked in the column assessment.

The professional misjudgment and incompetence seem to be manifested in the confusion and equation of the use of condoms as a general category of family planning. The euphemism of "comprehensive sex education" practically means condom promotion / distribution in the schools, with condomization of the nascent sexuality of the schoolgirls, the youngest generation(s) of the American population, with unknown grave consequences / sequels.

As a young congressman, George H.W. Bush may have sponsored the 1970 public health program of family planning services which, almost certainly, may have included condoms, but, as President, he is recorded at a series on ABC television stations, in 1990, as rejecting distribution of condoms: "Not for me and not for the federal government... I don't think that just passing out condoms, giving up on lifestyle, giving up on family and fundamental values is correct... In terms of just national passing out of condoms to people, I am not in favor of that." So, President George W. Bush seems to be actually continuing the family roots. His energetic condom-paradigm shift and the potential of curbing the current breast cancer epidemic with the new anti-condom reproductive policy are anticipated to achieve an impending 'eradication' of the dreaded epidemic disease to the levels of sporadic cases in the country and far beyond."

NOTE: In less than a month, on Dec. 5, 2006, the New York Times run an article entitled; "All the signs of pregnancy except one: A baby," by Elizabeth Svoboda (Svoboda, 2006). Apparently, the NYT editors have investigated the above critique, confirming the information of false pregnancy which was repeatedly termed by its ancient Greek name, *pseudocyesis*. By quoting certain medical authorities, a skepticism was underlined that "human pseudocyesis will never be completely scientifically understood," and another assertion that it is "one of the classic examples how the mind affects the rest of the body." In fact, the condomization of female sexuality (pseudocyesis) may prove to be one of the classic examples of how the injured body affects the mind, rather than the way around. The issue of false pregnancy is associated with the condom-related "reproductive freedom" fallacy (Gjorgov, 1980, 1996a).

4.8 Anorexia-bulimia ('eating') disorders

The literature of Anorexia-Bulimia (conveniently called "eating") disorders match only that of breast cancer. The number of new cases of anorexia and bulimia disorders rose rapidly worldwide in the past three decades, 1980s, 1990s, and 2000s, the rampant condition is rising ever since, continuing its rise in the 2000s, especially in the developed West, such as, the U.S. and the E.U.

A descriptive study was conducted in young female patients in mid-200s, at the Psychiatric outpatient clinic at the Faculty of Medicine of the University Sts. Cyril and Methodius, in Skopje, Macedonia, in order to assess the sub-hypothesis that (illicit) barrier contraception (condom use and withdrawal practice) is a risk factor of anorexia-bulimia disorders in schoolgirls, college female students, and other young women and brides (Gjorgov, 2009a). The main results indicated of the study indicated that the anorexia-bulimia patients [with mean age of 23.3 years (sd= 3.1)] used overwhelmingly condom device and equally practiced withdrawal technique for contraceptive purposes, during most of their young sexual experience and initial reproductive lives, as opposed to negligible use of OC pills.

On the basis of the prior observation (the sub-hypothesis), a confident communication along with a suggestion was forwarded almost 14 years ago to the **Swedish Royal Family**, concerning the announcement of the worrisome 'eating' disorder condition in the future Queen of the country, as follows:

M-me Elisabeth Tarras-Wahlberg, Spokeswoman, Skopje, December 10, 1997
The Royal Palace, Stockholm, Sweden

Dear Madam,

This is a humble attempt to try to address, as a physician and researcher, the reported news in the media of a heavy body-weight loss of Her Royal Highness Princess Victoria and to try to suggest a new possible approach in the efforts for solving this worrisome situation.

In my opinion, the heavy body-weight loss, so called *Anorexia nervosa*, is secondarily related to the problems of nutrition and diet. Rather, there is circumstantial evidence, that the life-threatening condition of *Anorexia nervosa* is perhaps causally related to the demands of reproductive and intimate life and to its applied technical barriers. The alternative hypothesis about the nature of *Anorexia nervosa* was deducted from a "byproduct" observation in my long research of the developmental processes in the field of breast cancer. Furthermore, the frequent condition of a prior excess body loss (and gain) in the affected, young, reproductive-aged women with breast cancer was controlled for and partially tested as a sub-hypothesis in my hypothesis-testing study of barrier contraception (the condom use and withdrawal practice) as an etiological risk factor associated to breast cancer in married American women.

During my field and ecological studies of breast cancer, it became obvious that the condom use in your country has been quite prevalent, with all the postulated subsequent consequences of the widespread misconception that "the use of condom has no side effects." On the other hand, breast cancer in Sweden has been reported and registered as one of the highest in the world, and still raising, mainly because of the widespread and long-term condom use in the general population, as postulated. In my separate study of the epidemiology and rising trends of breast cancer in Sweden, in 1992, the potential for prevention and control of the current breast cancer epidemic in the country was elaborated and suggested. Because the study could not be publish, copies of it were sent from Kuwait University to a number of health and political authorities and institutions in Sweden, as a personal communication.

Based on my research experience, I do believe that the exposure to the condom use (i.e., to technically induced sterile stimulation) induces some devastating effects to a normal, young, vivacious, healthy woman, among which the life-threatening response of *Anorexia nervosa* seems to be one of the most frequent condition in the advanced countries, such as Sweden. The assessment of H.H. the Princess' condition is done on incomplete information and on certain assumptions, which might not be correct. Nevertheless, the possible way out of the anorectic danger for such a lady, in my opinion, would be the absolute elimination of the condom as a fertility-control device, by reverting to any of the non-barrier contraceptive methods (the pills, diaphragm, rhythm, IUDs, creams-jellies), in order to be able to preserve the healthy reproductive and inter-human life, and to prevent neoplastic phenomena.

Enclosure: Clipping from the daily newspaper. Respectfully submitted, …

(The letter was acknowledged with thanks for the 'wish to help.')

A similar communication was submitted recently to the Chairwoman of the **White House Council on Women and Girls** and Special Advisor the President, on December 10, 2010, concerning the rampant "eating' disorders cases in the U.S. and other developed countries of the West, as follows:

Dear Madam Special Advisor: Re: Eating Disorders Prevention

"Along with the Best wishes to Rep. Alcee L. Hastings and Patrick J. Kennedy and 34 Members of the Congress for their initiative to incorporate the global eating-disorders issue into the First Lady Michelle Obama "Let's Move Campaign" and the "Federal Response to Elimination of Eating Disorders (FREED) Act 2010."

Just to reiterate that there are no greater "strong environmental, cultural, and social factors" associated to or causing eating disorders, as mentioned in the letter to the First Lady (July 21, 2010), but the condomization of the nascent sexuality of schoolgirls, college and other women in the population. An all-inclusive approach to women's health and the new research of both the breast cancer epidemic and the rampant anorexia-bulimia disorders has identified as the main root cause of the specific sex- (gender-) diseases in women the misconceived and deadly, false belief of condom as a "safe" device for fertility-control and family-planning use.

My concern is, yet, that the blackout history of the past three decades may repeat itself, to continue stocking the unabated breast cancer epidemic in middle-age women (mothers), and extending the ill effects to the helpless anorexia-bulimia bewildered young women (daughters). The strongly reinforced, misleading, renewed condom-use offensive, oblivious of the greatest ill-health consequences to the half of the population, is poised to persist with the discrimination against women, girls and couples, by withholding the potentially life-saving information of a primary (non-chemical, non-profit) prevention / protection against the grave female-specific diseases at personal, familial and community levels. "

4.9 Osteoporosis

Osteoporosis far exceeds in frequency (incidence and prevalence) all other conditions in the female populations. During the past decades, since the early 1980s, osteoporosis and its sequels rapidly rose and continued its unabated rise, reaching excess epidemic proportions. As a "silent epidemic," osteoporosis has become highly prevalent as a great clinical and societal burden, and a heavy public health problem of highest priority, especially in the affluent North American, European and other communities. A systemic disease, affecting 7.8 million women in the U.S. and worldwide, osteoporosis is diagnosed by low bone mass than average and steadily deteriorating bone tissues, leading to bone fragility and increased fracture risk. In the U.S. and Europe, 1 in 3 or even 2 women over 50 years of age will develop the disease, and more and more affecting premenopausal women. Presently, there is a gap in the efforts to control, treat and prevent the osteoporosis. The predominant theories of diet, calcium and vitamin D deficiency, and other macro-environmental factors have advanced no progress in the etiology, treatment and prevention of the osteoporosis in women. The traditional and doctrinaire approaches have neither identified the etiological causes of the osteoporosis epidemic nor defined the ways of preventing the disease in the community and at individual and family levels. Within the framework of the Bone and Joint Decade 2000-2010, an attempt was made by submitting a project proposal to test a new hypothesis of an etiological relationship between the barrier contraception and the risk of osteoporosis development in women. The proposed hypothesis of the etiology of osteoporosis (and osteopenia) and of the potential of primary prevention of the condition in women postulates that the osteoporosis is a late, delayed and/or a prolonged consequence of the marital exposure to (use of) barrier forms of contraception (specifically, condoms and/or withdrawal, and male/family infertility) during the reproductive, pre-menopausal age span of women (Gjorgov, 2006).

Once again, various manifestations of affected bone health, such as the low back pain, showed distinct increase in prevalence the U.S., after the 1980s, the same alleged time period during all other ill-health developments occurred in women (**Figure 17**).

Osteoporosis, and its initial stage, osteopenia, are perplexed with misinformation and misconceptions. First, the proportion of women with osteoporosis over men with osteoporosis is almost nine times greater in women than in men, which fact is not always underlined for further considerations; Second, the condition fall into the setting of so called sex- (gender-) specific diseases in women (like breast cancer, in proportion 100:1 females to males; Third, the grave condition do not 'naturally' come with age (look at the Sybille figures of the Michelangelo frescoes); Fourth, not all women carry the same risk of osteoporosis; Fifth, the (mystified) "FRAX" osteoporosis / osteopenia risk assessment tool from the osteoporosis associations, consists of majority of the same spurious and secondary risk factors of breast cancer; Sixth, a primary (natural) prevention of the conditions has neither been mentioned nor considered. Since the idea of potential breast cancer prevention is that it should start long before the malignant tumors are diagnosed, it could be safe to suppose that the "natural" (non-chemical) prevention of the crippling conditions of osteoporosis/osteopenia should be attempted at the same time along with the prevention of the other gynecological lesions, or even earlier, during the peak of the reproductive lives of women. Information for prevention seems far superior to pharmaceutical marketing concerning the chemical control and 'treatment' of osteoporosis and osteopenia in women.

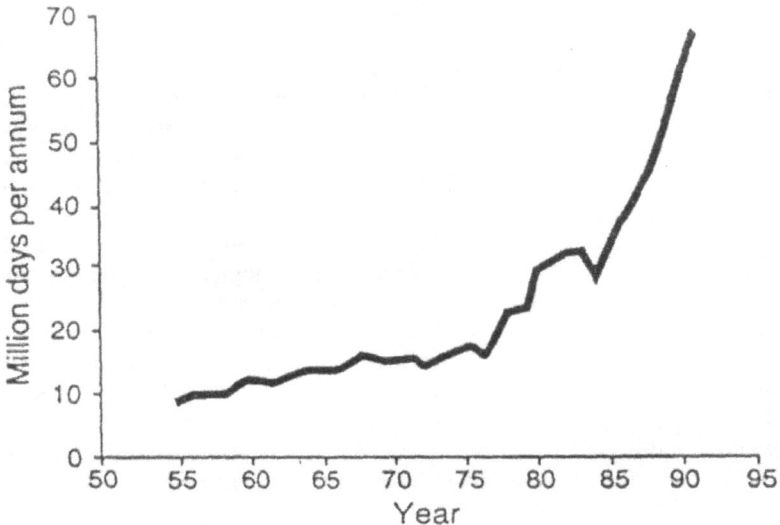

Fig. 17. Low back pain increasing trend in the U.S., 1955-1995.

5. Social and demographic consequences

5.1 Condomization adverse effects in marriage and divorce

The issues of contraception, marriage and divorces have been speculated upon frequently, mainly in the denominational quarters, in the U.S and elsewhere, under the sign of "controversial" issues and in some instance under feministic tendencies of interpretation. In the numerous judicial and social literature of the causes of divorce, some findings seem novel, such as he information that more women seek divorce than men nowadays (Ambekar, 2009) that divorces take husbands by surprise (Peatlng, 2005), that sex is a reason for divorce and that "dissatisfied women are less likely to have sex" (Kimbal, 2010). Some older sources of religious discussion were practically out of reach (Peters, 1998). It was early warning that the divorce rates have much risen recently. Hardly any of the recent studies in marriage, divorce and sexuality ever considered condoms as an impediment to marital relations.

Other recent reports confirmed the rapidly increasing divorce rates in the U.S., with a distinct jump at the end of the 1970s and the beginning of the 1980s, greatly surpassing any divorce rates in the U.S. over the recorded past 150 years (Stevenson & Wolfers, 2007a, 2007b; Wolfers, 2010). The surprising rise of the divorce rate, greater than that recorded after WWII, and subsequently fluctuating and slowly declining trend was presented in the first figure in the text. The explanation of the truly distinct changes of the divorce rates, with the mass and still high jump in divorce rates was not fully explained in the report. (Figure 18). The presumed 'driving forces' of divorce talked about a variety of conventional causes, such as, importance of marriage has changed, rising age at first marriage, high remarriage rates, rise of cohabitation, rise of out-of-wedlock fertility, and other social and economic reasons.

In a response to the authors, Betsey Stevenson and Justin Wolfers, a critical commentary of the missing biological dimension in their scholarly analysis of national data of divorce and marriage, underlying the following points:

"It seems we could not really know about the break-up of marriages, "long" or "new," if only the "broader economic and social consequences" are being considered, by forgetting the simple biological causes of the events.

By looking into the primary source of the news ("*Marriage and Divorce: Changes and their Driving Forces*," by B. Stevenson & J. Wolfers, 2007 & 2009; Brining & Allen, 2000), besides the scholarly done review and presentation of official registry, raw data, the way of thinking, heavily influenced by the old-time feminism, seems very one-sided and insufficiently interpreted. The woman is analyzed manly as a technological, social, economy- and business- oriented personality, with no reference whatsoever to her (their) biological individuality.

It was rightly emphasized in the study that marriage and divorce laws and regulations along with technical changes in the family do not explain the rise of divorces over the past few decades. And yet, the women "who suffer" are those who in majority file for divorce. The figure 1 in the aforementioned study, presenting the rates of marriages and divorces (per 1000 American people), stretching for 145 years (1860-2005) is truly revealing. It seems to explain to a great extent the missing references to the most critical period of rapidly rising and still on-going period of exceptionally high-divorce rates in the country in the decades of 1980s, 1990s, and first part of the 2000s: the mass CONDOMIZATION of female sexuality. While the contraceptive pills and their impact upon the society have been studiously explained, the destructive impact of the promoted use of condoms over the past three decades has been strangely overlooked, with an utter oblivion to the current, excess breast cancer epidemic, the greatest scare, dread and real risk of women, along with the widespread gynecological tumors and other afflictions.

Given the corroborated evidence that the condom use is significantly associated with the breast cancer development in American and other married women, it is not a wonder that many a woman is filing for divorce and, supposedly looking for a "new partner." Intimate condomized relations induce technical effects of absolute sterile husband in the marriage, perhaps worse stressor than other ones mentioned in the debate blog, such as "poor health, poverty, and unemployment." If in the biological struggle the wife is not supported (by a fertile husband), it is a general belief / observation, and she is turning against him. (The racial differences in rates of divorce are also consistent with the differences in breast cancer incidence and prevalence rates, the levels of condom-use acculturation.)

The figure 1 in the study seems circumvented in the analysis of the causes of the sudden bulge of skyrocketed rates of divorces ever since the end of 1970s and still on-going (in 2005). (The condomization started with rumors at the end of the 1970s.) It may be safe to assume that it is the most likely a response of women "who suffer" and try to escape (mainly by divorce) from the unknown but felt devastating and carcinogenic effects of sterile mating, and the incremental bodily and breast-cancer changes. Since the figure 1 with unusual trends of divorce trends is rarely seen in the literature, it may be worth following up the trend data, to witness the probable rapid fall of the divorce rates along with the information of the root cause(s) for and elimination (fall) of the epidemic breast cancer incidence rates and the main risk factor, the condom-control of women, perhaps at the earliest anticipated date, after the year 2010."

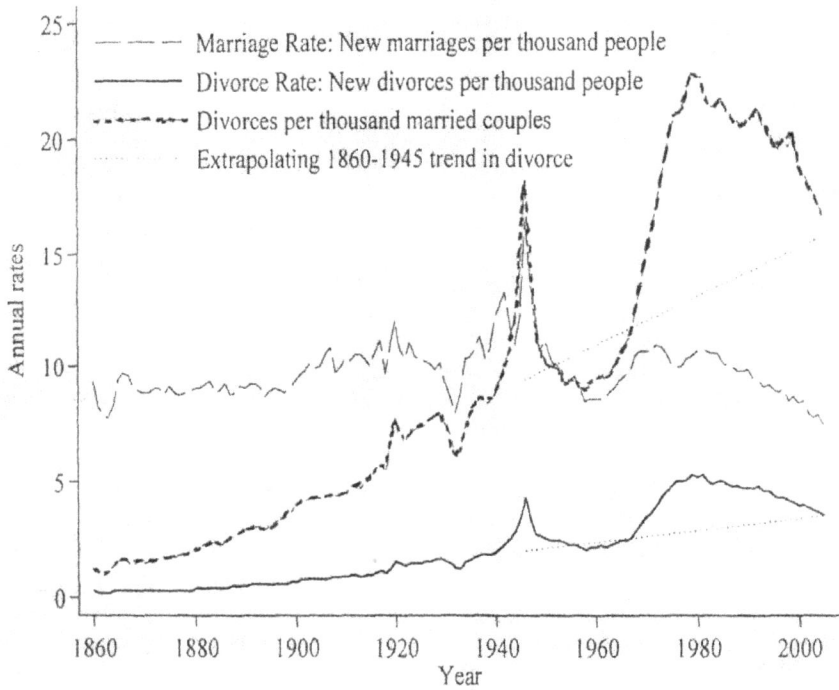

Fig. 18. Marriage and divorce rates in the United States, 1860-2000.

The unexplained changes in divorce rates reflected in other parts of the developed and affluent world. In **Australia**, a highly dramatic upsurge of divorce rates was recorded around 1978-1979, with a subsequent sharp decline and fluctuating changes afterwards (**Figure 19**) (Australian Historical Statistics, 2001). In the **UK**, the sudden almost threefold rise of the number of divorces was recoded somewhat earlier, in the mid-1978, and did not show appreciable decline for the next several years, until 2000 (**Figure 20**) (Office on National Statistics UK, 2004)...

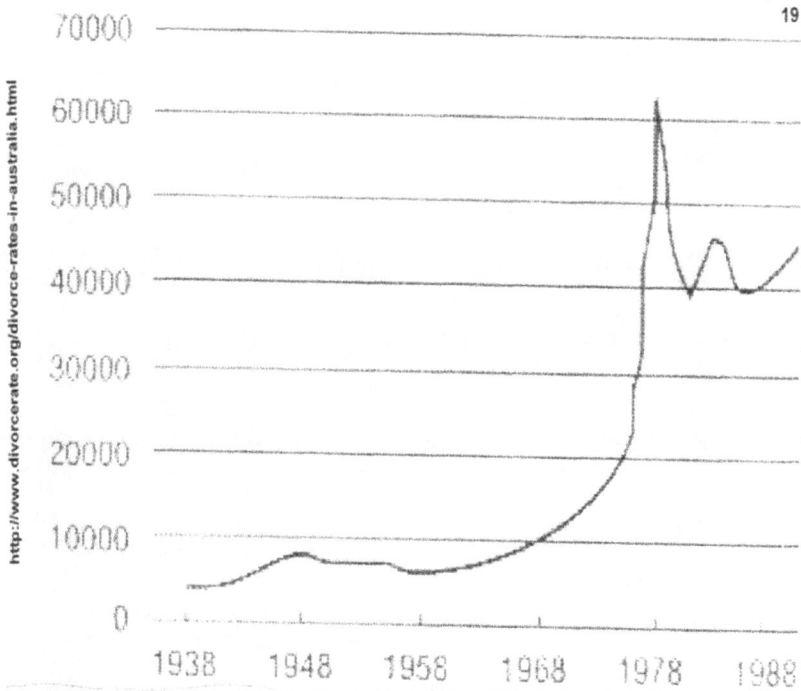

Source: Australian Historical Statistics and ABS

Fig. 19. Number of divorces in Australia, 1938-1991.

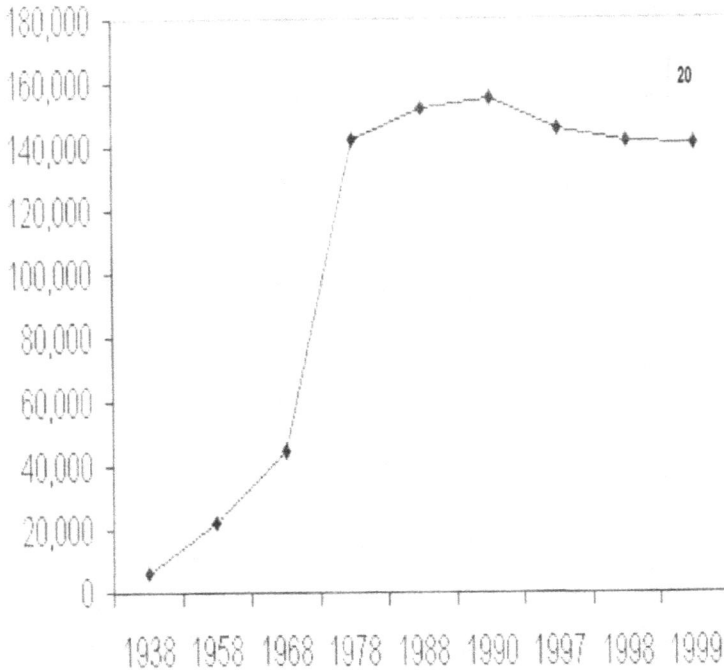

Fig. 20. Divorce rates in the UK, from 1938 to 1999.

In **Japan** there was also a wave of increased divorces as well (**Figure 21**) (Japanese Ministry of Health, 2002). However, the increase of the divorce rate in Japan showed at least three different demographic features: the increase was incremental and relatively lower, less than two rates (per 1000 population), against the increase in the U.S. (reaching more than 5.5 rate); and the peak of the divorce rates occurred about five years later than in the U.S. It is assumed that the changes in the divorce incidence rates may have the same driving force, stretching within a time period of several years, at the beginning of the 1980s.

The attempt for explanation of the observed social phenomena of high divorce outbreak did not reach considerations of condomization as a possible root cause of the observable fact. An attempt was made to address the issue of condoms as newly introduced environmental pollution in the inter-human intimate relations, in a comment to the article "Contraception and Divorce: Insight from American Annulment Cases," of 1998, by Dr. Edwards N. Peters, Edmund Card. Szoka Chair in Faculty Development, Canon of the Law Blog, Christmas 2010

"What prompted me to (belatedly) comment your article of 12 years ago is the ongoing routine of addressing condom as "contraception." In the mid-1970s, I conducted a hypothesis-testing study (jointly at two American universities) of the barrier contraception (condom use and withdrawal practice) and the development of breast cancer in American (and other) married women. The results corroborated the hypothesis and showed evidence of a significant condom and breast cancer association, together with the defined potential of primary (non-chemical) prevention of breast cancer as an epidemic disease. One of the main inferences was that marriage along with sexuality, love and family is a profound biological union between woman and man, along with the conventional definition of marriage as a social, economic, psychological, and legal unit.

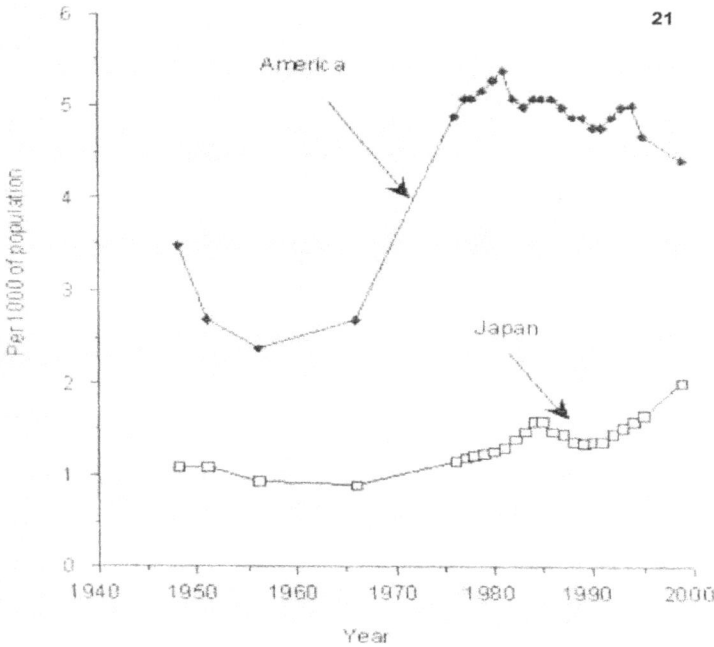

Fig. 21. American and Japanese divorce rates, from 1940 to 2000.

In a nutshell, condom is not a contraceptive method. This old/new (high-tech) barrier-device is literally a marriage-killer (divorce and a variety of psychosomatic phenomena and unhappiness) and woman-killer (breast cancer in mothers, and anorexia-bulimia disorders in young daughters). Condomization of female sexuality has been defined as the main and perhaps sole root cause of the unabated, excess breast cancer epidemic and other accompanying disorders of women and girls in the modern world. No other method of 'contraception' has been linked with the apparent natural experiment of the current breast cancer epidemic, or has shown the distinction to induce carcinogenic consequences on women on unprecedented scale in the country and societies globally. It seems that the study provided a basis of new understanding of contraception, and an attempt to use some of the (non-barrier) methods in preventive/therapeutical ways. In my view, the condomized control of women, rather the 'contraception' is the main causal factor for divorce, by which women supposedly try to escape from the deeply felt cancer-initiation process.

A real concern may present, time and again, the newly reinitiated, so-called "Rubber Revolution," the renewed, forceful and reckless condom promotion, entirely oblivious to the unabated, excess breast cancer epidemic, worldwide, and insensitive to the plight of the half of population, exposed to the highest risk of developing and suffering of the malignant epidemic disease(s) and other morbid phenomena."

The so-called Marriage calculator- divorce360 (Stevenson, 2010) could hardly fulfill its intended predictive purpose, since the analysis was based mainly on the educational levels and other social profiles of the spouses, and the failure (bias?) to consider the biological (sexual) dimension of marriage. Besides the calculator seems incomplete, because it lacks the necessary putative external risk factor quantified exposure, in order to serve as a Bayes' probability theorem requirements (Gjorgov, 2009b, 2010).

The dilemma of the official, but mistaken emphasis on strict promotion of use of condoms (in all sexual relations) in the U.S. House of Representatives (Lincoln, 1979) is given in the following personal communication to the **Honorable James H. Scheuer**, Chairman of the House Select Committee on Population, on May 29, 1979, in Philadelphia, PA:

"In reference to the conclusions of your Committee on Population concerning family planning policy, as reported by Richard Lincoln in *Family Planning Perspectives*, March/April 1979, the promotion of the "barrier" methods of contraception become an objective of first priority in the contraceptive research "of methods that are not known to be associated with hazardous side effects." No definition of "barrier" methods was presented in the journal's report (Lincoln, 1979) of the conclusions of your Committee. This is to inform you and your Committee that there are indications that some forms of barrier contraceptive methods are perhaps the most inadequate and hazardous methods for fertility regulation. This is also to present to you the available evidence of a recently completed study, indicating an association between the use of barrier contraceptive techniques and long-term health hazards in women. A barrier contraceptive, as defined in the study, is one which obstructs the passage and resorption of seminal content during sexual contact, such as the condom and withdrawal. The results of the tested hypothesis of the study corroborated the evidence that there is a significant relationship between barrier contraceptive practice and the development of breast cancer in women. The final findings corroborated the research hypothesis and the preliminary results of the study that women who used barrier contraceptive methods for extended periods of time in their marriages have a risk of developing breast cancer that is 4.6 – 5.2 times the risk of women who used other forms of fertility control. The results of the research also indicate that there is a potential for preventive action against the disease for a sizeable proportion of women in the population. It is estimated that by eliminating barrier contraceptive techniques, specifically the condom, and the incidence of breast cancer among married women in the United States could be reduced by as much as 50 percent. The results of the study consistently showed that the effects of a number of other reproductive and biological factors, such as age at first birth, parity, menarche, and others, had non-causal associations with the disease; The carcinogenic effect of the barrier contraceptive use was operative within a five-year exposure to condom use in marriage, with a cumulative effect; The study helps explain the increasing incidence of breast cancer, the international variation of the disease, and most of the reproduction-related risk indicators.

The final report, which is my dissertation, along with some other documents and material of the study would be gladly submitted to you and your Select Committee, if necessary. It is my belief that until further work in this field is done and confirmatory studies are conducted that this information of the devastating effects of condom use on woman's health should be made available to the users in community without unnecessary delay."

The recent report of the "Use of Contraception in the United States: 1982-2008" (Mosher and Jones, 2010) provided an abundance of data offering the opportunity to interpret the contraception figures, rates and trends in another way. There are a number of important findings which may shed a different light on the current discussion of the adverse impact of condomization upon society, and could be underlined, as such.

- It was stated in the Report that "in 2006-2008, 93 percent had ever had 'a partner' who used the male condom; 82 percent had ever used the oral contraceptive pill; and 59 percent had ever had 'a partner' who used withdrawal."

- The greatest increase of contraceptive methods recorded between 1982 and 1995 was for condoms, 79.5 percent of those who ever used the device, in comparison to OC pill, of only 7.9 percent increase. The increase of the condom 'ever used' prevalence in 1982 was 51.8 percent, and in 1995 82.0 percent, while the OC pill use remained virtually at a plateau, from ever-used prevalence of 94.5 percent in 1982 to 96.2 percent in 1995. For the next 13 years, until 2008, the increase of partners who have ever used condom was 93.0 percent (with 79.5 percent increase from 1982), while the OC pills ever used 82.3 percent (with 7.9 percent increase). The data may indicate that a combined (dual) use of condoms and OC pills might have been practiced, or an intermittent, non-consistent condom use.

- Changes in use of condom, pill and other contraceptive methods between 1982 and the subsequent years until 2008 clearly showed higher increases of all methods in certain ethnic groups in the U.S., corroborating the notion of condom acculturation as well. Thus, condom use by Hispanics at first sexual intercourse rose for 70.9 percent, for Afro-Americans 65.2 percent, and for whites 26.9 percent. OC pill dropped by -44.5 % for the Afro-American women, and withdrawal technique dropped by –17.3% for whites and -52.3% for Afro-Americans, but not for the Hispanics (which was low). The condom-use campaigns were not mentioned in taking place during the intervening years.

- Condom use by women aged 15-44 showed a declining trend after 1995, when the number of users (in thousands) declined from 13.1 to 11.1 in 2002, and to 10.0 in 2006-2008. The qualification of "persistent" condom use, which is considered practically impossible, because of the early adverse effects, use was not mentioned in the report.

- Prevalence of contraception use, both condoms and OC pills, was higher in younger groups up to age 30-34 than in the older groups 35-44, what is to be expected. The data of use of condom has obviously shifted to women of younger age which helps explain the "debut" breast cancer age-specific incidence peaks. The pill was used almost twice as much than condoms by women aged 20-24 (26.2 versus 13.4 by age, respectively); the condom was used in average of 10.0% by young women, and between 8.4 and 6.8 percent in older age groups 35-39 and 40-44. It looks like the ancient Roman "decimation" penal code is still powerful enough to make a strong impact on the community.

- Female sterilization was assessed at 27.1% in the 2006-2008 periods. There was age gradient of increase, showing a prevalence rate of 50.3% in the 40-44 age group. However, the unexpected high rate of "female sterilization" was not specified, in terms of proportion of elective tubal ligation and non-elective sterilizing surgical procedures. Tubal ligation is an established contraceptive method, but the hysterectomies and/or oophorectomies (one- or double-sided), are salvage surgical procedures carried out for survival in many cases of breast, ovarian and other gynecological cancers. The blurred category of "female sterilization" showed a gradual increase of rates by parity, to highest proportion, of 58.7%, in women with three or more children. Once again, the purpose of the "sterilization" has not been specified, but helps explain the increasing survival rates of breast cancer in younger patients. (The male sterilization, vasectomy, assessed at 9.9% in the studied population sample, in 2006-2008, is still considered too controversial a method of contraception for pertinent comments.)

- Reasons for discontinuation of ever used contraceptive method, included prominent concern for the OC pill. To the question of "You had side effects," the pill users responded positively in 63.7 percent, while only 12.0 percent of condom users responded positively; to the question "Did not like changes to menstrual cycle," positive answer provided 10.6 percent of the pill-users, and none (zero percent) of the condom users. There was no side effect either recorded for condom use, even after more than 30 years of the condom - breast cancer link evidence first published.

The Scriptures and other classic literature throughout history seem to give ground for validity of the debates on the perennial issues of sexual relations, marriage, woman, love, conception, human seed, the "sin against nature" of sterile acts (coitus interruptus), prostitution, adultery and other human matters. A consensus in the polemic seems to be the belief that "husbands are the chief persons responsible for dissipation of their wives" (Flandrin, 1975; Gjorgov, 1977/1998). Many writers (Leo Tolstoy, Honoré de Balsac, Stefan Zweig, and many others), and other artists seem to have been ahead of the contemporary medical experts in assessing the natural forces of human intimate (sexual) relations. The Gustav Klimt's artistic vision of "Medicine" was unfairly discarded by the professors of the famous Faculty of Medicine of Vienna at the beginning of the 20th Century. The apotheosis of "Medicine" was angrily discarded by the professors, most likely because the artist portrayed superiority of nature (physical love) over medicine, and depicted his idea of the role of man as a biological complement and the key to functioning of (impact on) the captured woman's life, health, reproductive processes, fate, and exquisite beauty (Gjorgov, 2003b). (Remember the strange slay of Biblical Onan because of his 'mortal sin' of spilling the seed on the ground in sexual relations with his "dissatisfied" second wife?). No wonder that there were confounding 'clusters" of breast cancer in various public institutions around the world (Australia, the U.S.), given the multitude of fashionable, politically correct, condom-promoting zealots.

One of the major conclusions from the studies on marriage and divorce could be inferred that condomization has been implemented long before the AIDS epidemic emerged, during the second half of the decade of 1970s. That was the time of ascendance of feminism, with its primary anti-marriage mission. The promotion of condoms seemed as an "ideal" technical device for the "Our Bodies Ourselves" health-promotion movement. Although condom-promotion started with whispers and rumors, it was quite fervent, distributing condoms at the entries / exits of some of the hospitals, in a somewhat confidential way. The semi-secretive distribution extended for several year until he the solemnization of the mass condomization in the summer of 1986 (Koop, 1986).

The popular belief of the sexual relations exerting biological impact and health gain between woman and man, and for the woman in particular, is strongly imbedded in the minds of the people in the Mediterranean and Balkan regions, especially among the isolated Macedonian rural, mountainous, population (Gjorgov, 2001). It seems that the popular belief of physiological marital inter-dependence on woman reflects possibly the remnants of the classical Hippocratic teaching on seed. The dramatic developments of the contemporary, ever-rising breast cancer epidemic and reproductive health and nature of women and girls may incite a renewed philosophical debate for better understanding as to what is in having sex for a woman, whether women need (drive for) sex for a different biological 'purpose' than men do, and to eventually reconsider the unanswered persistent question "What the women want?" which Freud failed to answer.

It should be mentioned here that in the meantime a fleeting attempt was made by the Israel Health Minister in the 1990s to ban AIDS campaign promoting condom as a prophylactic against the HIV infection, recommending divorce instead for the healthy wife, rather than use of condoms (Siegel-Itzkovich, 1999). More importantly, on December 19, 2002, the U.S. agency CDC (Centers for Diseases control and Prevention) in Atlanta, GA, proclaimed official news, entitled: **"CDC Fact Sheet Not Promoting Condom Use Anymore"** (Meckler, 2002), which was enforced by the American President, who acted on extra information about the ill-effects of condom use. The CDC declaration seems to have had an immediate but short-lived impact on decline of the breast cancer epidemic in the U.S. in the 2003-2004 time period.

5.2 The hidden impact of condomization on life expectancy of women

A few years ago a series of reports appeared simultaneously indicating an unexpected decline in the life expectancy of American people (Ezzati et al., 2008; Brown, 2008; Danaei et al., 2010). The main point in these and other reports was that after a long while a shift in the in U.S. demography has happen, from the customary decrease to sudden increase of mortality The 'reversal of fortunes' as the shift was termed of the increasing mortality has happened in the last three decades, exactly after 1983. The fall of women's life expectancy was more pronounced than in men – of "one in five women" now experiencing lesser longevity and dying younger than before the beginning of 1980s. Although admitting that that the root causes for the downward trend is "impossible to know exactly," the search for causes was directed primarily on "modifiable behaviors and exposures," such as smoking, diet, and lack of exercise, along with the mortality of certain conditions of both sexes. "This is a story about smoking, blood pressure and obesity," was one of the over-confident statement of one of the Harvard researchers (Ezzati, 2008). Besides, the investigation included also diabetes, obesity and AIDS as possible causes of the fall in the life expectancy. The AIDS mortality, while insignificantly linked with the male life expectancy decline, did not relate to that of women.

A more recent background source, 'Explaining Divergent Levels of Longevity in High-Income Countries' review (Crimmins et al, 2011), offers more detailed information on the subject matter of declining life expectancy in the country, and in other comparative countries as well. The evidence in the review, indicated that: (1) the life expectancy is falling in the U.S., (2) the observable fact of falling life expectancy is particularly pronounced among women, (3) the new phenomenon of falling longevity occurred in the last 25 years (during the period 1980-2005), and (4) no risk factors, disease, or any other reason for the falling life expectancy in the U.S. and elsewhere has been determined for the evident, unexpected decline in life expectancy, especially in women (**Figure 22**).

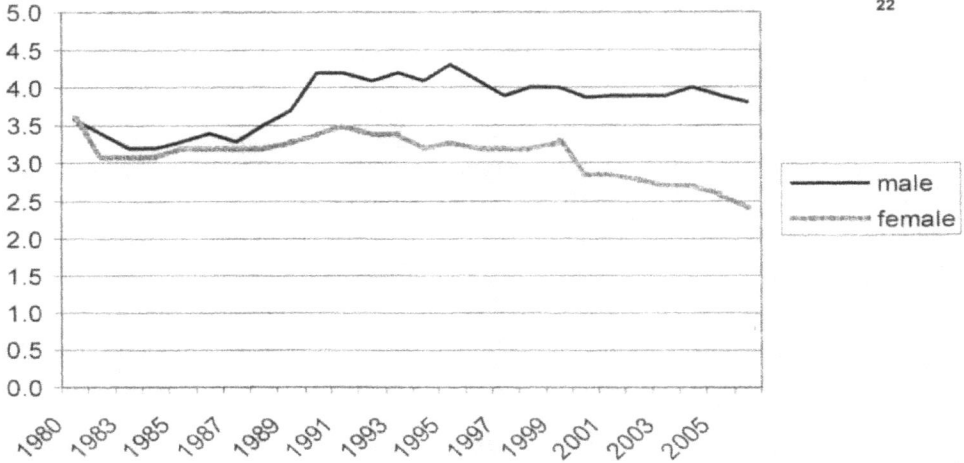

Fig. 22. Gender differences in declining life expectancy at age 50 for U.S. men and women, 1980-2006.

There must be some better way than unconvincing explanation of the confounding smoking and obesity factors, imparting them as the main culprit factors for the slashed longevity of American (and other) women. Missing factors in the review seem to be the unspoken breast cancer epidemic and the mass condomization of female sexuality. Breast cancer is generally treated in the analysis as a passing reference throughout the review. Conspicuously, the unabated and excess epidemic disease of breast cancer is hardly mentioned in the analysis. In the Chapter 8 of the review, entitled Hormone Therapy (in women), the main point of considerations was given on Coronary heart disease and Stroke, and Lung cancer, rather than on Breast cancer. Instead, Lung cancer was sited uncritically as a mortality factor for the decline of longevity even of men and women, because of neglected information that metastases of breast cancer to lungs account for more than 21 to 25 percent. The transmission of HIV/AIDS virus has not been found in the review as a risk factor for the enduring, 25-year decline of women's life expectancy.

The condomization of women's sexuality has been defined as a root cause of the current breast cancer epidemic along with the widespread, accompanying gynecological diseases, tumors and lesions of the organs of reproductive system and other phenomena in American women. The consequences, however, of the general condomization of women's and girls' sexuality in the mainstream population, in a misconceived attempt to stem the emergent AIDS epidemic by barrier birth-control device, has changed the demography of the American society, perhaps the most in the world. The never before experienced change of decline in longevity in of the people has been achieved by a profound corruption of the nature of the intimate (sexual) ecosystem of people, due to elimination of the biologically protective, primordial physiological impact of mutual woman-man relations. That is the change has been achieved by inducing technical effects of absolute male sterility in the marital and inter-gender micro-environment. Namely, the evidence of a significant association between condom use and breast cancer development in the population at large, rather than the transmission of HIV/AIDS virus in any high-risk group, or hormone therapy (for breast cancer) for that matter, may better explain the decline of longevity of American women. It is almost certain that the extent of condom promotion / distribution in the U.S. has been more persistent and more indiscriminate than in the other high-income, comparable countries.

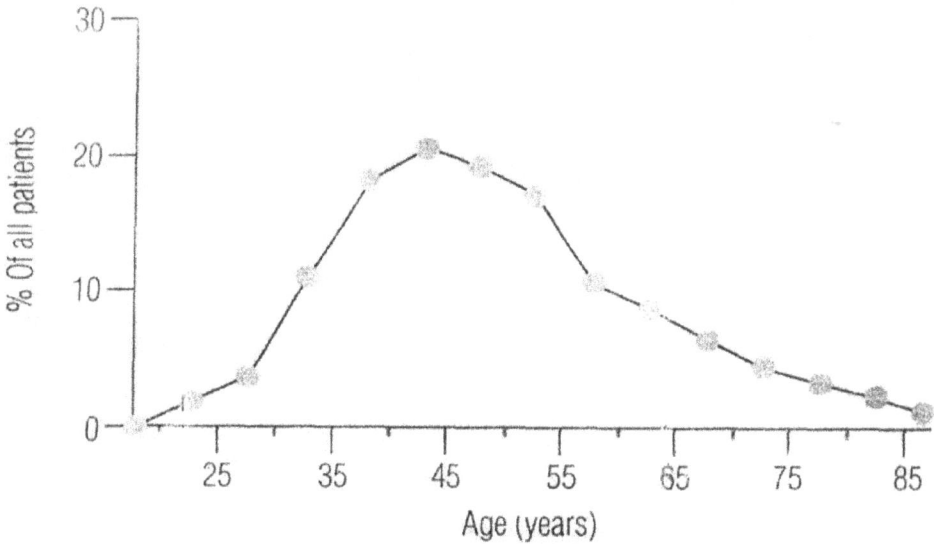

Fig. 23. Percentage of all deaths in women attributable to breast cancer (in 1990s).

The breast cancer epidemiology in the **U.K.**, in the mid-1990s (McPherson et al, 2000), included mortality figures of percentage of all deaths in women attributable to breast cancer (**Figure 23**). The proportion of breast cancer deaths was more than 20 percent in young women aged 40-45, and around 20% in the adjacent age groups 35-39 and 45-49.

In fact, the remarkable, long-term decline of life expectancy in American women may become a unique proof and testimony for both the medical, and perhaps political, misconception of social benefit of the indiscriminate, mass condomization, associated with the breast cancer epidemic, and the wrong-for-long misleading, deadly false belief of condom use as a "safe" hi-tech device for fertility-control and family-planning purposes. [The data of parallel decline on a lesser scale of male longevity might indicate that the devastating and carcinogenic effects of condomization on women's health and lives, resulting in epidemics of breast-ovarian-gynecological cancers, might exert some reciprocal, unknown social or any other biological effect on men as well.] The hope remains, however, that the elimination (practical 'eradication' to levels of rare, sporadic cases) of epidemic breast cancer, by elimination of the sole breast-cancer risk of condomized control of women's sexuality, to reflect rapidly on both decline of the breast cancer epidemic, and restoration of rising women's life expectancy, in a fast manner as the disease entered human race, after the point of departure of all events at the beginning of the 1980s.

6. The future: Prevention of the breast cancer epidemic

In the perspective of breast cancer, the future is present. The answer is the primary, non-chemical prevention of the breast cancer epidemic, although the idea about prevention seems lost and no-existent in the West (Ferlay et al, 2010; EuropaDonna, 2010). Based on 2002 to 2006 trend of increase, the projected future trend of breast cancer increase was estimated at 53% by 2030. Similar disturbing forecast of breast cancer increase of 66.3% in the England and Wales by 2025 has been computed by using a mathematical model based on abortion prevalence rates and several other secondary reproductive factors; the predicted increase being from 39,229 in 2004 to 65,252 in 2025 (Carroll, 2007). Other projected/predicted increase of breast cancer of 32.9% in the U.K., from 2005 till 2024, the present number of 41,900 new cases annually to 55,700 new breast cancer cases in 2024 was assessed by Cancer Research UK (2007). The basic assumption being that the present, sad situation of the breast cancer epidemic in the country will stretch helplessly in the next 20 years, and beyond, into infinity.

To the contrary, the breast cancer epidemic could change by a dramatic decline in the UK, by not less than -80%, from both the forecasted by Carrol excess number of 65,252 cases to eventually 13,050 in 2024, and the forecasted by the Cancer Research UK organization (2007) also excess number of 55,700 cases to 11,140 or less, by 2024, provided primary prevention is implemented in the meantime. The mentioned number of in-situ (DCIS) cases, defined as non-breast cancer (0-zero stage), is expected to decline to a level of one-third (1276 in-situ cases) or less, of the 3,827 cases in England & Wales in 2004 (Carroll, 2007), provided, again, primary prevention is initiated. This is just for laying the groundwork for testing *in vivo* the two opposite theories of breast cancer preventability in the near future.

The following comment was conveyed to **Nicholas D. Kristof**, the New York Columnist as a reply to his article "The secret war on condoms," NYT, Jan. 12, 2003:

"**The War On Condoms Is The War Against Breast Cancer**
With reference to your article, "The Secret War on Condoms" (NYT, January 10, 2003), your bitter denigration of the efforts and the politics of the U.S. President, George W. Bush, for dismissal of the condom use as a device for contraceptive, fertility-control and family-planning purposes is misplaced, one-sided and seemingly rational. Apparently, Mr. Bush is in command of extra information of the devastating, adverse and carcinogenic effects of the consistent condom use in married American and other women. It is not your fault, of course, that you might have been ignorant of a hypothesis-testing study, which defined and corroborated the true etiology of breast cancer in the country, determined a potential of a primary (non-chemical) prevention of the breast cancer epidemic in the community, predicted the imminent epidemic rise of the malignant disease and, I believe, provided ANSWER for solution and creation of a public health policy in the field of breast cancer and other accompanying diseases. The study was initiated, supported and completed during the mid-1970s, at the University of North Carolina School of Public Health, at Chapel Hill, NC, and at the University of Pennsylvania School of Medicine and Hospital, in Philadelphia, PA. The final report of the aforementioned study was published in the distant 1980, as well as in 1979 by the Michigan University Dissertation International, Ann Arbor, MI.
However, there are strong indications that the research study has been concealed and secretly suppressed by the previous ("liberal") administrations, dealing with researchers

---

discovering other approaches with unemployment, academic and professional uprooting and deportation; very soon afterwards, the breast cancer epidemic suddenly and sharply rose and unabated continued its ever-rising increase. The estimate of the U.S. Senate has been that about 2,000,000 women became breast cancer victims during the decade of the 1990s, with 500,000 deaths of the disease. Nowadays, it has been reported that one million of new American breast cancer cases (most of them affluent victims) are registered in four years (rather than in five years, like in the 1990s). The incidence of breast cancer in the United States (as well as in Europe) has been at least seven times higher than the spread of AIDS, the deadly twin epidemic disease. Based on the available WHO data, during the two-decade period, 1981 till 2000, in the U.S have been registered 500,000 (accumulated) cases of AIDS, with about 150,000 deaths (and not less than four million women afflicted with breast cancer, including in-situ cases, with mote than a quarter of the affected women perished).

Apparently, by this backdrop of massacre of women, shattered families, widespread fear, real threat and tragedy in the Country and worldwide, the promotion of the indiscriminate, absolutistic and persistent exposure to (use of) condom in the mainstream population had to be reassessed and amended. The previous administration (at the highest possible levels), regretfully, missed the opportunity to properly address and entirely eliminate the breast cancer epidemic in the country and beyond, and to make the American women happy. With the resolute campaign of President George W. Bush against condom education among the teenagers in the schools, the ultimate objective of condomization of the society has been terminated and the cornerstone of a condom culture has been removed, I hope. In addition, I wonder as to whether a solution of the present gloomy breast cancer emergency or a sustainable prevention of breast cancer could be reached in the Country or elsewhere as long as an American study in primary breast cancer prevention and etiology, such as my monograph "Barrier Contraception and Breast Cancer" (1980), is effectively banned from public view, professional scrutiny and clinical assessment for a possible basis of a new breast cancer policy and efficient public health action in the field.

cc: Dr. Andrew C. von Achenbach, Director of the National Cancer Institute, January 12, 2003

cc: The Editors of the New York Times, February 12, 2003

The breast cancer epidemic has remained a perplexing epidemic, and is the case in point of a gender-specific, malignant disease, replacing the routine models of traditional epidemics of contagious, infectious diseases in the general population of both genders and all age groups. The traditionally known in the human history epidemics of infectious diseases have had defined source(s) of the contagious agent, are known to take a course of three main phases (slow or explosive beginning, reaching acme (the peak), and a protracted self-decline ('tail') of the natural end of the epidemics. It seems that the incidence, new HIV/AIDS cases, globally, have reached the peak at the beginning of the 1990s, and are presently showing sings of gradual, protracted, steady decline ever since (McNeil, 2010; USAIDS, 2010). Contrary to the medical experience, the breast cancer epidemic emerged fast, continued its unabated rise, never reached its culmination (acme), and never subsided in expected, tailed decline in the last three decades, since the beginning of 1980s. To the contrary, the new epidemic of breast cancer and other malignant disease(s) in women is not expected to vanish 'naturally,' by its own. Almost certainly, the current breast cancer epidemic is to be terminated by deliberate and conscious human intervention only. The data indicate that the increase of the 'cancer' epidemic in the West, and in other parts of the world, is fueled up mainly by the cancer of the breast and its steady epidemic increase. Apparently, to try to eliminate the current, unabated and excess breast cancer epidemic, a new way of thinking may be needed. The misconception about the breast cancer etiology and community burden hinders the efforts to understand, prevent and control the epidemic malignant breast disease. "What is of concern...is the way the medical-industrial complex uses the research. They would have us believe that because of various findings, such as cancer genes, the cure lies just around the corner. The truth is, however, it doesn't make much difference if a cure ever emerges. The search is a splendid money generator," by quoting other authors, declared the unheeded UK Working Group on the Primary Prevention of Breast Cancer (2007) and, in addition stated, that "there is no sign of leadership from government regarding... (prioritizing).. primary prevention" of breast cancer.

In the last three decades, breast cancer epidemic has spread to other, developing countries of Africa, South Asia, Latin America and elsewhere, as expected. The emerging breast cancer epidemic in the "poor" countries is attracting increasing attention in western countries, with projects and programs relied on old science, and the failing strategy of "palliative care" and "no cure" attitude to continue to be applied against the epidemic disease(s) everywhere. Practically, the inner nature and hormonal balance of woman is still considered to be at fault, which should and could be 'corrected' by chemical agents and human interventions.

The basic strategy of a breast cancer prevention is chemoprevention, particularly with the obsolete *tamoxifen* and other 'selective estrogen modulators,' conducting "downstream" clinical activities of early detection with mammographic screening, so-called 'preventive' mastectomies and oophorectomies, and ineffective counsels for "lessening" spurious risk factors of breast cancer, among which the condom use as a contraceptive method is never considered and maybe still suppressed (Mills, 1987; Bray et al., 2004; National Cancer Policy Board, 2005; Anderson, 2008; WHO-PAHO, 2008; Frenk, 2009; Lancet Editorial, 2009; Meriman, 2010; .Miller, 2010; European Breast Cancer Network, 2010).

Several years earlier, a communication was directed to **Dr. Mitra Roses Periago,** Director of the Pan-American Health Organization-PAHO, Washington, DC, February 14, 2006, regarding the "*Guidelines for International Breast Health and Cancer Control,*" *Breast Journal* Suppl., January-February 2006, conveying the following critical comments (fragments):

"First and foremost, NO PREVENTION of breast cancer was ever mentioned in the PAHO Guidelines. The long-standing, tested evidence (Barrier Contraception and Breast Cancer," 1980), strongly indicating a potential of primary (non-chemical) prevention of breast cancer in American married women, was not taken under consideration in the Guidelines. The evidence, neither disputed nor rejected, showed that breast cancer is a preventable epidemic disease.

The PAHO Guidelines documented the fact that the expected epidemic wave of breast cancer, expanding from the affluent and prosperous Western World (North America and Europe, and others), has already reached the shores and lands of the developing world of Latin America, Africa, and Asia. The Guidelines displayed the growing rates of breast cancer in 'low-resource countries' as an equally serious, rapidly emerging political crisis and a grave public health issue and burden in both developed and developing world. The PAHO Guidelines for breast cancer control in developing countries, however, have relied heavily on the efforts and experience of the inefficient and fruitless breast cancer control measures in stopping breast cancer before it starts in the developed countries of the West and the WHO. The added rhetoric and new terminology in the Guidelines about the new approaches, innovative research, stratification of the levels of needs, community-based programs, social support, and other envisioned activities against the epidemic of the cancer of the breast, may only replicate the conceptual vacuum and futility in understanding of the etiology and prevention of breast cancer (along with other tumors of the reproductive organs and ill-health phenomena in women) in new settings around the world...

The recent, dramatic "condom paradigm shift" entailed by the U.S. Government (2002) in favor of an "anti-condom" reproductive policy was, most probably, imposed by no accident... Informed observations seem to indicate that race might play a more lethal outcome to married 'non-white' women (Afro-American, Hispanics, Asian-American), exposed to absolute-sterile mating (condom use), than to 'white' women, in terms of breast cancer development, earlier death, shorter survival and physical devastation. If anything, empowerment of women and their husbands / partners with information of the real breast cancer risk would prove to be more useful in preventing the disease at individual, familial and community levels, than the planned regulations and guidelines..."

The following **Table 5** is an attempt to define and elaborate the proposal of the hypothesis 1978 (Gjorgov, 1978a,b, 1979, 1980) of the etiology of breast cancer, and a likely shift of the conceptual framework of the epidemic disease:

Old Paradigm	New Paradigm
1. No Prevention of Breast Cancer (BC)	1. Yes, Primary (non-chemical) Prevention of Breast Cancer
2. Public-health emphasis on mammography screening and early BC detection; Epidemiologically: (unreported) *in-situ* cases	2. Public-health emphasis on primary prevention; Instead of exposure to the BC risks; the *in-situ* cases counted as BC cases;
3. The risk factors of BC are not amenable	3. The main risk factor readily amenable; BC is preventable
4. Treatment and chemical prevention of the BC epidemic	4. Primary (non-chemical) prevention of BC as epidemic disease
5. Nutritional presumed causes (fat, alcohol, smoking, diet, environmental chemicals, toxins, etc), and Reproductive causes: Early menarche, Late births (>30 yrs), Family history, Low parity, No breast-feeding, OC pill use, Late menopause, Lack of exercise, 'Marital' Infertility issue, and other risk factors; Genes and mutations	5. Semen-factor deficiency tested hypothesis: The main etiological cause: the widespread use of Barrier methods: of contraception: Condom devices, Withdrawal practice and male sterility/infertility in marriages. Condom-use technical effects of absolute male sterility: condomization of female sexuality due to Sterile mating
6. Environmental toxic substances & Industrial waste as BC causes, Polluted living settings (home, food, water, working place, streets); Radiation; Gene mutations	6. Inverse environmental factor of BC: absence or elimination of putative protective factors in the intimate (sexual) ecosystem and inter-human micro-environment

Old Paradigm	New Paradigm
7. Toxic environmental waste as direct cause of BC	7. Toxic waste: Indirect cause of BC *via* male infertility
8. Estrogen-Progestin model; 'Toxic-loaded' bodies, HRT, Ignored carcinogenic effects of external steroids, 'Endocrine disrupters' as causes of the current BC epidemic	8. 'Deficiency' of Prostaglandins, seminal fluid; Inner endocrine imbalance in women-related to causes of BC; Foretold BC carcinogenicity of "exogenous hormones"(HRT)
9. Marriage as a social, psychological, economic & legal unit only. Biological independence of spouses-genders	9. Marriage (along sex & love): a biological union w/ profound physiological impact; Sex (gender) inter-dependence
10. BC: poorly known, 'random' disease; local treatment	10. BC a systemic disease, No known cure
11. Hopes & trials in BC chemoprevention (*Tamoxifen*)	11. High-tech devices (condoms, HRTs) gone wrong
12. BC: poorly understood disease, treated as a local one	12. BC: Systemic disease with no known cure
13. Focus on selected BC figures & emphasis to find cure	13. Research-based, hypothesis-tested evidence & data
14. 'Heroic' treatment procedures, endurance of women, learned helplessness and ignorance for self-protection against BC; Decisions of BC 'reduction' at the top, governmental levels	14. Empowerment of women and couples with information of the root cause & BC prevention; Cause-effectiveness assessment for protection made 'at the bottom,' personal and family levels
15. BC as a political crisis, because of progressively rising epidemic spread of the malignant disease in the society	15. Solution/answer to the current, excess BC epidemic, subject to the will and commitment of highest political level
16. The risk of BC unknown; Early detection & treatments as secondary prevention of early death, longer survival	16. Evidence-based definition of the main BC risk: Marital and persistent (long-term) exposure to (use of) condoms
17. Focus on selected BC figures and prejudiced data	17. Evidence-based and hypothesis-tested results / data
18. Long latent period of BC: between 10-20 years or, starting even "in the womb" (both unsubstantiated)	18. Short BC latent period: between 2½ to five years; Evidence confirmed / verified by forecasted BC natural experiment
19. No comprehensive theory (conceptual vacuum) of BC & women's ill health and associated BC equivalents of tumors of the reproductive system; BC linked to ovarian cancer mainly	19. Comprehensive approach to women's health: BC, Ovarian cancer / cysts, uterine cancer/lesions, thyroid cancer / nodules. Anorexia disorders; female osteoporosis; Body-mind phenomena
20. BC prevalent in older, postmenopausal women (>50)	20. Shift to young women (<50); debut peak condom users
21. Current BC epidemic-rapid rise: Denial / artifact claims	21. Rise of the BC epidemic predicted; Verified by events
22. Officially, not recognized & nonexistent BC epidemic	22. Evidence of rapid, unabated & ever-rising BC epidemic

Old Paradigm	New Paradigm
23. 'Second' most common malignant disease in women	23. BC - the commonest malignant disease in women
24. Competing high rates of Lung Cancer in women	24. Fueled by >20% BC metastases to the lungs
25. Higher BC incidence rates in white women	25. Higher BC rates in women of higher living standards
26. Ostensibly, BC mortality decline due to early detection and BC screening programs; (Consensus: *in-situ* cases not to be included in the total annual number of BC figure)	26. If there is a BC mortality decline, then probably due to therapy and surgical modalities, particularly hysterectomy, (with or without one-sided or two-sided oophorectomy)
27. Promotion of condoms as "safe" device for fertility-control and family-planning method	27. Elimination of condoms for contraceptive purposes in population as the main etiological risk of the BC epidemic
28. Priority: 'downstream' activities: screening for more cases & clinical salvage of BC affected women;	28. Priority: Prevention of the risks & cause(s) of current BC epidemic: shift to non-barrier birth-control methods
29. No definition of female response to sterile mating	29. Inner imbalance (Pseudopregnancy), Missed abortion
30. Primary (non-chemical) prevention of the BC epidemic not considered, despite the failed chemoprevention trials	30. Primary prevention ('eradication'), w/ estimated >80% reduction at individual, family and community levels
31. Chemo-prevention of BC: assuming "wrong" female nature to be corrected by Tamoxifen / Raloxifene & drugs	31. Nothing wrong with women's nature subject to chemical correction: Misconceived toxic-substance prevention of BC
32. Ovarian, endometrial and thyroid cancers and other gynecological diseases as unrelated to BC entities	32. Ovarian, endometrial, thyroid & gynecological cancers, lesions of same etiology, condomization of women all ages
33. Silence and suppression of the information of the potential for prevention of the current BC epidemic	33. Decision (pending?) for non-mutually exclusive primary prevention against the twin epidemics of BC and AIDS
34. Plan for action: Search for cure, better therapy, and new drugs and 'better armamentarium' for BC screening	34. Needed plan for action for BC prevention: Elimination of condom use for contraceptive purposes.
35. Overlooked impact of condomization upon issues of marriage, divorce, and women's mortality and life expectancy	35. Considerable protective impact upon social issues of marriage, divorce, and women's mortality and life expectancy

Table 5. Breast cancer hypothesis 1978 and shift of the conceptual framework. (Updated: March 2011)

In the strategy for the global Millennium Development Goals 2015 (MDGs) decisions, a similar situation presented itself regarding condomization of women in less-developed regions. In a letter to the United Nations Secretary-General, the **Hon. Ban Ki-moon**, on September 25, 2010, the following message about the harmful effects of condom-use programs was conveyed:

"As a former United Nations Fellow, Fulbright Scholar, physician and researcher, I like to take the liberty of trying to draw your attention to the grave consequences on women's and girls' reproductive health and lives of continuation of the fallacious condom policy in pursuing the future global Millennium Development Goals 2015 (MDGs).

The condomization of female sexuality, defined long ago as the root cause of the current breast cancer epidemic worldwide, is going o be perpetuated by the UN global MDG Plan for Action. The Plan is apparently oblivious to the global twin epidemic of breast cancer along with AIDS, and is projecting the mass condomization as the main critical plan for action for the Goal 5 and Goal 6 in particular. The breast cancer epidemic has been superseding manifold the HIV/AIDS epidemic in the developed, affluent world of the West, including the U.S., UK, and other EU countries, from the outset, in the early 1980s.

From the affluent, rich western world, the breast cancer epidemic is rapidly spreading to the so-called developing, 'poor' world of Africa and Asia, as anticipated. The typically affected by the disease young / younger women (the main condom users), testify in favor of the defined etiology of the raising breast cancer crisis in the developing regions of the world... Besides breast cancer, there is a myriad of accompanying gynecological tumors and diseases increasingly afflicting women of all races and age-cohorts during their reproductive life-span. It is anticipated that another, more fatal category of female suffering may soon appear, of women affected by both HIV/AIDS and breast cancer diseases combined.

The main culprit of the on-going global breast cancer crisis is the deadly false belief of the use of condom is a "safe" device for fertility-control and family-planning purposes. (By this token, let me mention some official data of the Korean women in the U.S. who have been and still are with the lowest recorded breast cancer incidence rates, which, in my experience, could be attributed to a traditionally low prevalence of condom use and, accordingly, to the assumed lowest condom acculturation in the new/old country.) Almost certainly, it was not by accident that the former President, George W. Bush, acting most likely on extra information, imposed a bold 'condom-paradigm shift,' in favor of an anti-condom reproductive policy, followed by a global ban on condom promotion and distribution, and termination of the unlimited condom funds to global agencies at home and abroad (including WHO, UNFPA, UNAIDS, World Bank and others)... At the present, I believe, the signs may seem encouraging that President Barack Obama would proceed with the same policy of non-condomization of the mainstream population, which policy is expected to prove to be extremely beneficial for elimination, i.e., for primary prevention (non-chemical, non-profit) of the current breast cancer epidemic, and for a better control of the other gender- (sex-) specific diseases in women of all ages. What seem to be happening now, instead, is that the United Nations and its agencies continue to sponsor / promote the relentless push of condoms, disguised as family planning methods, with lingering ill-effects and inevitably up-dating and transferring the current, breast cancer epidemic and other harmful experience of the West into poor world regions...

Ii is my belief that your post of UN Secretary-General embodies a unique opportunity to be able to try to help reassess the new scientific evidence about the epidemiological and social consequences of the never openly debated, arbitrary silenced issue of condomized control of women's and girls' sexuality, a deceptive protection of their reproductive health in the UN sponsored MDGs 5 & 6."

E-mailed and AIRMAILED

7. Conclusion

The perplexing worldwide breast cancer epidemic, defined as unintended consequence of widespread condomization of women's sexuality, carried out in fervent campaigns for both contraceptive and prophylactic (anti-HIV/AIDS) purposes continue to reign supreme, globally. It is the quintessence of a deadly female sex- (gender-) specific, malignant disease. The data indicate that the increase of the 'cancer' epidemic in the West, and in other parts of the world, is fueled up almost entirely by the breast cancer epidemic and its steady increase. The breast cancer epidemic is thriving mainly because of lack of commitment to eliminate the disease(s) to rare, sporadic cases, at personal, familial and community levels. The condomization of women's and girls' sexuality is directly related to multitude aspects of female ill health, disturbed functions, specific and accompanying diseases, life, death, marital malfunctions, and reduced longevity.

Most of the researchers in the field of cancer research and birth control seem to refer to a "recreational" value of sex, by searching only for technical aspects ("frequency") of intimate encounters and utterly ignoring the biological aspects and barriers to the primordial 'gender' communication, sexual relations. It is amazing that the authors have consistently missed the opportunity to consider barriers to sex as a part of life, particularly of women. The new epidemic of breast cancer and other malignant disease(s) in women is not expected to vanish 'naturally,' by its own. The data indicate that the increase of the breast cancer epidemic in the West, and in other parts of the world, is fueled up mainly by the deceptive condomization of female sexuality in mainstream populations. Almost certainly, the current breast cancer epidemic is to be terminated by deliberate and conscious human intervention only. To try to eliminate the current, unabated and excess breast cancer epidemic, a new way of thinking may be needed.

The answer to the current breast cancer contingency is to undertake a primary, non-chemical, no-profit, prevention of the epidemic. Since information in public health actions is superior to legislation, it seems better to take the first steps with subtle, nonjudgmental attitude. Perhaps the true information of the devastating and carcinogenic effects of condom use should be communicated to the consumers and displayed on the commercial product.

The information (warning) of the breast cancers risk being included in condom labeling. No doubt that women and couples, empowered with preventative, potentially life-saving information, will be able to make correct assessment of the risks and benefits values on matters of life and death, at a bottom, personal and familial, rather than at the detached at the top decision-making level.

8. Acknowledgments

Thanks to Ing, Emil Gjorgov, from the University American College Skopje, and Ing. Dr. Kosta Mangaroski, from the University St. Cyril and Methodius, Skopje, for the technical support.

9. References

Ambekar A. (2009). Causes and Effects of Divorce. Article. January 12.   Internet web: www.articleswave.com/divorce-articles/causes-and-effects-ofdivorce.html

Anderson, BO., Yip, CH., Smith. RA. et al. (2008). Guideline implementation for breast healthcare in low-income and middle-income countries: overview of the Breast Health Global Initiative Global Summit 2007. Cancer 2008 Oct 15;113(8 Suppl):2221-43. Web: http://www.guideline.gov/content.aspx?id=13344#Section420

Australian Historical Statistics (2001). Divorce rates in Australia. Web: http://www.divorcerate.org/divorce-rates-in-australia.html

Bray, F; McCarron, P. & Parkin, DM. (2004). The changing global patterns of female breast cancer incidence and mortality. *Breast Cancer Research* 6: 229-239. Web. http://breast-cancer-research.com/content/6/6/229

Brining MF, Allen DW (2000). 'These boots are made for walking': Why most divorce filers are women. *American Law and Economics Review*, Vol. 2, pp. 126-169. Web: http://papers.ssrn.com/so13/papers.cfm?abstract_id=713110

Brown D (2008). Life Expectancy Drops for Some U.S. Women. Historic Reversal, Found in 1,000 Counties May Be Result of Smoking and Obesity. *Washington Post*, April 22. Internet web:
http://www.washingtonpost.com/wp-dyn/content/article/2008/04/21/AR2008042102406_pf.html

Carroll, PS. (2007) 'The breast cancer epidemic: modeling and forecasts based on abortion and other risk factors', Journal of American Physicians and Surgeons, 12(3): 72-78. Web: http://www.jpands.org/vol12no3/carroll.pdf

Cirado MP, Edwards B, Shin HR, Storm H, Ferlay J, Heanue M, Boyle P. Eds. (2007). *Cancer Incidence in Five Continents*, Volume IX, WHO-IARC, Sci. Publ. 160, Lyon, France. (Digital data edition on Internet)

Cancer Research UK. (2007). Breast cancer – UK incidence statistics. Web: http://info.cancerresearchuk.org/cancerstats/types/breast/incidence/

Crieger, N. (2002). Is breast cancer a disease of affluence, Poverty or both? The case of African American women. *American Journal of Public Health* 92:611-612.

Crimmins EM, Preston SH, Cohen B (2011). Explaining Divergent Levels of Longevity In High-Income Countries. National Research Council of the National Academies. January 25. *National Academies Press*. Web:
http://www.nap.edu/catalog/13089.html

Dinse, GE.; Umbach, DM.; Sasco, AJ. et al. (1999). Unexplained increases in cancer incidence in the United States from 1975 to 1994: Possible Sentinel Health Indicators. *Annual Review of Public Health* 20:173-209.

Danaei. G., Rimm, ER., Oza, S., et al. (2010). The promise of prevention: The effect of four preventable risk factors on national life expectancy and life expectancy disparities and county in the United States. PLoS Medicine, March, 7(3); e1000248. Web: http://www.ncbi.nlm.nih.gov/pmc/articles/PMC2843596/?tool=pmcentrez

Ehrchardt AA (1992). Trends in sexual behavior and the HIV pandemic. Editorial. *American Journal of Public Health* 82(11):1459-1461, November.

EuropaDonna. (2010). More women get breast cancer than any other cancer. (See Ferlay, J. et al., 2010) Web: http://europadonnaireland.ie/content/more

European Commission. (2006). *European Guidelines for quality assurance in breast cancer screening and diagnosis.* Fourth Edition. Perry, N. et al Editors. Health and Consumer Protection G.D., pp. 416.

Ezzati M, Friedman AB, Kulkarni SC, Murray CGL (2008). The reversal of fortunes: Trends in county mortality and cross-County mortality disparities in the United States. *PLoS Medicine*, April 22;5(4):e66, Web: http://www.plosmedicine.org/article/info%3Adoi%2F10.1371%2Fjournal.pmed.0 050066

Ferlay, J.; Parkin, DM. and Steliarova-Foucher, E. (2010). Estimates of cancer incidence and mortality in Europe in 2008. Eur J Cancer, 46(4): 756-81. Web: http://www.ejcancer.info/article/S0959-8049(09)00926-5/pdf

Flandrin, J-L. (1975). Contraception, Marriage, and Sexual Relations in the Christian West. In: R. Foster & O. Ranum, Eds. Biology of Man in History, Chapter 1. Selection from the Annales Economies Societes, Civilisations. The John Hopkins University Press, Baltimore & London, 23-47.

Fox, MF. (2004). Robert King Merton. Life time of influence. Scientometrics, Vol. 60, No. 1, 47-50. Web: http://www.spingerlink.com/content/m0822078639422vu/bodyRef/PDF/11192_ 2004_Article_5149145.pdf

Frenk, J. (2009). Cancer is on the rise in developing countries. The shadow epidemic. Harvard School of Public Health. November 25. Web: http://www.hsph.harvard.edu/news/hphr/fall-2009/shadow-epidemic.html

Gjorgov, AN. (1978a). Barrier contraceptive practice and male infertility as related factors to breast cancer in married women. *Medical Hypotheses* (Montreal, Canada) 4(2): 79-88. Medline - Abstract # 03590510/78224510. Web: http://www.sementherapy.com/mirror/sciencedirect.com_002.htm

Gjorgov, AN. (1978b). Barrier contraceptive practice and male infertility as related factors to breast cancer in married women. Preliminary results. *Oncology* (Munich, Germany) 35: 97-100, Medlars II - Popline PIP/783908.

Gjorgov, AN. (1979). Barrier Contraceptive Practice and Male Infertility as Related Factors to Breast Cancer in Married Women. A Retrospective Study, pp 325. University of Michigan Dissertation International, Ann Arbor, MI 48106; UMI publication # 79-14352. Dissertation Abstract: Vol. XV, No. 1. Abstract: Web: http://www.hsc.edu.kw/vpo/library/theses/Author.asp?view=Gjorgov,%20Arn e%20N#

Gjorgov, AN. (1980). *Barrier Contraception and Breast Cancer*. S.Karger Publ., Basel-Munchen-Paris-New York-Sydney: x+164.

Gjorgov, AN. (1986). Breast cancer in Kuwait, 1974-1983. An epidemiological study. *Journal of the Kuwaiti Medical Asso*ciation 20: 75-88.

Gjorgov, AN. (1989). Risk factors of female thyroid cancer in Kuwait. Retrospective study. (Leading article.) *Libri Oncologici* (Zagreb) 18(1-2):5-22. (Received for publication September 12th, 1988)

Gjorgov, AN. (1990). Breast cancer risk from use of condom: Interim evidence of an unplanned natural experiment. *Child and Family* (Oak Park, Illinois) 21: 97-101.

Gjorgov, AN. (1991). Breast cancer death rates in Yugoslavia, 1979-1987: An attempt to explain the new rising trends. *The Journal of the Medical Association of Macedonia*. 45(3-4): 67-73. (Summary in English).

Gjorgov, AN. (1993). Emerging worldwide trends of breast cancer incidence in the 1970s and 1980s: Data from 23 cancer registration centres. *European Journal of Cancer Prevention* (London) 2: 423-440.

Gjorgov, AN. (1994a). History of the condom: the overlooked adverse effects. *J Royal Society of Medicine* (London) 87: 570, September 1 (Opening of the Int'l Conf. on Population and Development, Cairo, Egypt, Sept. 2-14 (ICPD-1994). Web: http://www.ncbi.nlm.nih.gov/pmc/articles/PMC1294789/pdf/jrsocmed00081-0090c.pdf

Gjorgov, AN. (1994b). Worldwide BC Incidence: An Attempt at Interpretation of the Ecological Rising Trends and of the Potential for Prevention. Kuwait University. Poster at the *Lancet Breast Cancer Challenge Conference 1994*, Brugge, Belgium, April 21-23.

Gjorgov, AN. (1994c). Rising breast cancer incidence worldwide, 1980-1990. A potential for prevention. *J Med Assoc Macedon* 48(1-2): 118-123. (Summary in English).

Gjorgov, AN. (1996a). *Breast Cancer: Rationale for an Etiologic Hypothesis.* A Reappraisal of the Clinical, Experimental, and Theoretical Aspects of Neoplastic Processes, Pseudopregnancy Complex, and the Possible Role of the Seminal Prostaglandins. University of Pennsylvania School of Medicine, Philadelphia, PA, 1980, and Matica Mak. Publ., Skopje, 1996.

Gjorgov, AN. (1996b). Prevention and eradication of the *bovine spongiform encephalopathy (BSE)*: A solicited response and proposal. *Macedonian Veterinary Review* (Skopje) 1996; 25(1-2): 97-101.

Gjorgov, AN. (1997/1998). Breast cancer death of Empress Theodora, wife of Justinian I of Byzantine, in the Sixth Century. *ASKLEPIOS, International Journal of History and General Theory of Medicine*, Vol. XI, pp. 117-121. Web: http://prodavnicanatajni.blog.mk/2006/11/30/seks-da-no-priroden/

Gjorgov, AN. (1998a). Ecological breast cancer incidence differentials and condom use prevalence worldwide, 1983-87: Corroboration of the potential for primary prevention. *Archive Balkan Medical Union* (Bucharest) 33; 111-123.

Gjorgov, AN. (1998b). Breast cancer and barrier contraception: Postulated and corroborated potential for prevention. Invited lecture. *Folia Medica* (Plovdiv) 1998; 30: 17-23. (PMID: 10205987 - MEDLINE.)

Gjorgov, AN.; Junaid, TA.; Burns, GR. & Temmim, L. (1999). Efficacy of preventive prostaglandin treatment of malignant mammary lesions in rats. An experimental trial. *Journal of the Balkan Union of Oncology (J-BUON)* – (Athens) 4:295-306. Ditto: (1996) *European Journal of Cancer Prevention* (London) 5(Suppl 2):104 (Abstract). Web: http://journals.lww.com/eurjcancerprev/citation/1996/12002/efficacy_of_preventive_prostaglandin_treatment_of.21.aspx and/or http://www.unet.com.mk/medics/mammary.htm

Gjorgov, AN. (2000). Continuing rise of the breast cancer epidemic worldwide, in the 1990s: Further evidence and corroboration of the potential for primary prevention. *Contributions of the Section of Biological & Medical Sciences of the Macedonian Academy of Sciences and Arts (MASA)*, Skopje, Vol. XXI, No. 1-2, pp 41-63.

Gjorgov, AN., Narod, S. et al. (2001a) Tubal ligation and risk of ovarian cancer. (Correspondence)   Lancet,   Sep.   8,   358:843-4.   Web:

http://www.thelancet.com/journals/lancet/article/PIIS0140-6736(01)05991-8/fulltext

Gjorgov, AN. (2001b). Biological Foundations of Human Sexuality: Personal Notes on the Discordant Popular and Modern Attitudes. (Medical History Congress presentation, October 2001); *Asklepios, International Annual of History and Philosophy of Medicine* (Sofia) Vol. XIV: 160-164.

Gjorgov, AN. (2003a). Condomization of Female Sexuality - The Cause of FSD. *British Medical Journal*-Online, 26 January, Web:
http://www.bmj.com/cgi/eletters/326/7379/45#29155

Gjorgov, AN. (2003b). Klimt's man-woman relation in his 'Medicine.' *British Medical Journal*-Online. Rapid response to 'Doctors versus artists: Gustav Klimt's Medicine'. 11 March. Web: http://www.bmj.com/cgi/eletters/325/7378/1506#30361

Gjorgov, AN. (2003c). Primary prevention of breast cancer versus the current policy of salvage treatment: Update of evidence and the proposition. *Macedonian Journal of Medicine* 49(1-2): 15-26.

Gjorgov, AN. (2006). A review of the osteoporosis in women and a new hypothesis for testing. *Macedonian Journal of Medicine* 52(1-2): 5-21.

Gjorgov, AN. (2008). Incomplete Study of 'Birth Control Pills Prevent Ovarian Cancer.' *The Washington Post* Blog, Comment, posted January 25. Web: http://digg.com/health/Birth_Control_Pills_Prevent_Ovarian_Cancer

Gjorgov, AN. (2009a). Anorexia and Bulimia Nervosa in Young Female Patients and Barrier Contraception Practice. *Asklepios, International Annual of History and Philosophy of Medicine* (Sofia) Vol. III New Series (XXII)::97-108.

Gjorgov, AN (2009b). Breast cancer risk assessment to barrier contraception exposure. New Approach. *Contributions Soc Biol Med Sci* MASA, XXX, 1, 217-233. (Macedonian Academy of Sciences and Arts), Web: http://e20.manu.edu.mk/prilozi/16ag.pdf

Gjorgov, AN. (2010). Reproductive Health of Women: An Attempt to Define Breast Cancer Prevention. *Macedonian Journal of Medical Sciences*, 3(2): 169-179, Jun. 15, Web: http://www.mjms.ukim.edu.mk/Online/MJMS_2010_3_2/MJMS.1857-5773.2010-0104v.pdf

Hinman, AR. (1978). The condom as prophylactic. Bull. N.Y. Acad. Med. 52(8):1004-1011. Web: http://www.ncbi.nim.nih.gov/pmc/articles/PMC1807317/?log$=activity

Japanese Ministry of Health (2002). Major causes of divorce – Japan gaining on USA and Canada. (Update 2007.) Web:
http://hubpages.com/hub/Major_Causes_Of_Divorce

Kimball, M. (2010). Why Americans divorce. Women cite abuse, men site sex as top reasons for divorce. Internet web: www.divorce360.com/divorce-articles/causes-of-divorce/information/why-americans-divorce.aspx?artid=169

Koop, CE. (1986). Surgeon General's Report on AIDS. U.S. Public Health Service. *JAMA* 256:2783-2789.

Lancet Editorial. (2009). Breast cancer in developing countries. The Lancet 374:1567. November 7. Web: www.thelancet.com Vol 374 November 7, 2009 1567

Lincoln, R. (1979). The Select Committee Reports. *Family Planning Perspectives* 11(2):101-4, Mar-Apr. PMID: 456481 (Mesh Terms: Adolescent, Contraception, Emigration and Immigration, Family Planning Services, Fertility, Financing, Government, Humans, Cooperation, Population, Population Control, Research, Social Sciences)

Lê, Monique, G.; Bachelot, Annie & Hill, Catherine. (1989). Characteristics of reproductive life and risk of breast cancer in a case-control study of young nulliparous women. *Journal of Clinical Epidemiology* 42: 1227-1235.

Linos. E.; Spanos, D.; Rosner, BA. et al. (2008). Effects of reproductive and demographic changes on breast cancer incidence in China: A modeling analysis. *Journal of the National Cancer Institute* 100(19): 1352-1360.

Meckler, L. (2002). CDC Fact Sheet Not Promoting Condom Use Anymore. CDC Center for HIV,   STD   and   TB   Prevention,   December   19.   Web: http://www.aegis.com/news/ads/2002/AD022455.html

McNeil, DDG. (2010). UN reports decrease in new HIV infections. *The New York Times*, November 23-24. Web:
http://www.nytimes.com/2010/11/24/world/africa/24infect.html and http://www.blueridgenow.com/article/20101124/ZNYT04/11243009

McPherson, K.; Steel, CN. & Dixon, JM. (2000). Breast cancer epidemiology, risk factor, and genetics. *BMJ* 321:1198-1206. 9 September. Web:
http://www.bmj.com/content/321/7261/624.full

Malta National Cancer Registry (2010). Incidence of breast cancer in Females (1998-2007). *Dep't of Health Info. & Research.*

Meckler, L. (2002). CDC Fact Sheet Not Promoting Condom Use Anymore. Prevention News Update. December 19. Internet web:
http://aegis.com/news/ads/2002/AD022455.html

Merriman, A. (2010). Emerging breast cancer epidemics: impact on palliative care. Breast Cancer Research 12(Suppl 4):S11. Web:
http://breast-cancer-research.com/content/12/S4/S11

Miller, WR. (2010). Controversies in breast cancer 2010. Breast Cancer Research 12(Suppl 4): S1. Web: http://breast-cancer-research.com/content/12/S4/S1

Mills, JL. (1987). Reporting provocative results. Can we publish 'hot' papers without getting burned? Commentary. JAMA 258(23): 3428, December 18.

Moynihan R (2003). The making of a disease: Female sexual dysfunction. *BMJ*, 4 326:45-47, January.

National Academy of Sciences. (2011) Women's Health Research. Progress, Pitfalls, and Promise. Ch. 3. Research on Conditions with Particular Relevance to Women. (pp. 95-170) Table 3-1.

National Cancer Institute-NCI. (2002). SEER Cancer Statistics Review 1975-2000. Female breast cancer (In Situ) - Table IV-6.

Mosher WD, Jones J. (2010).Use of contraception in the United States: 1982–2008. *National Center for Health Statistics. Vital & Health Statistics* 23(29). Web:
http://www.cdc.gov/nchs/data/series/sr_23/sr23_029.pdf

Muir, C., Waterhouse, J., Mack, T., Powell, J., Whelan, S., Eds. (1987). *Cancer Incidence in Five Continents*, Volume V, WHO-IARC, Publ. 120, Lyon, France.

National Cancer Policy Board-NCPB. (2005). Saving Women's Lives: Strategies for Improving   Breast   Cancer   Detection   and   Diagnosis.   Web: http://books.nap.edu/openbook.php?record_id=11916&page=269

Office of National Statistics (2004). Divorce rate in UK. Web:
http://www.divorcerate.org/divorce-rates-in-uk.html

Parkin, DM.; Muir, CS.; Whelan, SL.; Gao, YT; Ferlay J. & Powell J. Eds. (1992). *Cancer Incidence in Five Continents*, Volume VI, WHO-IARC Sci. Publ. 120, Lyon, France.

Parkin DM, Whelan SL, Ferlay J, Raymond L, Young J. Eds. (1997). *Cancer Incidence in Five Continents*, Volume VII, WHO-IARC Sci. Publ. 143, Lyon, France.

Parkin DM, Whelan S, Ferlay J, Teppo L, Thomas DB. Eds. (2002). *Cancer Incidence in Five Continents*, Volume VIII, WHO-IARC, Sci. Publ. 155, Lyon, France. (Digital data edition on Internet).

Peatling, S. (2005). Divorce takes husbands by surprise. Article, March 17. Internet web: www.smh.com.au/news/National/Divorce-takes-husbands-by-surprise/2005/03/16/1110913668722.html

Peters, EN. (1998). Contraception and Divorce: Insights from American Annulment Cases. *Family Foundations (Nov.-Dec.)*. CanonLaw.info. Web: http://www.canonlaw.info/a_contraceptionanddivorce.htm

Pikhut PM, Levshin VF, and Moskaleva LI. (1991). Methods of contraception and the risk of breast cancer development. *Sovyetskaya Medicina*, issue 12, pp. 70-72.

Siegel-Itzkovich, j. (1999). Israel health minister bans AIDS campaign promoting condoms. BMJ 319 (7223):1455 (December 4). Web: http://www.bmj.com/cgi/content/full/319/7223/1455/b?maxtoshow=&HITS=1 0718/05/01

Stevenson, B. & Wolfers, J. (2007a). Marriage and Divorce: Changes in their driving forces. *Journal of Economic Perspectives* Vol. 21, No. 2, pp. 27-52. Web: www.hartonupenn.edu/betseys/papers/JEP_Marriage_and_Divorce.pdf

Stevenson, B. & Wolfers, J. (2007b). Marriage and Divorce: Changes in their driving forces. NBER Working Paper Series, No 12944. National Bureau of Economic Research, Cambridge, MA. March. Web: http://www.nber.org/papers/w12944.pdf

Stevenson, B. & Wolfers, J. (2009). The paradox of declining female happiness. *American Economic Journal: Economic Policy* 1:2, 190-225. Web: http://www.aeaweb.org/articles.php?doi=10.1257/pol.1.2.190

Stevenson, B. (2010). Marriage calculator. Web: http://www.divorce360.com/content/getthedivorcecalculatorwidget.aspx

Storm, HH. (2011). Johannes Clemmesen – a pioneer and founder of Danish cancer epidemiology, has passed away on December 20, 2010, at the age of 102. Web: http://www.iarc.fr/media-centre/iarcnews/pdf/JohannesClemmesenEng.pdf

Svoboda, E. (2006). All signs of pregnancy except one: a baby. Article. *The New York Times*, December 5.

UK Working Group on the Primary Prevention of Breast Cancer. (2007). No More Breast Cancer. December. Web: http://www.nomorebreastcancer.org.uk/assets/main_v.1.pdf

UNAIDS (2010). Report on the global AIDS epidemic 2010. Web: http://www.unaids.org/globalreport/Global_report.htm

United Nations Secretariat. (1994). *Key issues in family planning, health and family well-being in the 190s and beyond*. International Conference on Population and Development, Cairo, 5-14 September. (ICPD, Cairo, 1994).

Valdiserri, RO. (1988). Cum Mastis Sic Clypeatis: The turbulent history of the condom. Bulletin of the N.Y. Academy of Medicine 64(3): 237-245.

Waterhouse, J.; Muir, C.; Correa, P. & Powell, J. Eds. (1977). *Cancer Incidence in Five Continents*, Volume III, WHO-IARC Publ. No. 15, Lyon, France.

Waterhouse. J.; Muir, C.; Shanmugaratnam, K. & Powell, J. Eds. (1982). *Cancer Incidence in Five Continents*, Volume IV, WHO-IARC Publ. No. 42, Lyon, France.

WHO-PAHO. (2008). Guidelines for International Breast Health and Cancer Control. Cancer - Volume 113, Issue Supplement 8 - 15 October (World Health Organization and Pan American Health Organization). Web:
http://www.paho.org/English/AD/DPC/NC/pcc-breast-cancer-guidelines.htm and

Wolfers, J. (2010). How marriage survives. Op-Ed. New York Times, October 12. Web:
http://www.nytimes.com/2010/10/13/opinion/13wolfers.html

Part 2

From the Clinic to the Patients: Transmission, Diagnosis and Therapies

9

Transmission of HIV Through Blood – How To Bridge the Knowledge Gap

Smit Sibinga, Cees Th and John P. Pitman
ID Consulting for International Development of Transfusion Medicine/
University of Groningen
The Netherlands

1. Introduction

1.1 HIV and blood transfusion – The current state of the art

Of all blood donations 65% are made in developed (very high human development index or VH-HDI) countries, home to just 25% of the world's population. In 73 countries, donation rates are still less than 1% of the population (the minimum needed to meet basic needs in a country). Of these, 71 are either developing (low HDI) or transitional (medium to high HDI) countries; 42 countries collect less than 25% of their blood supplies from the safest source: voluntary non-remunerated blood donors. However, less than 50% of these donors donates regularly, the other half just one time only. In 2007, 31 countries (19%) still reported collecting paid donations, which is more than 1 million donations in total, where 41 countries (25%) were not able to screen all blood donations for one or more of the following transfusion-transmissible infections (TTIs) – HIV, hepatitis B, hepatitis C and syphilis (WHO 2010a).

Blood transfusion as a supportive haemotherapy contributes to saving lives and improving health, but millions of patients needing transfusion do not have timely access to or can afford safe blood. In 2007, 162 countries provided data to WHO on 85.4 million blood donations (World Health Organization [WHO] 2010a). These data come from countries that account for a total of 5.9 billion people, representing 92% of the global population. The report covers around 8,000 blood centres. In developed countries, the average annual collection per blood centre was 13,600 (range 49–289,075), in transitional countries 6,000 (range 20–499,212) and in developing countries 2,800 (range 114–23,251).

1.1.1 Blood supply

While the need for blood is universal, there is still a major imbalance between developing and advanced countries in the level of access to safe blood. It is estimated that blood donation by 1% of the total population (10 per 1,000 population) is generally the minimum needed to meet a nation's most basic requirements for blood; the requirements are higher in countries with more advanced health care systems and medical interventions.

Of the 85.4 milion donations in 2007, about 65 % were collected in developed countries. Blood donations per 1,000 population, which also reflect the general availability of blood in a country, vary widely and the lowest levels of availability are found in developing and transitional countries (WHO 2010a). The average donation rate in developed (VH-HDI) countries is 38.1 donations/1,000 population (range 4.92–68.01); in transitional (H and M-HDI) countries this rate is 7.5 (range 1.07–35.18) and in developing (L-HDI) countries an average of 2.3 (range 0.40–7.46) donations per 1,000 population were collected. In 2007, 73 countries (45%) reported collecting fewer than 10 donations per 1,000 population. Among them, 71 (97%) are either developing or transitional countries. Due to relatively high TTI marker prevalence the drop out of collected blood varies between 11 and over 20%, reducing the clinical availability substantially.

1.1.2 Blood donation

There are three major types of blood donation: voluntary unpaid donations (non-remunerated/altruistic), family/replacement donations (coerced), and paid donations. Donors who give blood voluntarily, regularly and for altruistic reasons have the lowest prevalence of HIV, hepatitis viruses and other blood-borne infections, as compared to people who donate for friends and family members or because of payment. Family and replacement donations are often hidden paid and seriously coerced. Sufficient supplies of safe blood can only be assured by regular donations from voluntary unpaid and anonymous donors. The 2007 WHO data reveal some improvements in such donations worldwide, but many developing and transitional countries still rely heavily on relatively unsafe one time only family/replacement donors and paid donors (fig 1).

This means a considerable gap in public awareness and knowledge about the essentials of blood donation as an act of social solidarity and blood transfusion as an integral element of the health care system.

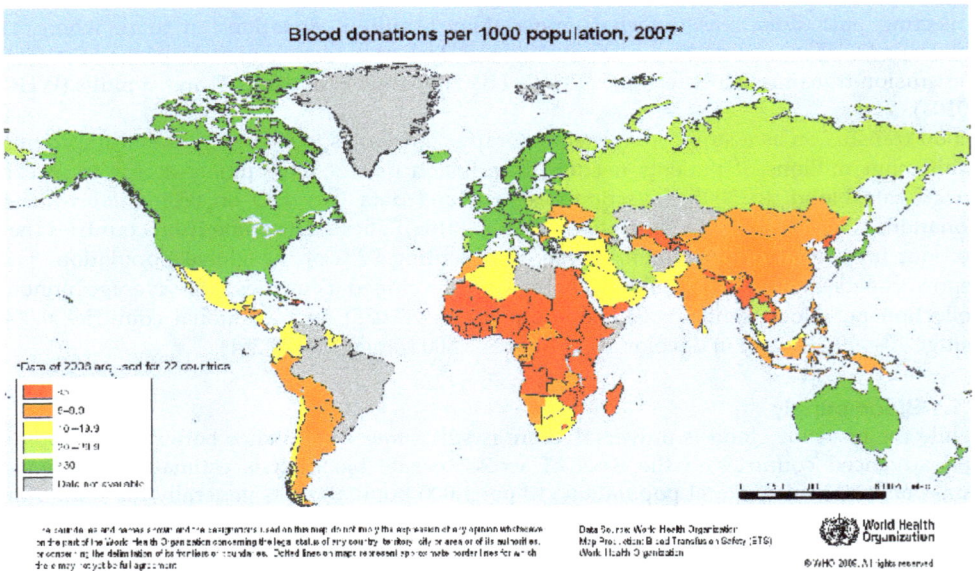

Fig. 1. Annual blood donations per 1,000 population, 2007. Source: Global Database on Blood Safety (GDBS), 2007 survey (WHO2010a)

1.1.2.1 Voluntary, unpaid donations

Of the 162 responding countries 57 (35%) report collecting 100% of their blood supplies from voluntary unpaid donors (fig. 2). Since World Blood Donor Day (14th June, birthday of Karl Landsteiner) celebration began in 2004, 111 countries (68.5%) reported an increase of the number of voluntary donations; 32 of these 111 (29%) have more than doubled the number of voluntary donations as compared to 2004 figures. All these 32 countries are developing or transitional countries. Additionally, 11 countries (Bosnia and Herzegovina, Burkina Faso, Cook Islands, Cape Verde, Kuwait, Guinea Bissau, Mauritania, Myanmar, Niue, Vanuatu and Vietnam) reported more than a 10% increase in voluntary unpaid donations in 2007, as compared to 2006 figures. However, a major problem remains the retention of voluntary non-remunerated blood donors.

1.1.2.2 Family/replacement donors and paid donors

Forty-two countries (26%) collect less than 25% of their blood supplies from voluntary unpaid blood donors. A significant amount of the blood supply in these countries is still dependent on family/replacement and paid blood donors. Thirty-one countries (18%) still report collecting paid donations in 2007, which represents more than 1 million donations in total.

The average donation rate in high-income countries is 45,400 donations per million people. This compares with 10,100 donations per million people in middle-income countries and 3,600 donations in low-income countries. If 1% to 3% of a country's population would donate blood, it would be sufficient to meet the country's needs. But in 77 countries, donation rates are still less than 1%.

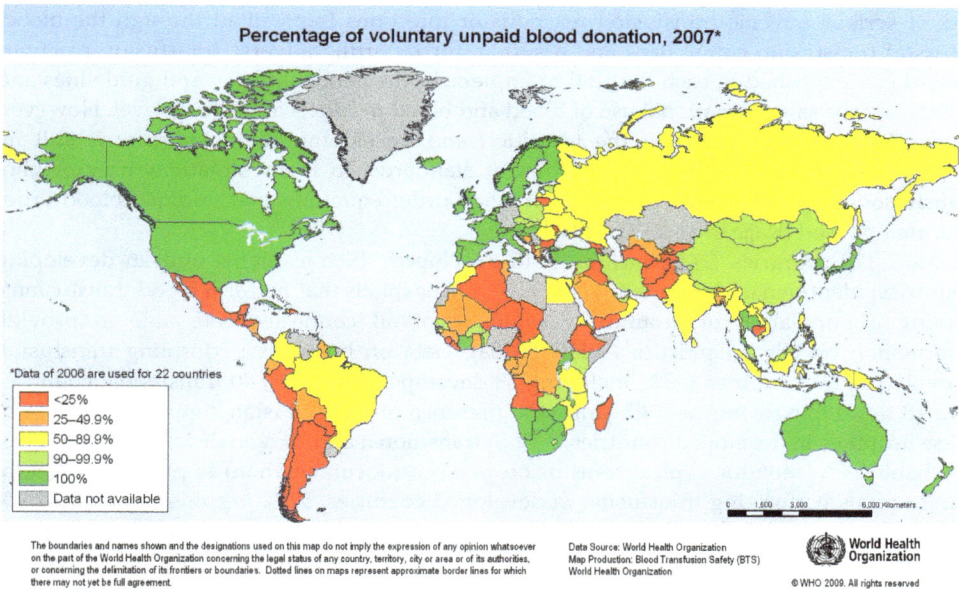

Fig. 2. Percentage voluntary non-remunerated blood donors, 2007. Source: Global Database on Blood Safety (GDBS), 2007 survey (WHO2010a)

1.1.3 Blood screening for transmissible infections

WHO recommends that all donated blood to be used for transfusion should be screened at minimum for HIV, hepatitis B, hepatitis C and syphilis (WHO 2010). Complete and accurate data on the screening of donated blood are not available from many developing countries, particularly those where blood services are not coordinated. Many countries do not have reliable testing systems because of staff shortages, lack of basic laboratory services, poor quality test kits or their irregular supply. Of the 162 countries that provided data on screening for transfusion-transmissible infections including HIV, hepatitis B, hepatitis C and syphilis, 41 (25%) are not able to screen all donated blood for one or more of these infections (fig. 3). The other 121 countries provided data on whether blood donations were screened in a quality-assured manner (use of standard operating procedures and participation in an external quality assessment scheme or EQAS). Overall, 88% of the blood collected are screened following these basic quality procedures: 89% in developed countries, 87% in transitional countries and 48% in developing countries. For the blood donations collected in the remaining 41 countries, which account for 22% of the global donations reported to WHO, the use of these basic quality assurance procedures for laboratory screening is still unknown. Additionally there is still a widespread mix of test kits used within countries, both ELISA and rapid test depending on availability and supply. Quality of performance and reliability of test results remain a problem of considerable concern.

1.1.4 Clinical use of blood

Data on the clinical use of donated blood is limited, but studies suggest that transfusions are often given unnecessarily when simpler, less expensive treatments can provide equal or greater benefit. Not only is this a waste of a scarce resource but it also exposes patients to the risk of serious adverse transfusion reactions or infections transmitted through the blood. Hospital transfusion committees and a system for reporting adverse transfusion reactions should be established in each hospital to implement the national policy and guidelines and to monitor the safe and rational use of blood and blood products at the local level. However, in a substantial proportion of the transition and developing countries there is still no national policy and no current guidelines or standards. In many situations haemoglobin transfusion triggers are high and surgical blood order equations and minimal blood order lists are not used (Kajja et al. 2010a, 2010b) .

In 2007, 120 countries (74%, including 46 developed, 48 transitional and 26 developing countries) identified and reported a total of 51,400 hospitals that perform blood transfusions, serving a population of around 3.6 billion. Not all countries were able to provide information on clinical practice (WHO 2010a). Data on hospitals performing transfusion provided by 96 countries (80%, including 38 developed countries, 40 transitional countries and 18 developing countries) illustrate the presence of a transfusion committee in 88% of these hospitals in developed countries, 33% in transitional and 25 % in developing countries. Mechanisms to monitor clinical transfusion practice (documentation) is present in 90% of the hospitals performing transfusion in developed countries, 52 % in transitional and 23 % in developing countries. However, a system for reporting adverse transfusion events (haemovigilance) in hospitals performing transfusion is found in 91% in developed countries, but only 46% in transitional and 23% in developing countries.

These 2007 WHO survey data illustrate a major gap in awareness and knowledge among policy makers and blood transfusion professionals, both in the procurement and the prescribing parts of the vein-to-vein blood transfusion chain in transitional (M-HDI) and even more prominent in developing (L-HDI) countries.

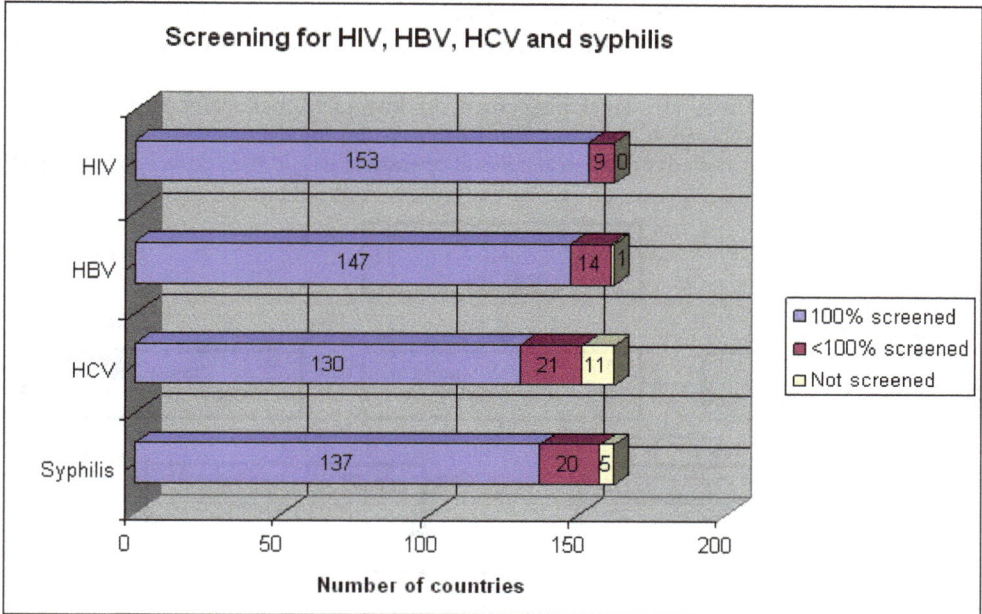

Fig. 3. Numbers of countries screening for HIV, HBV, HCV and syphilis Source: Global Database on Blood Safety (GDBS), 2007 survey (WHO 2010a)

1.2 Basics of the blood supply

Since UN together with its health organization WHO became operational in 1948, universal principles have been laid down in the UN Declaration of Universal Human Rights (UN 1948). For the health care and blood transfusion chain art. 25.1 – Right of Health through securing food, clothing, shelter and health care, and art. 26 – Right of Education, elementary and access to vocational education, are paramount.

In1975 the WHA passed a Resolution 28.72 (Utilization and Supply of Human Blood and Blood Products), indicating that blood is a national resource, to be 'shared' voluntarily and altruistically and to be given as a social act of solidarity, and that human blood and tissue should never be subject to commerce (WHO 1978)

These principles have been worked out by e.g. the International Society of Blood Transfusion (ISBT) in the Code of Ethics (ISBT 2000), but also by the EU in the Directives related to blood transfusion (EU 2003, Directive 2002/98/EC).

Blood transfusion in its vein-to-vein structure should be seen as a part of a larger project to develop a safe, sustainable, high quality and efficacious blood supply and transfusion system that is fully integrated into the health care system. Ensuring the safety and availability of blood and blood products is an essential public health responsibility. Measures to ensure blood safety also play a major role in preventing the transmission of HIV, hepatitis viruses and other blood born pathogens in health care settings. The Ministry of Health (MoH) should provide effective leadership and governance in developing a national blood system that is fully integrated into the health care system. First the foundation, then the construction of the organization and the necessary infrastructure (Quality System and Quality Management System, facilities, etc), will need to be developed. These will be followed by the development of the human capacity needed at all levels, including in the hospitals (medical and paramedical staff).

In principle, the approach for developing such an integrated nationally supported and organized country wide blood supply and transfusion system for the future, and in line with internationally accepted and advocated principles of operation, would then be as follows (fig. 4)

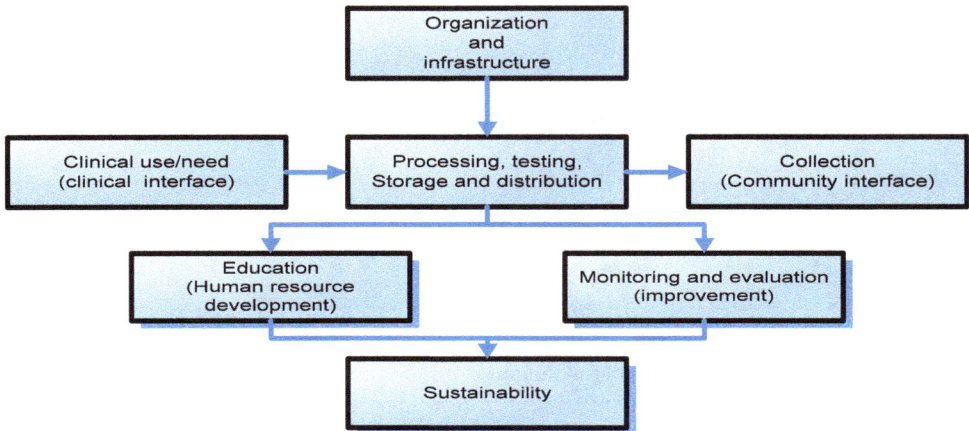

Fig. 4. Development scheme blood supply organization.

The set up should be based on a solid country specific legislative and regulatory system with sufficient authority to license operations according to international quality principles (cGMP, cGLP and cGCP)[1] supported by appropriate and standardized management principles based on ISO9001:2008. It starts with a clinical needs assessment to be followed by the logistics of the procurement and supply chain that has its roots in the community (public awareness) (Smit Sibinga 2006, WHO 2008c, Smit Sibinga et al 2009a,).

The implementation is not limited to public or private blood centres or establishments. The limitation is in the fragmentation with insufficient critical mass and economy of scale to guarantee quality and cost-effectiveness, nation wide access and affordability. National coordination and consistent and sustained governmental responsibility and support to protect citizens from unjustified and maleficent practices are the more important (Smit Sibinga 2000).

A nationally coordinated and integrated blood supply system needs competent and committed leadership and an appropriate budget to allow accessibility and affordability of haemotherapy, based on a proper and documented needs assessment. The financing system should be an integral part of a national health financing system based on cost recovery and a healthy insurance policy accessible and affordable for all citizens (WHO 2008, van Hulst et al. 2006).

---

[1] GMP = Good Manufacturing Practice, GLP = Good Laboratory Practice, GCP = Good Clinical Practice

The framework of such an integrated blood supply system could be based on the seven key elements (figure 4) as follows:

1. Organization and structure, including the necessary infrastructure to be strengthened and further developed. This element includes the development of an appropriate and implementable formal regulatory structure, development of a system of regional blood banks based on a sufficient economy of scale to become cost-effective. These institutions preferably should be part of a nationally coordinated blood transfusion service responsible for policy making, design of the necessary strategies, annual planning, the development of a national quality and quality management system based on internationally accepted standards and product specifications. Such quality and quality management system will have a uniform documentation system, which allows for the possibility of instituting a nation-wide ICT system for data management. The organization should have sufficient autonomy to operate its services. As the organization produces products (collection, processing and testing, storage and distribution) for clinical use, it is automatically product liable and should therefore operate independently from hospitals. Hospitals use the products for specific haemotherapy in patients and therefore have the legal obligation to protect consumer rights, which cannot be combined with product liability under the same final responsibility (conflict of interest). Another aspect of this first element is the need to develop appropriate and cGMP compliant working facilities, that guarantee a working environment that allows high quality operations to be performed by staff.

2. Clinical use needs full attention to develop evidence based transfusion practices all over the country. That means assessment of the current clinical practices and development of an in-hospital transfusion quality and quality management system. Hospitals will be supplied by regional procurement centers (blood centres) with a working stock that will be based on an inventory of actual needs per discipline – paediatrics, obstetrics, surgery and traumatology and haemato-oncology. The development of a well functioning clinical interface will lead to the change from the currently prevalent supply driven system to a demand driven system, based on mutual respect and understanding and key to the supplier-customer principle of quality operations (Kajja 2010).

3. Processing and testing of all units of blood collected will allow an efficient use of the blood collected and contribute to rational use of blood through component therapy. Testing for the key TTI markers (HIV, HBV, HCV and Syphilis) needs to be instituted with appropriate and standardized technology and methodology. Here, economies of scale are paramount to guarantee consistency of performance and cost containment. Where epidemiology indicates, additional tests can be considered such as brucellosis, Chagas or malaria. As screening tests focus on sensitivity, a system for confirmation needs to be developed at the national level – a reference laboratory that also could perform test kit and reagent validation before implementation is needed. Along with the development of component production, in-process quality control of the produced half and finished products (testing for standardized and uniform product specifications) will be part of the program.

4. Collection of source material – human blood or plasma – from voluntary non-remunerated and preferably regular blood donors, motivated and mobilized from identified low-risk groups in the community. This requires development of public awareness based on social marketing. The currently prevalent supply driven system of

the blood supply needs to be developed into a demand driven system, which means the availability of motivated potential donors willing to be mobilized to allow a balanced blood stock that is managed and the development of a contingency plan. Donor selection needs to be standardized and adjusted to internationally recommended minimum requirements for donor suitability.

5. Education (teaching and training) is the cornerstone of capacity building. A national assessment and inventory of available education (institutions, curricula) needs to be carried out to allow the development of an effective approach towards capacity building and human resource development at all levels involved. The in-country approach will focus on leadership development (senior and middle management) and development of operational competencies (professional knowledge and skills) through various education methodologies to allow larger groups of staff to benefit.

6. Monitoring and evaluation follows the implementation of a national quality and quality management system based on uniform documentation of what is being done, both at the management level (management information system) as well as at the operational level through an automated data processing system (ICT) with communication between all centres and the national Head Quarter and Ministry of Health. Use of simple statistical evaluation technology such as statistical process control (SPC) and application of Six Sigma (Gygi et al., 2005) will allow proper benchmarking focused on improvement through trend analysis. A nationwide compatible ICT system would allow proper quality management through coordinated monitoring and evaluation of uniform data collected through regional centres and hospitals (vein-to-vein).

7. Sustainability is not only dependent on financial resources, but comprehensively relates to all six elements as described above – organizational structure and infrastructure, competent and adequate human resources, a reliable and regular voluntary blood donor panel, a standardized procurement process, evidence based rational use of blood components and alternatives, and quality assurance through proper monitoring of set indicators and their evaluation through benchmarking focused on improvement. This follows the principle of the Deming cycle of improvement – **plan** (policy and strategies), **do** (implementation of managerial and operational processes), **check** (monitoring of the indicators/specifications and accurate data collection through documentation), **act** (evaluation of the collected data and the benchmarking).

1.3 Basics of the clinical use of blood

The clinical use of blood represents both the starting and the closing end of the demand and supply loop. Therefore, it does not make much sense to develop only the clinical interface if the basics of proper procurement (collection, processing and testing, storage and distribution), based on international principles (1948 UN Declaration of Universal Human Rights, 1975 WHA28/72 Utilization and Supply of Human Blood and Blood Products, International Red Cross and ISBT Code of Ethics) are not in place.

The in-hospital transfusion chain should include process analysis, process descriptions, related SOPs and operational documents such as a standard (national) blood request form, a standard compatibility test form, a transfusion outcome form, clinical guidelines and a haemovigilance report form (Kajja 2010).

The in-hospital transfusion chain consists of three distinctive processes, each containing a number of procedures, critical control points (CCPs/decisions) and documentation. (figure 5)

Each of these processes has a series of procedures and related documentation that needs to be developed:

1. The *blood ordering process* (ward/bedside) starts at the bedside with indication setting and decision making resulting in a standardized request and accompanying blood sample for compatibility testing. Traceability (documentation) is paramount to prevent adverse transfusion reactions due to clerical errors of identification (wrong blood in tube). It consists of six steps or procedures (diagnosis, indication, decision to transfuse or use alternatives, ordering, sample taking and transportation) and two operational documents (blood request form and sample label);

2. The *blood selection process* (laboratory) of blood components as requested and compatibility testing. It should be noted that compatibility testing is a laboratory diagnostic procedure. The blood selection process consists of four steps or procedures (reception and registration of request and sample, selection of blood, compatibility testing and transportation) and two operational documents (logbook and cross match form);

3. The *bedside transfusion process* (ward/bedside) of the selected units at the bedside, which needs careful identification of units and recipient (match), and the technical handling and observation of the transfusion, carried out by nursing staff and based on proper and uniform standard operating procedures with appropriate documentation to allow evaluation necessary to develop evidence based practice. It consists of two sub-processes:

   a. The preparation of the patient and the unit of blood before the transfusion – three steps or procedures (reception at the ward, patient and unit identification, vital signs);

   b. Transfusion and observation of the patient – four steps or procedures (connection to the patient, immediate observation, transfusion or discontinuation, observation of outcome).

These processes are closely interrelated, though distinctly different. The following steps are involved in the process:

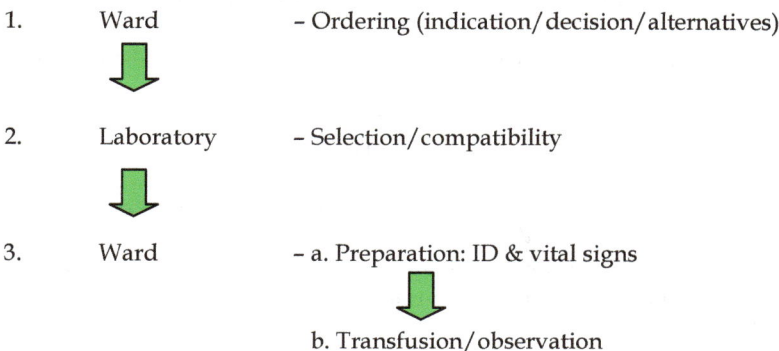

1.   Ward   – Ordering (indication/decision/alternatives)

2.   Laboratory   – Selection/compatibility

3.   Ward   – a. Preparation: ID & vital signs

                         b. Transfusion/observation

Fig. 5. In-hospital transfusion flow of steps.

Clinicians and nursing staff need to be trained in these steps and the related quality assurance and documentation to develop a proper and standardized monitoring and evaluation evidence based transfusion practice. To create ownership among the prescribing clinicians and nursing staff education should focus on consensus on items such as a uniform blood request form, terms of reference of a Hospital Transfusion Committee (HTC) and the outline of clinical guidelines (general and per prescribing discipline).

1.4 Gaps in the blood supply and clinical use

In many developing countries blood transfusion in the vein-to-vein concept is still in its first or second generation stage. This means that blood is most often collected and transfused in the absence of a formal policy environment and without adequate regulatory controls or standards. In such systems, blood collection and utilization are fragmented, often dependent on independent factors limited to specific hospitals, such as the availability of trained and competent staff, funds for procurement, and a population of blood donors willing to come on a voluntary and regular basis.

Following the vein-to-vein transfusion chain, major gaps exist in the following areas:

1. Organization and infrastructure -
   a. Legal and regulatory frameworks are often outdated or do not exist.
   b. Commitment of health authorities is lacking or isolated in fragmented centres.
   c. Management capacity to sustain blood collection, storage, testing and transfusion services differs from routine hospital or laboratory management.
   d. Organization and infrastructure for blood services requires national and facility-specific assessments and inputs.
   e. Chain of command and clear job descriptions contribute to quality control, stock management, and career development.
   f. Quality culture and professional discipline are dependent on successful pre-service and on-going in-service training opportunities.
   g. Poor hygiene and waste management may contribute to broader infection control problems within a facility and the local community.
2. Clinical use –
   a. Clinical awareness and accountability among clinicians is essential to avoid unnecessary transfusions and preserve limited blood stocks.
   b. Improper indication setting and decision making may increase transfusion recipients' risk.
   c. Informed consent of patients can create additional ethical and legal challenges for a facility when not obtained properly (Kajja et al. 2011)
   d. Poor documentation and traceability contribute to wastage; may facilitate fraud, and; create barriers to appropriate epidemiological follow-up and tracing in the event of an adverse transfusion event.
   e. Communication and understanding between suppliers and users is essential to ensure that suppliers (i.e., blood donors) contribute based on a humanitarian impulse, not one based on personal gain, and that users (patients and clinicians) recognize and consent to the risks related to transfusion.
3. Processing and testing –
   a. Standards of processing and quality control are a crucial line of defense in patient safety and preventing unnecessary wastage.
   b. Inconsistent supply logistics can interrupt quality-associated work routines, contribute to unnecessary wastage (out-dating and cold chain spoilage) and promote unequal service between regions or facilities (Kajja et al. 2010a, 2010b)

4. Collection of source material (community interface) –
    a. Community awareness about the need for blood and the risks of disease transmission via transfusion are essential to mobilize a safe donor pool.
    b. Types of blood donors must be actively motivated, selected and screened for safety.
5. Education –
    a. Education and staff competency: The basis for a quality assured and sustained system. (Smit Sibinga, 2009a)
6. Monitoring and evaluation –
    a. Applied research in the field of transfusion medicine through proper monitoring and evaluation (M&E) and continued statistical process control (SPC) can contribute to improved operations as well as global understanding of risks, barriers and best practices (Smit Sibinga, 2009b).

2. Principles and ethical aspects of blood donation and transfusion - How do these elements promote blood safety?

Like other medical specializations, the practice of transfusion medicine is bound by the ancient Greek Hippocratic mandate *Primum est non nocere* (first, do no harm). However, for transfusion specialists, this principle is not limited to the transfusion itself or to the recipient of the transfusion. Rather, it applies to a long chain of ethical decisions that stretches from the motivation of potential donors whose blood is used for transfusions to post-transfusion follow-up. This section will describe and explain how each link in this chain contributes to a safe blood supply and to safe transfusion practice.

2.1 Ethical aspects of blood donation

A brief history of blood donation and transfusion ethics

The ethical principles that govern the modern vein-to-vein transfusion system were developed relatively recently, that is to say, largely within the second half of the 20th century, when the science of transfusion medicine became an accepted and routine part of medical practice. (American College of Physicians [ACP], 1984) Indeed, from the 17th century, when physicians began experimenting with transfusing animal blood into humans, through the late 19th and early 20th century when blood groups were discovered and coagulation factors described, the field of transfusion medicine was marked by experimentation, trial and error, and few human subjects protections. (Feldschuh, 1990; McCullough, 1998; Kendrick, n.d.) The 1948 Nuremburg Code established a global framework for medical ethics following the atrocities committed by Nazi doctors during the Second World War. In Europe and North America, laws covering ethical concepts such as the requirement that patients give informed consent prior to medical procedures began to emerge in the 1950s and 1960s. (ACP, 1984) In the mid-1930s, the founding of the International Society of Blood Transfusion (ISBT), created a global forum for the development of specific ethical guidelines for the practice of blood transfusion. Two decades later, in 1955, the International Federation of Blood Donor Organizations (FIODS) was established to focus attention on ethical guidelines for the donation of blood and plasma. Both entities, as well as authors such as Richard Titmuss (The Gift Relationship: From Human Blood to Social Policy, 1971) (Titmuss, 1971), contributed to a body of ethical work that lead to the 1975 World Health Assembly resolution containing global recommendations

for ethical blood donations and transfusions (WHA 28.72). Those recommendations included the following key elements of transfusion ethics:
1. Blood donations should be voluntary and unpaid.
2. Countries should collect an adequate supply of blood to be self-sufficient.
3. Countries should develop legislation and supporting regulations to monitor and control the quality of blood collections, blood service laboratory operations (infectious disease screening, compatibility testing, production of blood products), and transfusion practice.

These recommendations seem especially prescient following the emergence of the HIV/AIDS epidemic in the 1980s, and the identification of blood transfusion as a significant route of HIV infection (US CDC, 1982). Between 1980 and 2000, the ISBT and WHO refined and adapted these original principles into a global code of ethics whose purpose was "*to define the ethical principles and rules to be observed in the field of Transfusion Medicine.*" The ISBT code of ethics is discussed in detail below. Most countries worldwide have blood policies based on these fundamental principles (WHO, 2011a). Since 2000, these principles have guided numerous global resolutions related to HIV prevention and the emerging donor-supported field of 'blood safety'. (PEPFAR, 2005-2010; WHO, 2011b)

'*Safe blood starts with me*'. This commonly used blood donor motivation slogan captures one of the principal ethical issues in blood donation, namely that donors share an equal burden of responsibility with blood services to ensure the safety of the blood supply (Grainger et al., 1997). As the sole source of blood for transfusion, donors are indispensible. Yet, donors also have rights that must be respected and are, more critically, the principal vector for transfusion-transmissible infections. Ensuring the safety of donated blood, therefore, requires a balanced, combination approach, including active, education-based and non-coercive social mobilization practices by transfusion services and donation centres, and the *active and honest* participation of donors in the pre-donation screening process.

The ISBT Code of Ethics (2000, 2006 revision) contains 11 principles that expand on these concepts, especially as they relate to donor health and safety, donors' right to anonymity or confidentiality during and after donation, and donors' *ethical responsibility* not to donate if they believe their blood may be infected with HIV or another blood-borne pathogen.

The ISBT code can be collapsed into a chain with four basic links. This pre-donation chain describes the individual links that protect donors and the recipients of donated blood. As noted above, each of these links contributes to blood safety in a different way.

Link 1: Mobilizing blood donors without coercion

Identifying, mobilizing, educating, motivating and retaining an adequate pool of eligible and willing blood donors is the primary challenge faced by blood transfusion services worldwide. The problem is especially serious in the developing world, where public awareness of blood transfusion is low (Elhence, 2006), traditional or cultural beliefs about blood may serve as powerful disincentives to blood donation (Umeora et al., 2005), and high population prevalence rates for HIV and other TTIs may be a barrier to blood donor appeals to the general public (McFarland et al., 1998). In countries with serious blood shortages, the impulse to pay or coerce blood donors can be powerful (Parry, 1984). But since the 1980s, prompted largely by concerns about transfusion-transmitted hepatitis and HIV, blood services in the developed world have largely adopted policies promoting voluntary and anonymous blood donation and prohibiting or limiting the payment of donors (ISBT,

2006b).[2] In the developing world, national blood policies developed since 2000 increasingly reflect World Health Organization recommendations that call for blood donors to act on an altruistic impulse, not in exchange for money or other kinds of compensation, and for blood services to mobilize *voluntary, non-remunerated* donors. The WHO Aide-Mémoire on establishing national blood transfusion services considers this practice '*the foundation of a safe and adequate blood supply.*' (WHO, 2011c)

The ISBT Code of Ethics (2006 revision)

Blood Centers: Donors and Donation

(International Society for Blood Transfusion [ISBT], 2006a)

1. Blood donation including haematopoietic tissues for transplantation shall, in all circumstances, be voluntary and non-remunerated; no coercion should be brought to bear upon the donor. A donation is considered voluntary and non-remunerated if the person gives blood, plasma or cellular components of his/her own free will and receives no payment for it, either in the form of cash, or in kind which could be considered a substitute for money. This would include time off work other than that reasonable needed for the donation and travel. Small tokens, refreshments and reimbursements of direct travel costs are compatible with voluntary, non-remunerated donation. The donor should provide informed consent to the donation of blood or blood components and to the subsequent (legitimate) use of the blood by the transfusion service.

2. A profit motive should not be the basis for the establishment and running of a blood service.

3. The donor should be advised of the risks connected with the procedure; the donor's health and safety must be protected. Any procedures relating to the administration to a donor of any substance for increasing the concentration of specific blood components should be in compliance with internationally accepted standards.

4. Anonymity between donor and recipient must be ensured except in special situations and the confidentiality of donor information assured.

5. The donor should understand the risks to others of donating infected blood and his or her ethical responsibility to the recipient.

---

[2] Exceptions exist to this general trend, most notably in paid plasma donations in the United States. Other developed countries provide financial or material compensation to donors, or have laws granting blood donors time off from work in exchange for donations. (European Commission, 2003, as cited in Farrugia et al., 2010; U.S. Food and Drug Administration, 2002) While the push for 100% voluntary, non-remunerated blood donations in developing countries has been shown to effectively screen out donors at high risk of infection with HIV or other transfusion-transmissible infections (Sarkodie et al., 2001), an emerging body of evidence suggests that some donors who act for reasons other than personal altruism – for instance, family members or others who donate in emergencies or to replace blood units – may present no greater risk to the blood supply than first-time volunteer donors (Allain et al., 2009; Diarra et al., 2009). Indeed, WHO and others stress the importance of motivating and retaining repeat donors '*who give blood regularly*', as the best way to screen out potential donors with a high behavioural risk profile. Yet, despite regular reinforcement of this global guidance, many services continue to provide or experiment with some forms of remuneration for blood donors, e.g., cholesterol screening (Glynn et al., 2003), distribution of lottery ticket (Stutzer & Goette, 2010), or transportation to and from the donation clinic (ISBT, 2006). These divergent findings pose a substantial ethical challenge for blood service managers faced with a limited pool of willing blood donors and unmet demand for blood.

6. Blood donation must be based on regularly reviewed medical selection criteria and not entail discrimination of any kind, including gender, race, nationality or religion. Neither donor nor potential recipient has the right to require that any such discrimination be practiced.
7. Blood must be collected under the overall responsibility of a suitably qualified, registered medical practitioner.
8. All matters related to whole blood donation and haemapheresis should be in compliance with appropriately defined and internationally accepted standards.
9. Donors and recipients should be informed if they have been harmed.
10. Blood is a public resource and access should not be restricted.
11. Wastage should be avoided in order to safeguard the interests of all potential recipients and the donor.

Link 2: Education is key

Worldwide, the public must be educated to understand that blood donation supports the collective good – that a unit donated today could save the life of a neighbour, a friend, a loved one, a stranger, or even the donor himself, tomorrow (*'today me, tomorrow you'*). But donors must also be educated about the risks associated with donation, both for the donor and for the recipient of donated blood. Education materials and programs should emphasize two main areas of risk and consent.

Risks to the donor and consent required prior to donation:

- The potential for syncope (fainting), hyperventilation, bruising or damage to veins during the veinipuncture process.
- Since most countries test or strive to test 100% of donated blood for pathogens such as HIV, hepatitis B and C, and syphilis, donors must be informed of these tests and given an opportunity to receive their results with appropriate counselling. In South Africa, the South African National Blood Service (SANBS) includes a clear statement about testing and the potential emotional impact on donors: *'Every blood donation is tested for HIV/AIDS. Persons testing positive must be aware that this may have a psychological impact and profoundly influence their lifestyle.'* (South African National Blood Service [SANBS], 2006)

Risks to recipients of donated blood:

- Transmission of infectious pathogens, including HIV.
- Other adverse transfusion events, e.g. circulatory overload, TRALI, mis-matched blood group, allogenic reactions.

Social mobilization and donor education campaigns will differ depending on the target audience. In many developing countries, youth, especially high-school students, contribute a substantial proportion of the national blood supply (Jacobs et al., 1994). However, it should be noted that donation camps at schools usually are based on coercion through the school authorities. (Los et al., 2009) In addition to confirming the voluntary nature of school-based donations, blood services must also study the epidemiology of HIV and other transfusion-transmissible infections among school-aged donors to ensure that this group actually carries a lower risk of infection compared to the general population. Over the last 10 years, several successful models to promote blood donation among youth have been established worldwide. These include the Club 25 model created by the International Federation of Red Cross and Red Crescent Societies (See: http://www.ifrc.org/en/what-we-do/health/blood-services/international-club-25-new-blood-for-the-world/) and the annual WHO-sponsored World Blood Donor Day on June 14, the birthday of Karl Landsteiner.

Link 3: Pre-donation counselling and behavioural risk screening

Pre-donation screening occurs after a donor has decided to make a donation, but before the blood is collected. The use of behavioural screening – also often referred to as self-exclusion screening – allows donors a confidential space in which to reflect on their behavioural risk profile and to weigh the consequences of a contaminated donation, especially donations that carry a high risk of infection with HIV. Behavioural questionnaires provide the blood service with information about lifestyle practices that could increase the donor's risk of carrying a TTI, and work-related information (e.g. do you operate heavy equipment?) that could create a safety hazard for the donor immediately after a donation. Questionnaires also provide information on medicines the donor is taking or other health conditions that could cause adverse reactions in the transfusion recipient or an adverse reaction for the donor (e.g. dizziness or fainting).

In most countries, pre-donation screening includes a written questionnaire and a face-to-face interview with a trained nurse or a donor counsellor. Questionnaires should ask donors simple, yet direct, questions about their general health and lifestyle, especially risky sexual practices. The following questions, drawn from the South African National Blood Service (SANBS) pre-donation questionnaire, are representative of the kinds of behavioural questions donors should be asked in confidence prior to a donation:

- Have you ever been refused as a blood donor, or told not to donate?
- In the past six months have you had sexual activity with or without a condom: With more than one sex partner? With a regular sex partner excluding your spouse? With someone whose sexual background you do not know?
- In the past six months have you: Had sexual activity with a prostitute or anyone else who takes money or drugs or other favours for sex? Received money, drugs or other payment for sex? Been a victim of a sexual assault?
- Male donors: In the past 6 months have you had oral or anal sex with another man with or without a condom?
- In the past 12 months: Have you had a sexually transmitted disease (STD) e.g. syphilis, gonorrhoea, genital ulcers, VD or 'drop'?
- Have you ever used needles to take drugs, steroids, or anything not prescribed by your doctor or a nurse?
- Do you think your blood is safe for transfusion to a patient?
- To your knowledge does your sex partner have other sex partners?

While the safety rationale justifies this kind of intrusive personal questioning, some automatic exclusion criteria, notably YES answers to questions about homosexual sex, have sparked ethical debates about the fairness of excluding donors on the basis of sexual orientation (Martucci, 2010).

Link 4: Laboratory screening

The WHO Aide Mémoire for National Blood Programmes encourages '*testing of all donated blood, including screening for transfusion-transmissible infections, blood grouping and compatibility testing.*' However, this WHO recommendation must not be viewed in isolation. Indeed, the Aide Mémoire and other WHO guidance stresses that laboratory screening must be part of an 'integrated strategy' that includes the mobilization of low behavioural risk voluntary, non-remunerated donors, a quality assurance system within the laboratory, and the reduction of unnecessary transfusions (WHO, 2011a). Research from high HIV prevalence countries in

Africa has shown this integrated approach can have a positive impact on reducing the number of donations with incident or 'window period' HIV infections that the antigen/antibody assays used in most developing countries might not detect (Basavaraju, 2010).

The 2010 WHO Guidelines on Screening Donated Blood for Transfusion-Transmissible Infections recognize that operational limitations (*'lack of coordination ... inadequate infrastructure ... shortages of trained staff ... poor quality systems'*) may prohibit some blood services from screening all donated units, or create barriers to the implementation of a coordinated, integrated laboratory screening program. The guidelines identify the following negative outcomes that may occur when laboratory screening systems do not exist or fail:

- Inefficient screening systems and wastage of resources owing to differing levels of operation at multiple sites
- Lack of quality assurance and quality management systems
- Use of poor quality test kits and reagents
- Unreliable, inconsistent supplies and transport conditions of test kits and reagents due to poor logistics
- Equipment failure
- Variations in laboratory procedures and practices
- Double standards due to a mix of technologies and methodologies
- Incorrect storage or inappropriate use of test kits and reagents
- Inadequate procedures for identification, leading to the misidentification of patient or donor blood samples, donations or processed units of blood and blood components
- Technical failure in testing
- Misinterpretation of test results
- Inaccuracies in the recording or transcription of test results.
- Higher error rates in test results
- Increased risk of failure to detect TTIs
- Unnecessary hold time due to poor access to confirmatory tests
- Unnecessary discard of non-reactive blood
- Blood shortages and use of unscreened blood in urgent situations
- Incorrect donor notification and stigmatization. (WHO, 2009)

2.2 Ethical aspects of blood transfusion

As noted in section 1.2, Article 25 of the 1948 UN Declaration of Universal Human Rights (DUHR) makes reference to individuals' *'right to security in the event of ... sickness, disability ... or other lack of livelihood in circumstances beyond his control.'* The principle of obtaining patient consent prior to performing a blood transfusion or other medical procedure is derived from the broad concepts of *health* and *security ... in the event of sickness* described in the DUHR. Subsequent codes of medical ethics, including the Council of Europe's 2007 revision of its Guide to the Preparation, Use and Quality Assurance of Blood Components; these codes expanded on this basic definition of 'security' to cover all of the decisions preceding, during, and following a transfusion: From confirming the appropriate diagnosis and prescription order, to correct patient identification and adverse event monitoring during the transfusion itself. (Council of Europe, 2007) Occasionally, prescribers of blood will encounter patients who refuse a recommended transfusion on religious grounds. Clinicians may also face difficult decisions with patients who are minors and patients for whom a transfusion may extend life but not necessarily improve the quality of the patient's life; the creation of institutional ethics committees within hospitals and transfusion centres is recommended to educate staff about ethical issues; support ethical decision-making; develop ethics codes and policies, and; counsel staff and conduct ethical reviews (Perlin, 2001; Kajja et al. 2011).

Ethical considerations continue even after a successful transfusion, most notably in cases where recipients become infected with a transfusion-transmissible infection, or are deemed at risk of infection because new information about the donor of the transfused unit comes to light (e.g. HIV sero-conversion in the donor).

The ISBT code of ethics for hospitals and patients contains seven key principles related to the transfusion of blood and blood products.

ISBT Code of Ethics for Hospitals and Patients

(International Society for Blood Transfusion [ISBT], 2006a)

1. Patients should be informed of the known risks and benefits of blood transfusion and/or alternative therapies and have the right to accept or refuse the procedure. Any valid advance directive should be respected.
2. In the event that the patient is unable to give prior informed consent, the basis for treatment by transfusion must be in the best interests of the patient.
3. Transfusion therapy must be given under the overall responsibility of a registered medical practitioner.
4. Genuine clinical need should be the only basis for transfusion therapy.
5. There should be no financial incentive to prescribe a blood transfusion.
6. As far as possible the patient should receive only those particular components (cells, plasma, or plasma derivatives) that are clinically appropriate and afford optimal safety.
7. Blood transfusion practices established by national or international health bodies and other agencies competent and authorised to do so should be in compliance with this code of ethics.

It should be noted that these seven principles are predicated on an assumption that the ethical principles related to blood donors and the screening of blood for transfusion-transmissible infections have been respected. As with the ethical framework for blood donations, these principles can contribute to reduced risks of transfusion-transmissible infections by reducing or minimizing the number of inappropriate transfusions.

3. Assessment techniques and methodologies: Identifying and addressing gaps and needs in blood safety programs and blood transfusion services

Understanding the roles and responsibilities associated with the various departments and job descriptions within a blood transfusion service is a complex task, involving layers of policy, science, human behaviour, risk, ethics, finances, and, ultimately, medical practice. Further identifying gaps, risks and needs within each (or all) of these layers, is an additional step that blood transfusion services must take in order to address weaknesses, strengthen services, recruit and/or retain staff, improve quality and evaluate the impact of services and products provided to transfusion centres or hospitals and patients. The ultimate goal of these objectives is to improve the safety of blood and blood products used for transfusion. The U.S. Food and Drug Administration cites the '*safety, purity, and potency*' of blood products as the main rationale for conducting blood service quality audits and assessments (Food and Drug Administration, 2010).

To accomplish assessment and evaluation objectives, blood services may use a number of assessment and evaluation tools, many of which are drawn from business practices (e.g. Six Sigma, Total Quality Management, SWOT analyses) or the field of risk analysis. International organizations (WHO, ISBT, the IFRCRCS), national blood transfusion services, regulatory agencies, and Red Cross/Red Crescent Societies, as well as multilateral and bilateral donors (e.g. the European Union, the U.S. President's Emergency Plan for AIDS Relief, the Japan International Cooperation Agency) have also developed assessment tools and indicators to assist with the development, implementation and monitoring of blood safety projects and programs.

The field of evaluation has evolved and expanded substantially in the last 20 years. A recent PubMed literature search found nearly 250,000 papers dedicated to public health evaluations or assessments within the last decade. Beyond the scientific literature, thousands of programme reports, guides and other documents in the 'gray literature' are published each year. This massive diversity of material includes many different methodologies, some of which have been used by blood transfusion services to monitor, evaluate, assess or audit (Chevrolle et al., 2000) human resource needs (Ferrera et al., 2001), blood banking, stock management, laboratory and transfusion practices (Fretz, 2003; Dosunmu & Dada, 2005), training curricula (Wehrli, 2011), epidemiological surveillance (Roussel et al; Linden & Bianco, 2001), and quality systems (Berte, 1997; Mintz, 1995; Smit Sibinga, 2001).

This chapter will review the basic elements these tools are designed off to assess, monitor and evaluate. Examples derived from specific tools and indicators, such as the WHO Global Database on Blood Safety, will be presented to highlight the utility of assessment and evaluation in the development of strong blood transfusion services, especially in areas with high burdens of HIV and other transfusion-transmissible infections.

As mentioned above in section 1.2, blood services worldwide are built around a framework with seven basic components, each of which can be evaluated through techniques such as SWOT analyses (Strengths-Weaknesses-Opportunities-Threats), and addressed with the principles of the Deming cycle of improvement (Plan-Do-Check-Act):

1. Structure and organization
2. Clinical use of blood
3. Processing and testing
4. Blood collections
5. Education and Training
6. Monitoring and Evaluation
7. Sustainability

Within each of these elements, WHO and other blood safety technical assistance programs have developed assessment indicators to help blood services identify needs, gaps and risks.

3.1 The WHO global database on blood safety

A good place to begin to make sense of the diversity of available materials is the WHO Global Database on Blood Safety (GDBS). The GDBS was developed by WHO with expert input through the Global Collaboration on Blood Safety (GCBS) and launched in 1998. WHO member countries are asked to submit data to the GDBS every two years. The indicators collected by the GDBS are periodically revised and increasingly reflect collaborative work between WHO and development partners supporting blood safety programmes in countries.

The GDBS questionnaire contains 253 process, outcome and output indicators clustered around eight operational and technical areas (WHO, 2011d) :
1. Administrative Information
2. Organization and Management
3. Blood Donors and Blood Collection
4. Screening for Transfusion-Transmissible Infections
5. Blood Group Serology Testing of Blood Donations
6. Blood Component Preparation, Storage and Transportation
7. Hospital Transfusion Process and Clinical Use of Blood & Blood Components
8. Fractionated Plasma Products

Since its launch, WHO has received and compiled three reports (1998-1999; 2001-2002; 2004-2005); data collection for a fourth report was begun in 2008.

3.1.1 Mind the gaps – Recent GDBS findings

The identification of blood transfusion as a significant vector for HIV transmission in Africa in the 1990s (Colbunders, 1991) led to increasing attention and financing for blood safety programmes via global health programmes focused on HIV prevention.[3] As noted above, the epidemiology of transfusion-transmitted HIV also drove the passage of World Health Assembly (WHA) resolutions on the blood safety, and the development, over the last decade, of WHO's catalogue of blood safety guidelines and recommendations. In many countries this increased attention to blood safety as part of a comprehensive HIV prevention strategy has strengthened the whole national blood service – from vein-to-vein – in addition to reducing the transmission of HIV through transfusion. Still, despite progress, transfusion systems remain weak in many countries, especially those in the lower income strata. The most recent GDBS report (2004-2005) highlighted a number of these weaknesses, including:

*   Less than 50% of countries report collecting blood exclusively from voluntary, non-remunerated blood donors.
*   40% of the 172 countries surveyed, reported having national haemovigilance systems.
*   53% reported having national regulatory bodies for blood transfusion.
*   80% of the world's population live in countries that collect only 45% of the global blood supply.

3.1.2 Addressing gaps – Achieving change

Experience and evidence from the field over the last decade has shown that blood services in countries with high prevalence HIV have been able to systematically reduce the prevalence of HIV in donated blood units by identifying and addressing gaps and weaknesses in their operations and structures. In 2008, the U.S. Centers for Disease Control and Prevention (CDC) presented data from the PEPFAR blood safety program that showed substantial gaps in the legislative and policy frameworks in 14 countries in sub-Saharan Africa and the Caribbean (US CDC, 2008).

Using indicators adapted from the WHO GDBS, CDC asked countries if a national blood policy was in place or if the national blood transfusion service (NBTS) was supported by a 'legislative framework' (e.g. laws and regulations). In 2003, only six of the 14 countries

---

[3] Half of the 101 countries that responded to a GDBS question about external support for their blood services indicated that they were receiving some kind of international assistance in 2004-2005.

reported having a national blood policy; the same year only four of the 14 countries reported having a 'legislative framework' to support NBTS activities. By 2007, all 14 countries had national blood policies in place or in development, and 10 of 14 countries had established or were developing 'legislative frameworks' based on WHO blood safety guidelines. (Table 1)

Country	Established national policy		Enacted legislative framework		No. of whole blood units collected					No. of whole blood units collected per 1,000 population†				
	2003	2007	2003	2007	2003	2004	2005	2006	2007	2003	2004	2005	2006	2007
Botswana	Yes	Yes	No	No	11,583	13,210	20,643	21,061	22,230	6.4	7.3	11.2	11.2	11.6
Côte d'Ivoire	Yes	Yes	Yes	Yes	67,780	77,972	86,321	86,082	92,009	3.8	4.3	4.6	4.5	4.8
Ethiopia§	No	Yes	No	No	17,208	17,941	19,203	21,019	22,220	0.2	0.2	0.2	0.3	0.3
Guyana	Yes	Yes	No	In development	4,008	4,896	4,531	5,192	5,475	5.4	6.6	6.1	7.1	7.5
Haiti	No	Yes	No	In development	8,711	9,513	10,823	13,622	17,094	1.0	1.0	1.2	1.4	1.8
Kenya	Yes	Yes	Yes	Yes	40,857	47,661	80,762	113,080	123,787	1.2	1.4	2.3	3.1	3.3
Mozambique	No	In development	No	In development	67,105	69,648	76,667	72,170	79,925	3.4	3.5	3.8	3.5	3.8
Namibia	No	Yes	No	In development	17,860	19,154	19,133	18,422	18,309	9.1	9.6	9.5	9.0	8.9
Nigeria¶	No	Yes	No	Yes	—	—	1,266	5,519	16,987	—	—	<0.1	<0.1	0.1
Rwanda	No	Yes	No	No	30,786	28,777	37,893	38,539	32,543	3.5	3.2	4.1	4.1	3.3
South Africa**	Yes	Yes	Yes	Yes	809,322	813,239	805,923	822,950	821,258	17.3	17.2	16.9	17.2	17.0
Tanzania¶	No	Yes	No	In development	—	—	12,597	63,411	109,471	—	—	0.3	1.6	2.7
Uganda	Yes	Yes	Yes	Yes	102,703	106,996	115,988	122,442	133,585	3.8	3.8	4.0	4.1	4.3
Zambia	No	In development	No	In development	40,616	38,477	61,982	54,308	68,056	3.7	3.4	5.4	4.6	5.7

* As described in: World Health Organization. Aide-memoire for national blood programmes. Geneva, Switzerland: World Health Organization; 2002. Available at http://www.who.int/bloodsafety/transfusion_services/en/Blood_Safety_Eng.pdf.
† Based on United Nations Population Division census estimates for 2003–2007.
§ Ethiopia Red Cross Society is the designated national blood transfusion service.
¶ Nigeria and Tanzania established their national blood transfusion services in 2004. The first year with 12 complete months of data available was 2005.
** Includes data from South Africa National Blood Service and Western Province Blood Service.

Table 1. Standards of national blood transfusion policies and legislative frameworks, number of whole blood units collected, and number collected per 1,000 population – U.S. President's Emergency Plan for AIDS Relief, 14 countries, 2003-2007

Country	% of persons with HIV infection*		% of blood collections reactive for HIV					% of blood collections received from voluntary, non-remunerated donors				
	2001	2007	2003	2004	2005	2006	2007	2003	2004	2005	2006	2007
Botswana	26.5	23.9	7.5	5.7	4.0	2.7	2.1	100	100	100	100	100
Côte d'Ivoire	6.0	3.9	1.6	1.4	1.5	1.4	1.2	100	100	100	100	100
Ethiopia†	2.4	2.1	—	3.6	3.4	2.5	3.0	38.8	27.5	23.2	28.1	28.4
Guyana	2.5	2.5	0.8	0.6	1.0	0.6	0.3	21.7	18.9	26.1	31.2	61.1
Haiti	2.2	2.2	1.7	1.8	1.6	1.9	1.4	5.2	5.4	14.9	27.4	51.9
Kenya	8.1	7.8§	1.5	1.7	1.9	2.5	1.2	99.0	95.3	97.6	98.9	99.5
Mozambique	10.3	12.5	8.6	6.9	6.4	8.3	7.2	58.0	58.3	59.6	52.0	72.3
Namibia	14.6	15.3	0.7	0.6	0.6	0.5	0.6	100	100	100	100	100
Nigeria¶	3.2	3.1	—	—	3.8	3.5	2.5	—	—	100	100	92.3
Rwanda	4.3	2.8	1.1	0.1	1.2	0.9	0.5	100	100	100	100	100
South Africa**	16.9	18.1	<0.1	<0.1	<0.1	<0.1	0.1	100	100	100	100	100
Tanzania¶	7.0	6.2	—	—	4.8	3.2	2.8	—	—	66.5	80.0	89.2
Uganda	7.9	5.4	2.0	1.9	1.6	1.5	1.3	95.5	96.3	99.0	99.9	100
Zambia	15.4	15.2	6.9	6.4	9.0	6.4	3.8	72.7	71.2	90.6	97.9	99.6

* Estimates from the Joint United Nations Programme on HIV/AIDS (UNAIDS), available at http://data.unaids.org/pub/globalreport/2008/jc1510_2008_global_report_pp211_234_en.pdf. Because UNAIDS methodology used to estimate 2003 prevalence was different from the methodology used for 2007, data are presented for 2001, the most recent pre-program year for which the same methodology was used as for 2007.
† Ethiopia Red Cross Society is the designated national blood transfusion service.
§ Preliminary estimate.
¶ Nigeria and Tanzania established their national blood transfusion services in 2004. The first year with 12 complete months of data available was 2005.
** Includes data from South Africa National Blood Service and Western Province Blood Service. Autologous donations and collections from designated donors are reported as donations from voluntary, non-remunerated donors.

Table 2. Estimated percentage of persons aged 15-49 years with human immunodeficiency virus (HIV) infection, percentage of blood collections reactive for HIV, and percentage of collections from voluntary, non-remunerated donors – U.S. President's Emergency Plan for AIDS Relief, 14 countries, 2003-2007

During the same four year period, all 14 countries reported lower or stable rates of HIV prevalence in donated units (Table 2).

Although a strict causal association cannot be derived (Noumsi et al., 2008) from these data, this report suggests a positive relationship between progress toward addressing policy and other operational gaps and improvements in the safety of donated blood for supportive haemotherapy.

4. Evidence based strategies to move from a supply-driven to a demand-driven blood transfusion system

4.1 Community specifics for tailor made solutions

In the majority of economically restricted countries the transfusion chain from vein-to-vein is determined by what happens to be available. The supply drives the system. When a clinical need occurs, either the scarce hospital or blood bank stock is being used and exhausted or family is urged to search for blood donors, whether family related, friends or what the market offers. Often that results in under-treatment of patients, unjustified use or no treatment at all. The data available for mother and infant death due to shortages illustrate this situation (WHO et al. 2010).

Most of these donors are seriously coerced, time pressure stimulates poor handling and the serious and realistic effect of transmission of infections such as HIV, HBV and HCV. Besides, it has been observed and documented that hidden stocks are being kept or just grow due to shortage in organization and poor logistics of the supply (Kajja I et al., 2010a). The chain quite often is interrupted at the clinical interface side, with a serious paucity of communication between producer/supplier and prescriber/consumer of blood and blood components. The root cause of this paucity is in limited and focused knowledge and related practices on either side of the chain. When regular need assessments are being done a better idea would grow about the epidemiology of blood transfusion in the hospitals, which then could lead to balanced and evidence based logistics of supply of human blood in anticipation of the needs.

As a consequence the blood supply and clinical use should be firmly embedded in the health care system with major involvement of the community to allow such anticipatory strategies. Community involvement means community education to understand why a continuous and not an incidental and *ad hoc* support is needed (Los & Smit Sibinga, 2001). It is the principle of *'today me, tomorrow you'* as a social act of solidarity. When the blood supply becomes a community issue, awareness and responsibility to support with healthy blood on a sharing principle, rather than being dragged into blood donation because of urgent needs of family and relatives who might die if you would not donate immediately (Los & Smit Sibinga, 2001). Questionnaires and testing, whether rapid or ELISA then move towards the edge of becoming a farce, seriously jeopardizing the safety of blood transfusion. To find out what the knowledge, attitudes and practices of a community are in relation to blood donation and transfusion, a KAP (knowledge, attitudes, practices) study could certainly be beneficial. KAP studies can be done broad, focused on the community by and large or target specific groups, such as presumed low risk categories, known or registered blood donors, and non-donors. Each such KAP study will need a careful analysis to unravel the underlying anthropological and psychological information needed to understand how the mind is set of those who participated and how that relates to community feelings and behaviour as a whole. KAP studies should not be incidental, but be part of a mechanism to follow up and study the changes in mind set and behaviour of the community. Only then will it provide a useful tool for benchmarking progress in attitude and related practices (Los & Smit Sibinga, 2009; Los et al. 2009).

4.2 Prerequisites – Leadership, awareness, willingness, environment/climate, access

Unsafe blood transfusions have contributed to the enormous burden of HIV infections in various developing parts of the world, in particular in sub-Saharan Africa and the Central Asian region (World Bank et al., 2008), and still continue to add to this burden. The risk of HIV, HCV and HBV infection through unsafe blood and blood products is exceptionally high (95–100%) compared to other common routes of exposure: For example, 11–32% for mother-to-child transmission of HIV and HBV and 0.1%–10% for sexual contact. Sub-Saharan Africa has a particularly high level of transfusion-associated HIV compared with other developing regions due to a higher risk of infected blood being transfused. This results from a combination of factors: High rates of transfusion in some groups of patients (particularly women during labour, and children in the malaria Season), a higher incidence and prevalence of HIV infection, dependence on unsafe blood donors and inadequate or even absence of testing of blood for HIV in some countries (WHO 2008a, 2010a, 2010b). However, also the poor education level and poverty among larger groups in the community play an important role. Women and children account for a disproportionate number of HIV, HBV and HCV infections through unsafe blood because they are the main groups of patients receiving blood transfusion. In developing countries around 50% of the blood is transfused to women and 25% to children, largely under the age of 5 years. Up to 20% of maternal mortality and 15% of child deaths have been attributed to severe anaemia due to malaria. Timely access to safe blood transfusion is a life-saving measure in many of these clinical conditions and can also prevent serious illness in these patients.

Besides the need for identified, competent and designated leadership (Smit Sibinga 2009a, 2009b), there is the holistic need for awareness – politicians and policy makers, community in all its diversity, health professionals and related stakeholders such as hospital managers, religious leaders and educators. The government is final responsible for the well being of the community and should create the environment and climate for education and professional infrastructure to allow awareness and willingness to grow and sustain. The organization of the health care should guarantee access and affordability to all in need, and the blood supply and clinical prescribers should use and optimize the professional and social climate and environment to allow proper, safe and justified practices of procurement and clinical use of blood and blood components to be developed and implemented.

It has been demonstrated that a well organized and structured nationally supported blood supply and transfusion system yields a better and safer transfusion practice with a minimum residual risk for transmission of blood born infections, in particular HIV/AIDS, as compared to a non-cohesive and fragmented blood supply. Any structure should find its anchor in an appropriate legal framework – documented principles of blood donation and transfusion, adequate regulations and an operational system for audit and inspection of compliance with the principles and related operational standards and technical requirements (Hollan et al., 1990)

4.3 Role of education and vocational institutes

As mentioned in section 2.1 the key factor is competent human capacity at all levels, which means education of the community to create public awareness, the professionals to create professional awareness and politicians to create political awareness. The awareness to be raised relates to the risks for contracting infectious diseases such as HIV/AIDS, hepatitis, malaria and tuberculosis. Additionally these infectious diseases may be spread through a variety of contacts, e.g. the blood supply. Education provides knowledge through information, which is stored in the brains. A major question and related process is how to convert the acquired knowledge into appropriate action. The process depends highly on how the information is presented and how the knowledge is perceived. The perception ultimately triggers the action needed (WI Thomas & Thomas DS, 1928).

Education and vocational institutes do play a paramount role in the presentation of information and the way the acquired knowledge is perceived individually and collectively, leading to individual behaviour and collective or group behaviour – the moral and ethics of a community. To bridge the existing knowledge gap, analysis is needed of both the way, the environment and the contents of the information offered, and the intellectual mechanisms of the perception of the knowledge necessary for the triggering of appropriate action (Los & Smit Sibinga, 2009; Kajja, 2010).

Potential teachers and parents therefore need to be educated on how to pack and present the information and how to monitor and evaluate the perception of the knowledge. This continuum should have a high rank on the priority list of any nation, filling in one of the key universal human rights – the right of education. Competence is the intimate twinning through matching of acquiring knowledge and developing skills to act appropriately, whatever is concerned. When the community or public understands the need for a healthy life style, for sharing regularly a bit of healthy blood with those in need, by donating blood on an altruistic and regular basis, when the professionals in the health care understand the need to appropriately deal with the collection, processing, testing, storage and distribution of human blood as a transplant and at the clinical side with the in-hospital processes of prescription and ordering, selection and compatibility testing, and the ultimate transfusion and its monitoring and evaluation, the gap will be substantially narrowed and shallowed. However, without a proper understanding of the policy makers, the gap will not be bridged completely.

Evidence-based strategies for blood safety and availability have been successfully implemented in most developed countries and some transitional and developing nations. However, despite the proven effectiveness of these strategies, many countries are making slow progress towards their implementation. There is ample evidence that a nationally supported blood supply and clinical use of human blood, well regulated and professionally implemented on an adequate economy of scale, leads to a significant reduction in risk of transmission of infectious diseases.

Such nationally supported approach covers the entire nation and is based on education of all parties involved, understanding the importance and relevance of the necessary and ongoing provision of information and related actions.

Such systems recognize and address the potential weaknesses and gaps as listed above in the 6 major areas of transfusion medicine - 1. Organization and structure; 2. Clinical use (clinical interface); 3. Processing and testing; 4. Collection of source material (community interface); 5. Education; 6. Monitoring and evaluation (research and development).

Such systems are based on the needs of the community to be met by the supply through anticipation, proper planning and adequate logistics (Smit Sibinga, 2000). The demand then will drive the supply and no longer the other way around.

5. Directions for improvement – Values and realities

Over the past few decades, since the outbreak of the HIV/AIDS epidemic, much work has been done to provide a better understanding of the routing of transmission of the virus. There are prominent differences in the various cultures in the perception of the risks related to behaviour, personal and collective. That relates to different standards of moral and ethics, of values of life and realities of human attitudes and behaviour. Education remains a key factor in the provision of knowledge and related perception needed for action to prevent transmission, both vertical and horizontal. Blood transfusion in the vein-to-vein concept lacks behind in its development despite the continuum of initiatives developed by organizations such as the World Health Organization (WHO), the International Federation of Red Cross and Red Crescent Societies (IRC), the International Society of Blood Transfusion (ISBT) and the World Federation of Hemophilia (WFH) (Smit Sibinga, 2002). The WHO Blood Transfusion Safety Programme at WHO-HQ, Geneva, evolved from the WHO Global Programme on AIDS and the Global Blood Safety Initiative (GBSI) of the late 1980s. The leadership role of WHO has become visible through the development of a number of tools for education, collecting data, and providing guiding documents such as the series of *Aide Mémoires* to support and advise Governments in their attempts to structure national blood supply systems on a cost-effective, safe and sustainable basis. The Global Blood Safety Initiative started to map the situation of the blood supply and clinical use in the world and provide a series of expert advises, including two documents on education in transfusion medicine (WHO 1992a, 1992b).

5.1 WHA resolutions
With the goal of ensuring universal access to safe blood, WHO has been at the forefront of the movement to improve blood safety as mandated by successive World Health Assembly resolutions. In 2007 an important global meeting took place in Ottawa, Canada, addressing in a global consultation crucial aspects of a universal access to safe blood all part of the identified gaps (WHO, 2008a). More than 30 years after the first World Health Assembly resolution (WHA28.72) addressed the issue of blood safety, equitable access to safe blood and blood products and their safe and rational use still remain major challenges throughout the world. While the demand for blood is growing in the advanced world with longevity of life and increasingly sophisticated clinical procedures, national blood supplies are rarely sufficient to meet existing requirements in the restricted economy part of the world with some 80% of the global population.

Since that first World Health Assembly Resolution, a series of Resolutions has been created, endorsed and signed by the Member State representatives in an attempt to stimulate implementation at national level (Table 3). A recent one, WHA63.12 on Availability, Safety and Quality of Blood Products, was endorsed in May 2010 and urges Member States –
1. to take all the necessary steps to establish, implement and support nationally-coordinated, efficiently-managed and sustainable blood and plasma programmes according to the availability of resources, with the aim of achieving self-sufficiency, unless special circumstances preclude it;
2. to take all the necessary steps to update their national regulations on donor assessment and deferral, the collection, testing, processing, storage, transportation and use of blood products, and operation of regulatory authorities in order to ensure that regulatory control in the area of quality and safety of blood products across the entire transfusion chain meets internationally recognized standards;
3. to establish quality systems, for the processing of whole blood and blood components, good manufacturing practices for the production of plasma-derived medicinal products and appropriate regulatory control, including the use of diagnostic devices to prevent transfusion transmissible diseases with highest sensitivity and specificity;

4. to build human resource capacity through the provision of initial and continuing education (teaching and training) of staff to ensure quality of blood services and blood products;

5. to enhance the quality of evaluation and regulatory actions in the area of blood products and associated medical devices, including in vitro diagnostic devices;

6. to establish or strengthen systems for the safe and rational use of blood products and to provide education (teaching and training) for all staff involved in clinical transfusion, to implement potential solutions in order to minimize transfusion errors and promote patient safety, to promote the availability of transfusion alternatives including, where appropriate, autologous transfusion and patient blood management;

7. to ensure the reliability of mechanisms for reporting serious or unexpected adverse reactions to blood and plasma donation and to the receipt of blood components and plasma derived medicinal products, including transmissions of pathogens (haemovigilance);

The red thread through all these resolutions is the prevention of further spread of HIV/AIDS through contaminated blood transfusions and improving patient care, addressing the major knowledge gaps.

The global need for blood safety and availability has been highlighted in the following WHA and Executive Board (EB) resolutions and regional resolutions (PAHO and AFRO) that provide specific direction on strategies and activities within individual regions:	
1975:	WHA Resolution WHA28.72: Utilization and Supply of Human Blood and Blood Products
1987:	EB Resolution EB79.R1: Blood and Blood Products
1995:	WHA Resolution WHA48.27: Paris AIDS Summit
1999:	DC-PAHO/AMRO Resolution CD41.R15: Strengthening Blood Banks in the Region of the Americas
2000:	WHA Resolution WHA53.14: HIV/AIDS: Confronting the Epidemic
2001:	RC-AFRO Resolution AFR/RC51/R2: Blood Safety Strategy for the African Region
2002:	WHA Resolution WHA55.18: Quality of Care: Patient Safety
2003:	WHA Resolution WHA56.30: Global Health Sector Strategy for HIV/AIDS
2005:	WHA Resolution WHA58.13: Blood Safety: Proposal to Establish World Blood Donor Day
2007:	WHA Resolution WHA60.24: Health Promotion in a Globalized World
	WHA Resolution WHA60.29: Health Technologies
2010:	WHA Resolution WHA63.10: Partnerships
	WHA Resolution WHA63.12: Availability, Safety and Quality of Blood Products
	WHA Resolution WHA63:18: Viral Hepatitis
	WHA Resolution WHA63:19: WHO HIV/AIDS strategy for 2011–2015
	WHA Resolution WHA63:20: Chagas Disease: Control and Elimination

Table 3. WHA Resolutions related to blood safety.

5.2 Millennium development goals

The United Nations Millennium Development Goals (MDG) are eight goals that in 2000 all 191 UN Member States have agreed to try to achieve by the year 2015 (UN, 2000). The United Nations Millennium Declaration, signed in September 2000 commits world leaders to combat poverty, hunger, disease, illiteracy, environmental degradation, and discrimination against women, all essential parts of the original 1948 UN Declaration of Universal Human Rights.

The eight MDGs are derived from this UN Millennium Declaration.

1. to eradicate extreme poverty and hunger;
2. to achieve universal primary education;
3. to promote gender equality and empower women;
4. to reduce child mortality;
5. to improve maternal health;
6. to combat HIV/AIDS, malaria, and other diseases;
7. to ensure environmental sustainability;
8. to develop a global partnership for development.

All eight goals have specific targets and indicators. Of these eight goals, the numbers 4, 5 and 6, and eight of the 18 targets relate directly to health and safe blood transfusion. The number 2 relates to education and the number 8 to the role of partnership for development, equally important to the development of safe and efficacious blood transfusion practices.

Some developing countries have made impressive progress in achieving the health-related Millennium Development Goals, targets and indicators. However, many more are still falling behind. Progress is particularly slow in sub-Saharan Africa but also in other developing and transition countries such as a number of the Newly Independent States (NIS), where knowledge gaps remain a major issue to address.

5.3 Success stories

There is a steadily growing number of success stories on bridging the knowledge gap and improving on the safety of the blood supply. We present just a few recent examples, largely from the African continent.

Eritrea (Baraki et al., 2010) - In 2006, despite the production of blood components in the National Blood Transfusion Centre (NBTC), about 90% of blood requests were for whole blood, an evidence of inappropriate use of blood and blood components in Eritrea. This could be the result of absence of proper and up to date guidelines and lack of training in appropriate use of blood and blood components, and alternatives. To change, the NBTC adapted clinical guidelines from the WHO document on appropriate use of blood (WHO, 2001). Copies of this document were distributed to all hospital staff in the country followed by training to the guidelines.

Objective of this Swiss Red Cross and Academic Institute IDTM (Groningen, NL) supported project was to assess the impact of distributing clinical guidelines and training (interventions) on knowledge, attitude and practice (KAP) of clinical prescribers in blood transfusion before and after the interventions. Correctly responded knowledge, attitude and practice (KAP) questions were collectively considered. Baseline: 3.8 percent of respondents correctly answered all KAP questions, which increased to 6.1 percent after the intervention. Of the total KAP questions, the average correct responses were 15.86 in the baseline and 17.45 in the follow-up assessment. The difference was positive and statistically significant ($p < 0.000$) demonstrating the intervention had a major impact in changing the overall knowledge, attitude and practice of these health workers. When certain tools were audited, the compliance was found to be 38.1 percent among the assessed hospitals, though the auditing was limited to seven (7) major hospitals. This shows the intervention has made an impact when compared with the pre-intervention status.

When blood and blood components utilization comparison was made before (2006) and after the intervention (2008), demand for whole blood had decreased whereas the demands for all blood components had increased significantly (except FFP which remained unchanged).

This shows the progress made in Eritrea through focused education in addressing safe transfusion practice, and the measurable improvements in that practice.

Malawi (courtesy Dr. Jean C. Emmanuel) – Malawi (population of ± 11 million) is a Low Human Development Index (L-HDI) country. The European Union EC EDF VIII Project document set out to develop an independent and sustainable National Malawi Blood Transfusion Service (MBTS) following the recommendations and guidelines of the World Health Organisation (WHO), International Federation of Red Cross and Red Crescent Societies (IFRCRCS) and the International Society of Blood Transfusion (ISBT). The MBTS project plan was based on sustainable and effectively managed and organised independent National Blood Services. The platform for development was the establishment of a Finance and Administration department, with an experienced chartered cost accountant (CPA) as Director; with facilities and trained staff. Effective collaborative networks have been established with Ministry of Health (MoH) and Ministry of Finance (MoF), ensuring incorporation of a sustainable budget into the national annual fiscal budget, negotiated 'fee for service' from the private health insurance schemes for the private sector, and an equitable career structure for all staff with social benefits to ensure continuous capacity building and retention of staff. MBTS Trust Board appointed an experienced CEO; Finance & Administration Director and Medical Director.

In February 2000 a financing agreement, MAI/7001/002, was signed between the Republic of Malawi and the European Commission (EC) for € 7.8m in order to support the Malawi MoH to establish an independent National MBTS under a formally constituted and independent Malawi Blood Transfusion Service Trust. Project funding was increased with a further € 1.3m following a successful mid-term review (MTR). The Project Manager was appointed in March 2003 and development commenced. The Board of Trustees is responsible for the effective operation of MBTS and drafted appropriate legal frameworks, comprising the Constitution for the Board of Trustees and Legislation of the Service. MBTS is an officially registered Non Government Organisation (NGO) with a legal seal. MBTS is managed and organised by a competent Chief Executive Officer (CEO) who has internationally recognised qualifications, a Finance and Administrative Director and Medical Director with a Deputy; together form the Senior Management Team reporting directly to the Board. Developing collaborative working partnerships with the relevant NGOs, stakeholders and bodies in the private and public sector in Malawi is an important and ongoing strategy.

The overall objective of MBTS is to provide safe blood and blood products, reduce the incidence of HIV, and other diseases transmissible by blood, ensuring equitable access and availability of blood and promoting appropriate clinical use of blood. The goal was achieved within the planned project timeframe a sustainable, national blood transfusion service providing a safe, adequate and accessible supply for all those in need in recognised health care establishments from 100% voluntary non-remunerated safe blood donors, which meets the needs of all hospitals in Malawi through the three centres specifically designed and built within the project framework.

The five-year project ended 2007. An independent Mid Term Review (MTR) Team contracted by European Commission (EC), concluded that the project had been successfully implemented. As a result EC agreed to an extension to the funding of € 1.3m through EDF IX, for the construction of 3 Blood Centres.

Key achievements of the project:

-   Establishment of an approved and effective Board of Trustees, CEO and Executive Team, with effective leadership, organisation and management, personnel (110 staff) all trained to international standards in all areas of work, with job descriptions, SOPs and implementing quality systems;
-   MBTS policy, plan and legal framework approved as official legal instruments;
-   Construction of 3 blood transfusion centres (completed 2008);
-   Equipment and vehicles for 8 mobile collection teams including a blood donor bus;
-   Recurrent expenditure secured in fiscal budget by 'subvention' from fiscal year beginning July 2006 to present;
-   Project Manager/Technical Assistance funded by EC responsible for development and training ended 31 March 2007;
-   All objectives, and planned outputs, were achieved on time;
-   All donated blood is tested for HIV I/ II, p24 antigen; Hepatitis B & C; Syphilis and malaria with the introduction of a quality management system, and good laboratory practices. Trained senior staff have become trainers of district hospital blood bank staff and future MBTS staff;
-   Blood Cold Chain (BCC) system in place for the transport of blood specimens for centralized testing and distribution of blood and blood products to all hospitals; provision of targeted hospitals with appropriate resources for the storage of blood and blood products for blood transfusion;
-   District Hospital laboratory staff have been trained using WHO Distance Learning Materials (every technician has a personal copy);
-   Training workshops, seminars and lectures on appropriate clinical use of blood facilitated by respective senior staff;
-   Research ongoing on knowledge, attitudes and practices (KAP) on blood donation issues; evaluating prevalence of Hepatitis C (HCV); on evidence based rationale for individual patient identification arm bands; research paper co-authored on Clinical Paediatric Transfusion Guidelines;
-   MBTS provides blood and products from 100% voluntary non-remunerated donors to all public and private hospitals;
-   MBTS is a sustainable and effective Service with an approved fiscal budget and a "fee for service" through private medical insurance.

Sudan (Hassan Ali et al., 2010) - In Sudan blood transfusion services were fragmented - hospital based with 85% of blood collected from family and replacement donors. More than 300 hospital blood banks practice blood collection and transfusion; 40% are rural hospitals with transfusion rate of 5-100 units of blood per month besides large central and specialized urban hospitals with transfusion rate of 100-300 units of blood per month. About 300,000 units of blood are collected annually; 56% is screened using rapid tests and 44% by ELISA technique, with a TTI marker prevalence of HIV - 2%, HBV - 6%, HCV - 2% and syphilis - 5%. Apart from a few solitary guidelines and SOP-like instructions no quality system was in place. Almost exclusively whole blood is being transfused and adverse events are poorly observed. In 2009, in close collaboration with World Health Organization and the Academic Institute IDTM (Groningen, NL), a project to improve quality in blood transfusion through an appropriate quality management system was established, focused on the creation of a solid national blood supply and transfusion framework. Objectives were to review existing quality management programme and identify gaps, assist in the development of a draft national quality policy and develop a plan for quality improvement including capacity building. Through a series of field visits to main blood transfusion centres in three main States, the establishment of a National Steering Committee to create full ownership, capacity building through basic education in quality management and clinical transfusion medicine (quality culture) and enhancement of a voluntary blood donation programme strategy, the following goals were reached –

1. Endorsed National Blood Transfusion Policy (Ministry of Health);
2. Voluntary Blood Donor Association established and registered;
3. 50 senior blood bank quality managers from 10 States educated in the basics of quality management. Committees from these trainers have worked on developing a draft national quality manual;
4. 6 seminars for prescribers conducted in 3 States, to improve clinical blood transfusion knowledge and practice (in-hospital transfusion chain).

This demonstrates that international collaboration (WHO/IDTM) can generate major achievements in establishing a national framework and improving quality blood transfusion services in developing countries to achieve the goals of safe and adequate blood supplies and clinical awareness and knowledge at national level.

Uganda (Kyeyune et al., 2010) - In 1957, a centralized transfusion service - the Uganda Blood Transfusion Service (UBTS), was started at Nakasero. This supplied blood to the entire country for the following 20 years. The period from 1977 to 1987 saw political unrest disrupt national infrastructures and aggravated the human resource crisis in the health sector. This resulted into reversion to the original unregulated hospital based transfusion service nationwide. Like any other low HDI country, Uganda is still challenged by a low availability of voluntary non-remunerated blood donors (VNRBD); insufficient transport and storage facilities; low capacities in testing of donated blood and quality assurance in testing laboratories. Through a step-by-step approach these problems are being reversed using locally and internationally sourced technical and financial support. In May 1987, Uganda with the assistance of the Global Programme on AIDS (GPA) of the World Health Organization (WHO) held a financial donor conference in Kampala. As a result, the Uganda AIDS Control Programme (UACP) was formed. The European Commission (EC) through its AIDS Task Force (ATF) made a pledge of 1.5 million Euros to rehabilitate the central blood bank at Nakasero and the collection, processing and distribution of 10,000 units of whole blood to be supplied to hospitals within 100 kms from Nakasero Blood Bank. In the period 1989-2004, further funding from EC together with adequate technical advice and support enabled the UBTS to improve its infrastructure by opening four regional blood banks in Mbarara, Fort-Portal, Gulu, Mbale and two satellites in Arua and Kitovu. This was accompanied by development and adoption of a National Blood Transfusion Policy, and organization and coordination of a national safe blood transfusion service based on voluntary non-remunerated blood donors. This period saw significant reduction of HIV and hepatitis B sero-prevalence among donors. A quality assurance programme was instituted in the UBTS establishment, and opportunities for human resource development in-service training were initiated. The EC fund was phased out in 2004 amidst increasing demands for safe blood for an increasing population. From 2004 to date UBTS has enjoyed technical (TA provision) and financial support from the US PEPFAR project, focused on strengthening of the national blood transfusion service. This has been followed by renovation of existing and establishment of new facilities, increased blood collection from 107,000 units in 2004 to 165,500 units in 2009. Blood testing for hepatitis C was started in 2005 in addition to HIV, Hepatitis B and syphilis testing. Hospital transfusion committees to oversee clinical use of blood are being created, and a major emphasis is on quality system essentials and capacity building in the regional blood banks.

Uzbekistan (Makhmudova & Smit Sibinga, 2008) - Project focus: development of a Republican Blood Supply and Transfusion System based on international standards – safe, efficacious, sustainable and affordable.

The Government of Uzbekistan initiated measures to reform the Health Care System. Government and Asian Development Bank (ADB) signed a Loan Agreement (2004) for a major project: Woman and Child Health Development (WCHD); part is used to improve blood services. The blood services situation requires radical improvement: Donated blood is not safe, majority is collected from paid donors with serious risk of HIV, HCV and HBV transmission. The country lacks a national blood safety policy, strategic plan, appropriate legislative and regulatory framework. The Blood Safety Program (component 3) of WCHD comprises a nationwide blood supply system, initiated in 2004 and substantiated in 2006, based on WHO and Red Cross principles. The programme is public health oriented, addressing the need for a nationally supported system, cost-effective, motivation and mobilization of the community to convert the current paid and replacement system into a truly voluntary and regular blood donor system, upgrading procurement operations (regional and economy-of-scale). It addresses the need for equitable access of safe blood to all citizens, appropriate clinical practices, and a national budget system to allow sustained and continuous operations. Using public education and social marketing campaigns with the support of NGOs, a voluntary and regular donor programme will be implemented stepwise. Another major point is in establishing appropriate clinical transfusion practices. With support of international expertise, MoH has created a Republican reform plan to reduce the number of inadequate hospital based blood transfusion units. The plan focuses on consolidation of core activities - blood collection, processing and testing, storage and distribution in 6 regional centres, strategically spread over the country to be able to handle logistics of demand and supply, and provide cost-effective operations. Implementation is in phases to allow proper adaptation and guarantee of continued supply of blood over the transition period. The WCHD conducts training needs assessments, develops training modules based on WHO guidelines and provides education for clinicians and transfusion medicine specialists (capacity building). Another example of how to bridge the knowledge gap.

This demonstrates that donor funding when appropriately utilized and supported by adequate provision of guidance and technical advice can improve blood transfusion programmes in the low human development index countries.

5.4 Lessons learned

To reduce the burden of morbidity and mortality through HIV infected blood transfusions of particularly the poor and marginalized populations, the focus should be on an increasing access to clinical and diagnostic technology, safe blood, blood components and medical devices. This could be achieved through reducing the leading risk factors to human health in which lack of education (knowledge) plays a major role. When a safe and professional environment for the vein-to-vein use of blood and blood components is created, the risk for transmissible and transfusion related diseases will be reduced. At the same time there should be developed a sustainable and integrated health care system by building competent leadership, management and operational capacity in the methodologies and technologies involved in the procurement and clinical use of blood and blood components as fundamental elements of a sustainable health care system.

That could only be achieved sustainably when enabling policies and an institutional environment are developed through appropriate national drug and blood policies (legal and regulatory framework), with all partners involved in the health technologies and within the framework of national health policies (integrated), which generate a common vision and a realistic and feasible plan for action.

6. Acknowledgement

The authors would like to acknowledge Dr. Yifdeamlak E. Baraki from Eritrea, Dr. Jean C. Emmanuel from Malawi, Dr. Abdul Hassan Ali from Sudan, Dr. Dorothy Kyeyune from Uganda and Dr. Mayya Makhmudova from Uzbekistan for their invaluable contribution to the success stories.

7. References

Adriani WPA, Smit Sibinga CTh. *How to develop a practical Quality Management System in resource limited countries,* Vox Sanguinis, Vol. 95, Issue 241 (Suppl), pp. 501

Allain JP, Sarkodie F, Asenso-Mensah K, Owusu-Ofori S. (2009). *Relative safety of first-time volunteer and replacement donors in west Africa,* Transfusion, Vol. 50, pp. 340-3

American College of Physicians Ad Hoc Committee on Medical Ethics (Eds.). (1984). *American College of Physicians Ethics Manual Part I: History of Medical Ethics, The Physician and the Patient, The Physician's Relationship to Other Physicians, The Physician and Society, Annals of Internal Medicine,* Vol. 101, Issue 1 (July 1984), pp. 129-137

Baraki Y, Swiss Red Cross, Smit Sibinga CTh. (2010). *The Impact of Introduction of Clinical Guidelines and Training in Appropriate Use of Blood and Blood Products (AUB) on Knowledge, Attitude and Practice of Blood Prescribers in Eritrea.* Transfusion, 2010;50 (2S):187A

Basavaraju S et al. (2010). *Reduced risk of transfusion-transmitted HIV in Kenya through centrally co-ordinated blood centres, stringent donor selection and effective p24 antigen-HIV antibody screening,* Vox Sanguinis, Vol. 99, Issue 3 (October 2010), pp. 212–219

Berte LM. (1997). *Tools for improving quality in the transfusion service,* American Journal of Clinical Pathology, Vol. 107, Issue 4 Suppl 1 (April 1997), pp. S36-42

Chevrolle F et al. (2000). *Blood transfusion audit methodology: the auditors, reference systems and audit guidelines,* Transfus Clin Biol, Vol. 7, Issue 6, (December 2000), pp. 559-62

Colebunders R et al. (1991). *Seroconversion rate, mortality, and clinical manifestations associated with the receipt of a human immunodeficiency virus-infected blood transfusion in Kinshasa, Zaire,* Journal of Infectious Diseases, Vol. 164, pp. 450–6

Council of Europe (2007). Chapter 30: Pre-transfusion Measures, In: Guide to the Preparation, Use and Quality Assurance of Blood Components, Accessed March 25, 2011, Available from:
http://books.google.com.na/books?id=huNgp2KJ-wQC&pg=PA47&lpg=PA47&dq=council+of+europe+2005+Preparation,+Use+and +Quality+Assurance+of+Blood+Components&source=bl&ots=l6T4a7MmBy&sig= gljoQKBPlhZXCZIUCh6yNeoFBMc&hl=en&ei=vtKMTZ-DNM33gAfJh9mfDQ&sa=X&oi=book_result&ct=result&resnum=5&ved=0CDQQ6 AEwBA#v=onepage&q=council%20of%20europe%202005%20Preparation%2C%20 Use%20and%20Quality%20Assurance%20of%20Blood%20Components&f=false

Diarra A, Kouriba B, Baby M, Murphy E, Lefrere JJ. (2009). *HIV, HCV, HBV and syphilis rate of positive donations among blood donations in Mali: lower rates among volunteer blood donors,* Transfusion Clin Biol, Vol. 16, pp. 444-7

Dosunmu AO, Dada MO. (2005). *Principles of blood transfusion service audit, African Journal of Medical Science,* Vol. 34, Issue 4 (December 2005), pp. 349-53

European Union. (2003). Directive 2002/98/EC of the European Parliament and the Council of 27 January 2003 Setting standards of quality and safety for the collection, testing, processing, storage and distribution of human blood and blood components and amending Directive 2001/83/EC Official Journal of the European Union 2003 I.33/30-39

Farrugia A, et al. (2010). *Payment, compensation and replacement – the ethics and motivation of blood and plasma donation,*Vox Sanguinis, Vol. 99 (June 2010), pp. 202-211

Feldschuh J, with Weber D. (1990). *Safe Blood: Purifying the Nation's Blood Supply in the Age of AIDS,* The Free Press, 0-02-910065-8, New York

Ferrera V et al. (2001). *Methodology for the development of a program for following and maintaining the competency of human resources,* Transfusion Clin Biol, Vol. 8, Issue 1 (February 2001), pp. 30-43

Fretz C. (2003). *Self-Assessment Tools,* Transfusion Clin Biol, Vol. 10, Issue 2 (April 2003), pp. 94-8

Glynn SA, Williams AE, Nass CC, Bethel J, Kessler D, Scott EP, Fridey J, Kleinman SH & Schreiber GB. (2003). *Attitudes toward blood donation incentives in the United States: implications for donor recruitment,* Transfusion, Vol. 43, Issue 1 (January 2003), pp. 7-16

Grainger B, Margolese E, Partington E. *Legal and ethical considerations in blood transfusion,* Canadian Medical Association Journal 1997; 156 (11 suppl)

Gygi C, DeCarlo N, Williams B. (2005) *Six Sigma for Dummies.* Wiley Publishing Inc. ISBN: 0-7645-6798-5, Hoboken, NJ, USA

Hassan Ali A, Abdellah YE, Smit Sibinga CTh. (2010) *International Collaboration: an Approach to Establishing Blood Transfusion Quality System in Sudan,* Vox Sanguinis 2010;99 (suppl 1):92

Hollán SR, Wagstaff W, Leikola J, Lothe F. (eds.). (1990) *Management of blood transfusion services.* WHO Press, Geneva, CH

International Federation of Red Cross/Red Crescent Societies (IFRC).

International Society of Blood Transfusion [ISBT]. (2006) *International Forum: Paid vs. unpaid donors,* Vox Sanguinis, Vol. 90, No. 1, pp. 63-70.

International Society of Blood Transfusion [ISBT]. (2006) ISBT Code of Ethics for Blood Donation and Transfusion, In: Documentation, Accessed March 23, 2011, Available from: http://www.isbt-web.org/documentation/default.asp

Jacobs B et al. (1994). *Secondary school students: a safer blood donor population in an urban with high HIV prevalence in east Africa*, East Africa Medical Journal, Vol. 71, Issue 11 (November 1994), pp. 720-3

Kajja I, Bimenya G, Smit Sibinga C. (2010b) *The interface between blood preparation and use in Uganda*, Vox Sanguinis 2010;98:e257-e262

Kajja I, Bimenya GS, Eindhoven GB, ten Duis HJ, Smit Sibinga CTh. (2010b) *Surgical blood order equation in femoral fracture surgery*, Transfusion Medicine; 2010: doi: 10.1111/j.1365-3148.2010.01033.x

Kajja I, Bimenya GS, Eindhoven GB, ten Duis HJ, Smit Sibinga CTh. (2010a) *Blood loss and contributing factors in femoral fracture surger*, African Health Sciences 2010;10:18-25

Kajja I, Bimenya GS, Smit Sibinga CTh. (2011) *Informed consent in blood transfusion: Knowledge and administrative issues in Uganda hospitals*, Transfusion and Apheresis Science 2011; 44:33-39

Kajja I, Kyeyune S, Bimenya GS, Smit Sibinga CTh. (2010a) *Bottlenecks of blood processing in Uganda*, Transfusion Medicine, 2010;20:329-336

Kajja, I (2010). *The Current Hospital TransfusionPractices and Procedures in Uganda*, PhD Thesis, GrafiMedia RUG, ISBN 978-90-367-4619-9

Kendrick DB. (n.d.). Blood Program in World War II, In: *Medical Department United States Army in World War II*, Accessed March 25, 2011, Available from: http://history.amedd.army.mil/booksdocs/wwii/blood/default.htm

Kyeyune D, Kataaha P, Kajja I, Smit Sibinga CTh. (2010) *The Success Story of Donor Funding to Uganda Blood Transfusion Service*, Vox Sanguinis 2010;99 (suppl 1):513

Linden JV, Bianco C (Eds.) (2001). *Blood Safety and Surveillance*, Marcel Dekker, 0-8247-0263-8, New York

Los APM, Mutegombwa SM, Gabra GA, Smit Sibinga CTh. (2009) *Liaison role of school teachers to support blood collection, donor motivation and retention at schools in Africa: Could the Uganda experience serve as an example for other African countries?* Africa Sanguine 2009;12:5-10

Los APM, Smit Sibinga CTh. (2001) Community involvement: The Development – the Past, the Present and the Future of Blood Donation as a Form of Community Involvement. In: Transfusion Medicine: Quo Vadis? What has been achieved, what is to be expected. Smit Sibinga CTh & Cash JD. (Eds.). pp21-29.

Los APM, Smit Sibinga CTh. (2009) *Social marketing tools to improve blood collection and donor retention*, Vox Sanguinis 2009;96 (suppl. 1):124 (abstract P-147)

Makhmudova MR, Smit Sibinga CTh. (2008) *Creation of a National blood program in Uzbekistan*, Vox Sanguinis, 2008;95 (Suppl 1):218 (P440)

Martucci J. (2010). *Negotiating exclusion: MSM, identity, and blood policy in the age of AIDS*, Soc Stud Sci, Vol. 40, Issue 2 (April 2010), pp. 215-41

McCullough J. (1998). Transfusion Medicine, McGraw-Hill, 0-07-045113-3, New York

McFarland W et al. (1998). *Risk factors for HIV seropositivity among first-time blood donors in Zimbabwe*, Transfusion, Vol. 38, Issue 3 (March 1998), pp. 279-84

Mintz PD. (1995). *Quality assessment and improvement of transfusion practices*, Hematol Oncol Clin North Am., Vol. 9, Issue 1 (February 1995), pp. 219-32

Noumsi GT, Schneider WH, Lachenal G, Smit Sibinga CTh. *Use of blood donor screening data to access HIV dynamics in Cameroun,* Vox Sang 2008;95 (Suppl 1):261 (P559)

Parry E.H.O. (Ed.). (1984) Principles of Medicine in Africa, 2d Edition, Oxford Medical Publications, 0192613375, Nairobi

Perlin T. (2001). TKTK, In: Ethical issues in transfusion medicine, Macpherson CR, Domen RE, Perlin T, Editors, pp. TK-TK, AABB Press, 978-1563951381, Bethesda

Roussel P et al. (2001). *Methodologic contribution to blood transfusion materials surveillance,* Transfus Clin Biol, Vol. 8, Issue 4 (August 2001), pp. 359-73

Sarkodie F, Adarkwa M, Adu-Sarkodie Y, Candotti D, Acheampong JW & Allain JP. (2001). *Screening for viral markers in volunteer and replacement blood donors in West Africa,* Vox Sanguinis, Vol. 80, pp. 142-7

Smit Sibinga CT, Los APM, van der Tuuk Adriani WPA. *Project management as a recommendable approach to improve donor management in restricted economy countries (preliminary results),* Vox Sanguinis, 2006;91 (Suppl 3):191 (P-405)

Smit Sibinga CT. *Needs and essentials for Nationally supported structure and organisation of the blood supply: the Sanquin model,* Transfusion 2006;46(Supplement):192A

Smit Sibinga CTh, Kajja I. (2009). *How to determine the needs for safe blood in Africa – expectations and realities.* Programme and Abstracts book 5th International Congress AfSBT, Nairobi, KY 2009: F56 p.97

Smit Sibinga CTh, van der Does JA, Los APM, Molijn HM, van der Tuuk Adriani WPA. (2009) *Opzet en ontwikkeling van de bloedvoorziening in ontwikkelingslanden. Hoe doe je dat?* Tijdschrift voor Bloedtransfusie 2009;2:87-92.

Smit Sibinga CTh. (2000). *Transfusion medicine in developing countries,* Transfusion Medicine Reviews 2000;14:269-274.

Smit Sibinga CTh. (2001) *Risk management: an important tool for improving quality.* Transfusion and Clinical Biology 2001;8:214-17.

Smit Sibinga CTh. (2002). *GCBS, ICBS and other initiatives; Will there be a 'toto pro partum'?* In: Transmissible Diseases and Blood Transfusion. Smit Sibinga CTh, Dodd RY (eds.). pp 195-202. Kluwer Academic Publishers ISBN 1-4020-0986-0. Dordrecht/ Boston/London

Smit Sibinga CTh. (2006). *Needs and essentials for Nationally supported structure and organisation of the blood supply: the Sanquin model,* Transfusion, 2006;46(Supplement):192A

Smit Sibinga, CTh. (2007). *Detecting and Monitoring Reactions in the Developing World,* In: Transfusion Reactions. Popovsky, MA, ed. 3rd edition AABB Press, Bethesda, MD, USA, 449-65

Smit Sibinga CTh. (2008). *The need for post-academic leadership development and transfusion medicine related health sciences research.* The Academic Institute for International Development of Transfusion Medicine. Transfusion Today 2008;77:9

Smit Sibinga CTh. (2009). *Is the need for safety of the blood supply in Africa different from other resource limited parts of the world?* Programme and Abstracts book 5th International Congress AfSBT, Nairobi, KY June 2009: T29 p.72

Smit Sibinga CTh. (2009a). *Filling a gap in transfusion medicine education and research,* Transfusion Medicine Reviews 2009;23;284-291

Smit Sibinga CTh. (2009b). *Pioneers and pathfinders – C.Th. Smit Sibinga: an autobiography,* Transfusion Medicine Reviews 2009;23:160-165.

South African National Blood Service [SANBS]. (2006) Donor Form, Accessed March 23, 2011, Available from: http://www.sanbs.org.za/new_donors/Eng_SEQ.pdf

Stutzer A & Goette L. (2010). *Blood donor motivation: what is ethical? What works?* ISBT Science Series, Vol. 5 (2010), pp. 244–248

Thomas WI & Thomas DS (eds,). (1928). The child in America. Alfred Knopf, New York USA

Titmuss R. (1971). The Gift Relationship: From Human Blood to Social Policy, New Press, 1565844033, New York

Umeora OU at al. (2005). *Socio-cultural barriers to voluntary blood donation for obstetric use in a rural Nigerian village*, African Journal of Reproductive Health, Vol. 9, Issue 3 (December 2005), pp. 72-76

United Nations. (1948) Universal Declaration of Human Rights. 22 March 2011 Avalailable from: www.un.org/en/documents/udhr/index.shtml

United Nations. (2000). Millennium Development Goals. 22 March 2011 Availble from: www.un.org/millenniumgoals/

United States Centers for Disease Control and Prevention [CDC]. (1982). *Possible transfusion-associated acquired immune deficiency syndrome (AIDS) – California*, MMWR Morbidity and Mortality Weekly Report, Vol. 31, pp. 652-654

United States Centers for Disease Control and Prevention [CDC]. (2008. *Progress Towards Strengthening Blood Transfusion Srvices – 14 Countries, 2003-2007*, MMWR Morbidity and Mortality Weekly Report, Vol. 57, pp. 1273-1277

United States Food and Drug Administration [FDA]. (2010). CPG Sec. 230.150 Blood Donor Classification Statement, Paid or Volunteer Donor (05/07/2002 new), In: Compliance Policy Guides, Accessed March 27, 2011, Available from: http://www.fda.gov/ICECI/ComplianceManuals/CompliancePolicyGuidanceMa nual/ucm122798

United States Food and Drug Administration [FDA]. (2010). Compliance Manual, Part I: Background, In: Inspection of Licensed and Unlicensed Blood Banks, Brokers, Reference Laboratories, and Contractors, Accessed March 25, 2011, Available from: http://www.fda.gov/BiologicsBloodVaccines/GuidanceComplianceRegulatoryInf ormation/ComplianceActivities/Enforcement/CompliancePrograms/ucm095226. htm

United States President's Emergency Plan for AIDS Relief. (2011) 2005-2010 PEPFAR Annual Reports, In: Annual Report to Congress on the President's Emergency Plan for AIDS Relief, Accessed March 23, 2011, Available from: http://www.pepfar.gov/press/c19573.htm

van Hulst M, Sagoe KW, Vermande JE, van de Schaaf IP, van der Tuuk Adriani WP, Torpey K, Ansah J, Mingle JA, Smit Sibinga CT, Postma MJ. (2008*). Cost-effectiveness of HIV screening of blood donations in Accra (Ghana)*, Value Health 2008;11:809-19.

van Hulst M, Smit Sibinga CTh, Postma MJ. (2009). *Health economics of blood transfusion safety – focus on sub-Saharan Africa*, Biologicals 2009;doi:10.1016/j.biologicals.2009:1-6

van Hulst R, Dhingra N, Smit Sibinga CT, Postma MJ. (2006). *Cost-effectiveness of interventions ensuring blood transfusion safety in Africa*, Transfusion 2006;46 (Supplement):169A

Wehrli J. (2011). *The nuts and bolts of curriculum and assessment*, Journal of Clinical Apheresis, Vol. 26, Issue 1 (ePub December 2010), pp. 29-46

World Bank in collaboration with U.S. CDC/CAR, USAID and WHO-EURO. (2008). *Blood Services in Central Asian Health Systems: A clear and present danger of spreading HIV/AIDS and other infectious diseases*. The International Bank for Reconstruction and Development/The World Bank, Washington DC, USA

World Health Organization. (1978). *WHA28.72 Utilization and supply of human blood and blood products*. WHO 1978, Geneva CH

World Health Organization. (1992a). *Report of the GCBS informal consultation on 'Assessment of Training Needs in Transfusion Medicine'*. WHO_LBS_92.6, 1992, Geneva, CH

World Health Organization. (1992b). *Report of the GCBS informal consultation on 'Collaboration in Training in Transfusion Medicine'*. WHO_LBS_92.71, 1992, Geneva, CH

World Health Organization (2001) *The Clinical Use of Blood. Handbook*. WHO/BTS/99.3, 2001, Geneva, CH

World Health Organization. (2008b). *Global Database on Blood Safety. Report 2004-2005*, WHO 2008 Geneva, CH

World Health Organization. (2008c). *Aide Mémoire for National Policy Makers. Good Policy Process for Blood Safety and Availability*. WHO/EHT/08.02. January 2008, Geneva, CH

World Health Organization. (2010a). *Global Blood Safety and Availability. Facts and figures from the 2007 survey*. WHO 2010, Geneva, CH

World Health Organization. (2010b). *Screening donated blood for transfusion-transmissible infections: recommendations*. World Health Organization. ISBN 978-92-4-154788-8

World Health Organization. (2008a). *Universal access to safe Blood Transfusion* WHO/EHT/08.03, Geneva, CH

World Health Organization. (2009). *Screening donated blood for transfusion-transmissible infections: recommendations*, In: Research Policy, Accessed March 26, 2011, Available from: http://www.who.int/rpc/guidelines/9789241547888/en/index.html

World Health Organization. (2011a). Blood Transfusion Safety, In: *National Blood Policies*, Accessed March 23, 2011, Available from: http://www.who.int/bloodsafety/transfusion_services/nat_blood_pol/en/

World Health Organization. (2011b). World Health Assembly/Executive Board Resolutions on Blood Safety, In: Blood transfusion safety documentation centre, Accessed March 23, 2011, Available from: http://www.who.int/bloodsafety/publications/en/index.html

World Health Organization. (2011c). Aide-Memoire on Blood Safety for National Blood Programmes, In: *Documentation*, Accessed March 23, 2011, Available from: http://www.who.int/bloodsafety/publications/en/index.html

World Health Organization. (2011d). *Global Database on Blood Safety, In: Blood transfusion safety*, Accessed March 25, 2011, Available from: http://www.who.int/bloodsafety/global_database/en/

10

Saliva Testing as a Practical Tool for Rapid HIV Screening

H. Blake[1], P. Leighton[2] and S. Sharma[3]
*[1]Division of Nursing, University of Nottingham, B Floor (South Block Link), Queen's
Medical Centre, NG7 2HA, Nottingham,
[2]Division of Primary Care, University of Nottingham, Room 2104, C Floor South 3Block,
Queen's Medical Centre, NG7 2UH, Nottingham
[3]Department of Psychology, University of Strathclyde, G1 1XQ, Glasgow,
[1,2]United Kingdom
[3]Scotland*

1. Introduction

Whilst the annual number of new HIV infections is steadily declining, levels of new infections overall are high and the number of people living with HIV has increased worldwide. An estimated 73,000 people in the UK are living with HIV, of which it is estimated that 24,000 are undiagnosed or unaware of their HIV status (Health Protection Agency, 2007). The prevalence of undiagnosed HIV infection would therefore seem a key driver for increased and routine HIV testing, both to lessen the potential for unwitting transmission of HIV and to support early detection and timely access to medical care in those infected. It has been shown that late diagnosis of HIV infection, resulting in delayed patient management, is associated with poorer survival (Losina et al., 2009). In the UK, the National Strategy for Sexual Health and HIV (Department of Health, 2001) aims to reduce the prevalence of undiagnosed HIV by increasing screening.

This is a rapidly advancing field and whilst it is beyond the scope of this chapter to encapsulate all the current evidence in this field, a brief overview is presented of saliva testing as a diagnostic tool, the benefits and the caveats. The contexts in which saliva testing for HIV are currently conducted is considered both in the UK and internationally. The evidence for the sensitivity and specificity of this method will be considered. Attitudes of recipients towards rapid HIV screening, in particular saliva testing, are considered together with attitudes towards the contexts in which testing is undertaken.

2. Diagnosis of HIV/AIDs

HIV screening is undertaken for a number of purposes, the UNAIDS/WHO summarise these as i) testing for screening blood, ii) testing for epidemiological surveillance and iii) testing for diagnosing infected individuals (UNAIDS, 1997). A variety of specific tests might be used to these ends. The British HIV Association (BHIVA) states that, "a potentially important mechanism for limiting the HIV epidemic is the widespread use of HIV testing in a variety of clinical settings," but provides no specific guidance on how the testing should be done (BHVA, 2005). The selection of the most appropriate test, and testing protocol, should not only be informed by test sensitivity and specificity, but also by a number of economic and logistic factors (Branson, 2003). The following sections outline some key information relating to procedures for HIV testing, categories of HIV testing, and HIV testing guidelines, and consider technical and process issues relating to HIV testing.

2.1 Testing for HIV

HIV testing has evolved from initial concerns, in the mid/early 1980s, for screening the supply of donated blood, to now reflect a broader range of concerns which include clinical diagnosis and strategic public health intervention (Branson, 2000a, 2000b). UNAIDS/WHO have identified four distinct categories of HIV testing: Diagnostic testing, Voluntary counselling and testing (VCT), Routinised testing in specific setting, and Mandatory testing. Diagnostic HIV testing is testing undertaken where signs and symptoms related to an HIV infection are observed in any individual. Testing is carried out to ensure timely clinical diagnosis, and to ensure the provision of adequate clinical support and services. People with certain diseases, such as tuberculosis and any other sexually transmitted disease, are also tested for HIV infection on a regular basis to this end.

Voluntary counselling and testing, also referred to as 'client focused testing', categorises those programmes of HIV testing which are designed to promote HIV awareness and to broaden access to HIV testing. Such testing is carried out in the absence of individual symptoms and is combined with group and individual counselling around HIV issues to raise awareness and educate in relevant health, and health behaviour, areas. This kind of testing programme is often undertaken with those who are perceived to be at high-risk of exposure to the HIV virus, or those who are concerned that they have been recently exposed to HIV. Testing is provided in local health and community settings, and pre and post-test counselling is offered to all those being testing. Pre-test counselling is often delivered in group settings, with post-test and follow-up counselling delivered on a one-to-one basis. UNAIDS/WHO identify VCT as the most effective approach to testing for achieving behaviour change to prevent HIV transmission in public settings.

Routine HIV testing of those accessing clinical or medical services is often carried out in those settings where high risk client groups are prevalent. Such testing is carried out with the purpose of early (asymptomatic) identification, with associated benefits for reduced risk of unwitting transmission of the virus. Carried out in community health centres, specialist clinics or hospitals settings such testing includes that undertaken in sexual health clinics with people who are undergoing diagnostic testing for other sexually transmitted diseases. It also incorporates the testing of intravenous drug users in primary and secondary care settings. Routine testing of this kind often utilises rapid HIV tests, which are described in more detail in section 3.

Mandatory HIV testing may be carried out for all donors prior to procedures involving transfusion of blood, bodily fluids or any organ transplant. In some countries, HIV testing is compulsorily carried out at the time of immigration, pregnancy and during routine medical check-ups of military personnel.

The individual, and health service cost, benefits associated with early detection and early medical intervention in cases of HIV infection offer a strong argument for routine testing, even amongst those populations where the incidence of HIV is low (Paltiel, 2006). Whilst evidence for screening programmes reducing the transmission of HIV is unclear (Paltiel, 2006), a range of studies indicate that those who are aware of their HIV status amend their behaviour so as to limit the risk of HIV transmission to others (Marks et al., 2005; Crepaz et al., 2006; Chou et al., 2005).

In the United States (U.S.) in 2006, in an effort to improve the identification of HIV-positive individuals, the Center for Diseases Control and Prevention (CDC) released their current HIV testing guidelines. These recommended routine testing for those age 13 to 64 years regardless of risk factors, unless testing is specifically declined by the individual (opt-out testing) (Branson et al., 2006). In the U.S. the following criteria apply: opt-out HIV screening is recommended for patients in all healthcare settings, with people at high risk for HIV infection screened for HIV at least annually. Here, separate written consent for HIV testing is not required; general consent for medical care should be considered sufficient to encompass consent for HIV testing. Finally, prevention counselling should not be required with HIV diagnostic testing or as part of HIV screening programmes in healthcare settings (Branson et al., 2006). Although one-third of people with HIV infection in the UK remain undiagnosed, current UK guidelines recommend opt-out testing only for pregnant women and people attending genitourinary clinics (Hamill et al., 2007).

2.2 HIV tests

HIV testing involves the detection of antibodies produced by the body in an unsuccessful attempt to fight HIV infection, such antibodies being more easily detected than the virus itself. Testing can be carried out on whole blood, plasma, serum, urine, dried blood spots and saliva samples, but might only be carried out after a 3-8 week period following infection (Schopper & Vercauteren, 1996). During this 3-8 week window the HIV antigen is rarely identified - bar in exceptional circumstances at the peak of high circulation of virus particles (Carne, 1988; Chin, et al., 2007).

Initial developments in HIV screening centred upon the need to ensure that donated blood remained free of the HIV virus. A *testing paradigm* thus emerged to protect the supply of donated blood, a paradigm marked by "tests with high sensitivity, suitable for batch processing of high volumes of specimens in centralised laboratories with specialised equipment." (Branson, 2000a). The enzyme-linked immunosorbent assay (ELISA) was indicative of this; a screening test for blood, efficient in large-scale hospital settings and reliant upon specialist laboratory equipment. The ELISA is the most appropriate, and most commonly used, screening test for samples greater than 100 per day; the ELISA is most appropriate for population level surveillance of HIV infection (UNAIDS, 1997). Performed by trained medical staff the ELISA test is reliable, but incurs substantial costs and might only offer results a few days after testing. Whilst this cost and delay are less important in screening donated blood, for other forms of testing they might act as a barrier.

During the late 1980s and early 1990s the benefits of *voluntary counselling and testing* were increasingly recognised and other testing algorithms were developed to meet this end (Branson, 2000a). Concerns about false positives from the ELISA test led the U.S. Public Health Service recommending secondary testing with the Western Blot (WB) to ensure accuracy. Although once again, the significant time delay associated with this combination of tests, of up to 2 weeks before test results are returned to patients, was a significant barrier. Also ELISA both in isolation and in combination with the WB test has limited suitability for remote or smaller clinical settings where resources are limited and access to adequate facilities is restricted (McCarthy et al., 1993; Owens et al., 1996). With particular concern for testing in the developing world, and to reflect a growing number of simple and rapid assays, the UN/WHO offers an informative typology of testing combinations (UNAIDS, 1997; Branson, 2000a, 2003).

For blood screening, population surveillance (of high risk groups) and diagnosis of individuals from high risk populations (who are displaying signs/symptoms of HIV infection) a single screening assay is adequate; and, a reactive test should be considered sufficient for a HIV positive diagnosis. For population surveillance (low and mid-risk groups), asymptomatic individual diagnosis (high risk group) and symptomatic diagnosis (low and mid-risk social group) a second screening assay should follow an initial reactive test; if both initial and second assays are reactive then the specimen is considered positive. For asymptomatic diagnosis (low and mid-risk social group) a third screening assay should be carried out following initial and second reactive tests; the specimen is considered positive if the third test is also reactive.

2.3 Technical and process issues

Above all, HIV testing should be carried in accordance with ethical principles designed to protect human rights. Testing should be carried out in a confidential manner and the person being tested should be fully informed about the nature and procedures of the test. Tests should be undertaken with caution since clinicians may be both civilly and criminally liable if they take a blood sample for HIV testing without disclosing to the patient (i) the nature of the test, (ii) the possible consequences of a positive result, and (iii) without obtaining informed consent (Sherrad & Gatt, 1987).

Further, where a positive HIV test manifests, appropriate psychological counselling should be provided to the diagnosed individual (WHO, 2004). Other technical and process issues include consideration of the cost-effectiveness of testing, of the quality of tests and testing procedures, and of the potential for home testing and the associated benefits and caveats.

Cost-effectiveness

Evidence from the U.S. suggests that routine, voluntary HIV testing is not only of crucial public health importance but is also economically justified (Walensky et al., 2007). The cost of HIV testing kits is variable, although this expenditure accounts for a substantial portion of the budget in national AIDS programmes. Selecting the most appropriate and cost-effective products for each particular setting therefore includes careful consideration of a range of factors including cost of test kit, storage, equipment maintenance and training of personnel.

Quality of testing procedures

Ensuring that quality is maintained and standard operating procedures are followed is critical to the generation of reliable results. The majority of HIV diagnostic products perform very well when used according to specific instructions. However, there is a risk that kits may be produced that do not meet exacting standards for quality, or make fraudulent claims for endorsement by WHO or the U.S. Food and Drink Administration (Kurtzweil, 1999). This remains an ongoing challenge.

Home testing

Home testing has positive implications for offering an alternative to people who might otherwise not seek testing in traditional health care facilities. For example, in some countries, a high uptake has been achieved by delivering both HIV counselling and testing at home, in the highest uptake in rural areas, in young people and groups with low educational attainment; this has resulted in substantial reductions in existing inequalities in accessing such services (Mutale et al., 2010). However, there are serious caveats associated with home testing which must be considered and balanced against any perceived benefits. Firstly, there is a potential that such kits may be fraudulent (e.g. Kurtzweil, 1999) or less accurate than those administered by trained staff. Secondly, there may be a risk of abuse if individuals are forced to take tests against their will. Finally, there a need for immediate confirmation of results and also access to counselling for those with a positive test result. In the UK little HIV testing is currently performed outside GUM and antenatal settings (Tweed et al., 2010).

3. Rapid testing and saliva testing

The introduction of rapid and 'point of care' testing in HIV was primarily to increase identification of HIV infected individuals, to enable inexpensive and convenient methods of testing amongst rural, outreach and at-risk populations, and to improve consumer experience of the testing procedure (Holt, 2009). Such rapid tests use finger-stick capillary whole blood (FSB) or oral fluid (OF), thus avoiding the need for venous blood sampling and centrifugation (Pavie et al., 2010). Specific benefits associated with rapid testing include immediate communication of test results (in standard tests between 25% and 33% of those tested do not return to receive their results), and advantages in immediate medical staff awareness of HIV status so as to limit the potential for HIV transmission during medical procedures (Kane, 1999; Branson, 2000a).

Rapid tests modified to use oral fluid samples obviate the need for either venepuncture or finger prick blood analysis (Hamill et al., 2007). Oral fluid HIV tests offer additional advantages due to their non-invasive nature, can be performed anywhere, do not require specialist phlebotomy training or equipment, and reduce biohazardous risk (Delaney et al., 2006). Rapid, reliable and affordable tests, requiring no equipment and minimal training, are now also available for HIV infection in developing countries (Peeling & Mabey, 2010).

3.1 Nature of rapid testing and saliva testing

In recent decades, a number of rapid test assays have been developed that enable HIV antibody status to be determined quickly, efficiently and less invasively than traditional forms of testing. Most rapid tests can be conveniently carried out 'on site' by someone with basic training and for this reason these are often referred to as 'point-of-care testing' (Kendrick et al., 2005). These tests are designed to detect antibodies in several different body fluids including whole blood from finger-prick blood, plasma, urine, or saliva. Rapid tests are simple to perform, can be conducted in rural settings without laboratory equipment, and remove the need to process and store specimens and transport them from the field (Pascoe et al., 2009).

Rapid tests rely on samples of blood taken from fingertip or saliva sample obtained by rubbing an absorbent pad across the lower and upper gums in the mouth. Obtained blood or saliva sample is then transferred into a plastic device already containing a developer solution, followed by the insertion of an assay test strip into the device. After a brief waiting period of approximately 15-20 minutes the appearance of two lines on the test strip is interpreted as a positive test result, indicating the presence of HIV-1 antibodies; however, a single line indicates a negative test result, and no visible lines imply an invalid test.

The speed with which test results can be produced make rapid HIV tests very popular and extremely useful particularly in public outreach settings (Spielberg et al., 2005). In such settings there may be limited access to a HIV test centre and furthermore, there may be a reluctance to be assessed for HIV infection amongst certain groups (e.g. sex-workers, drug-injectors). Moreover, it is not uncommon that individuals who have agreed to take a HIV test, do not return for their conventional laboratory blood test results and thus remain unaware of their HIV virus carrier status, presenting a danger to society as potential HIV transmitters (Galvan et al., 2004). Use of rapid saliva tests also have the potential to prevent HIV infections occurring in health workers due to handling of blood during standard ELISA, WB or rapid blood tests.

The unique features manifested by all rapid tests are their non-invasive testing procedure and the immediacy of producing results. Another advanced characteristic of rapid tests is the level of anonymity offered since the saliva, blood or urine specimen can be collected at home, sent to the laboratory for testing and results declared via the telephone, without a need to visit the clinic in person.

3.2 Diagnostic accuracy of HIV rapid tests

All diagnostic tests have limitations and sometimes their use may produce erroneous or questionable results. The accuracy of tests is often described in terms of 'sensitivity' (the percentage of results that will be positive when HIV is not present) and 'specificity' (the percentage of results that will be negative when HIV is not present). False positives occur when the test incorrectly indicates that HIV is present in a non-infected person. Conversely, false negatives occur when the test incorrectly indicates that HIV is absent in an infected person.

In a review of the risks and benefits of HIV screening, the U.S. Preventive Services Task Force concluded in 2005 that, "...the use of repeatedly reactive enzyme immunoassay followed by confirmatory Western blot or immunoflourescent assay remains the standard method for diagnosing HIV-1 infection. A large study of HIV testing in 725 U.S. laboratories reported a sensitivity of 99.7% and a specificity of 98.5% for enzyme immunoassay, and studies in U.S. blood donors reported specificities of 99.8% and greater than 99.99%. With confirmatory Western blot, the chance of a false-positive identification in a low-prevalence setting is about 1 in 250,000 (95% CI, 1 in 173,000 to 1 in 379,000)" (Chou et al., 2005).

The specificity rate outlined above for enzyme immunoassay screening tests indicates that, in every 1,000 positive HIV test results, there will be around 15 false positive results. However, confirming the test result (e.g. repeating the test, if this option is available) may reduce the likelihood of a false positive to just 1 result in every 250,000 tests. The sensitivity rating outlined above indicates that, in every 1,000 negative HIV test results, there will be 3 false negative results. Nevertheless, the high negative predictive value of these tests is extremely high, meaning that a negative test result will be correct more than 9,997 times in 10,000 (99.97% of the time). Due to the high negative predictive value of HIV screening tests, the CDC recommends that a negative test results be considered conclusive evidence that an individual does not have HIV.

Non-specific reactions, hypergammaglobulinemia, or the presence of antibodies directed to other infectious agents that may be antigenically similar to HIV can produce false positive results. Auto-immune diseases, such as systemic lupus erythematosus, have also rarely caused false positive results. Most false negative results are due to the window period; other factors, such as post-exposure prophylaxis, can rarely produce false negatives (Hare et al., 2004).

Rapid tests have been used for more than two decades to test serum and plasma, particularly in developing countries and for emergency diagnosis. They are simple to use and have high specificity, however, false positives do occur and they have been criticised in previous years for lacking in sensitivity relative to reference enzyme immunoassays (EIA/ELISA), particularly during primary HIV infection and infection by variant strains (Makuwa et al., 2002). There is, however, research evidence to indicate that rapid HIV tests produce results of comparable sensitivity and specificity to the ELISA test (Franco-Paredes et al., 2006; Greenwald et al., 2006; Branson, 2000a). Laboratory testing of 1266 specimens at rural peripheral laboratories of varied combinations of seven rapid HIV tests even showed a specificity of 100% (Stetler et al., 1997). Empirical studies have shown promising findings in a range of settings and populations including HIV positive individuals (DeBattista et al., 2007), HIV negative individuals (Makasso, 2005), sexual health clinic attenders (DeBattista et al., 2007), pregnant adult women in Namibia (Hamers et al., 2008), acute care (Lee et al, 2011) and adults presenting for voluntary testing elsewhere in the developing world (Pascoe et al., 2009).

Furthermore, whilst some early work has suggested that salivary testing should be recommended only for epidemiological studies (Mortimer & Parry, 1992), more recent studies have continued to demonstrate that rapid oral fluid tests show a high standard of sensitivity and specificity (e.g. Debattista et al., 2007; Hamers et al., 2008; Delaney et al., 2006). Independent performance data for 4 FDA approved rapid HIV tests (Franco-Paredes et al., 2006) and a wider range of rapid tests (Branson, 2000a) highlight product testing with both sensitivity and specificity outcomes of 100% (Oraquick and Retrocell HIV-1/2) (Branson, 2000a). Data from 2006 showed that in testing, sensitivity and specificity exceeded 99% in 4 FDA approved tests (with the exception of Reveal G2 Plasma test where specificity is 98.6%) (Franco-Paredes et al., 2006). Comparisons between rapid HIV tests are inconsistent. It has been suggested that there may be differences in diagnostic accuracy, with tests being less sensitive on oral fluid than on finger-stick whole blood and less sensitive on finger-stick whole blood than on serum (Pavie et al., 2010). More recently, in a direct comparison of the performance of all 6 tests currently approved by the FDA for use in the U.S. (using whole blood, oral fluid, serum, and plasma specimens), it has been shown that *all* rapid tests have statistically equivalent performance characteristics, based on overlapping confidence intervals for sensitivity and specificity, compared with conventional ELISA (Delaney et al., 2011).

It should be noted that although rapid tests using saliva have been shown to have high sensitivity and specificity parameters (Delaney et al., 2011), these are essentially brief screening tests and it has long been recognised that in cases where the first screening test utilised saliva, the diagnosis should be reconfirmed through a rapid test that involves blood testing (Andersson et al., 1997). In fact, it is now generally accepted that a second confirmatory test which detects the presence of a specific type of antibody to HIV 1/2 *must* follow (Franco-Paredes, et al., 2006). WHO recommends that for diagnostic purposes, two assays be used with a third test for discrepant results (Strategy II and III); the first test must have the highest sensitivity and the second test a similar or higher specificity (UNAIDS/WHO, 2004). Accuracy may be altered in pregnancy, and to improve diagnostic accuracy and to reduce false-positive results it may be necessary to use two rapid tests during labour and delivery (Pai et al., 2007). Some further limitations have been identified with oral fluid assays (e.g. unlikely to detect those in early stages of HIV infection or with reduced viral load) these limitations also apply to other rapid assays (Pascoe et al., 2009).

A large number of studies have been published to date on various aspects of test performance specifically for oral mucosal transudate (OMT) and saliva tests. A number of brief narrative reviews published between 1994-2006 have focused predominantly on the description of oral rapid test technologies, although this early work has not evaluated diagnostic accuracy. Two more recent systematic reviews on diagnostic accuracy have been conducted (Wesolowski, 2006; Pai, 2007). These include a review undertaken by the CDC as part of a post-marketing surveillance of one rapid test (Wesolowski, 2006) and a systematic review focused exclusively on performance of all rapid tests in pregnant women (Pai, 2007). A recent meta-analysis has evaluated OMT, saliva based rapid and point of care tests in at-risk populations worldwide from 1986-2011 (Balram & Pai, 2010). This data provided evidence of good overall performance of oral fluid-based HIV tests in global settings. The authors recommended these oral rapid tests as first line screening alternatives to blood-based rapid test and suggest their enhanced use in global expanded HIV testing initiatives (Balram & Pai, 2010). Furthermore, rapid testing is deemed to be suitable for use in community-based clinical research settings, to assess eligibility both for trial participation and for the provision of on-site voluntary counselling and testing services (Everett et al., 2009).

3.3 Acceptability of HIV rapid tests

Non-invasive rapid HIV tests have been consistently shown to be a preferred method of testing amongst varied population groups in both youth (Peralta et al., 2001; Pugatch et al., 2001) and adults, including men who have sex with men (MSM) (Sy et al., 1998; Chen et al., 2010) and injecting drug users (Colfax et al., 2002; Greensides et al., 2003; Spielberg et al., 2000). Recent research has also considered the acceptability of testing amongst healthcare professionals.

Youth populations

Although universal testing of adolescents is currently recommended in the U.S., previous studies have demonstrated that only 41% to 61% of adolescents offered a non-rapid HIV test agree to testing (Mehta et al., 2007; Goodman et al., 1994). Furthermore, only between one and two-thirds of adolescents who are tested return to receive their results and post-test counselling (Goodman et al., 1994; Ilegbodu et al., 1994; Lazebnik et al., 2001; Tsu et al., 2002). A recent study by Mullins et al. (2010) showed that 70% of adolescents preferred rapid to traditional HIV testing, and that rapid testers were more likely to receive their results within the follow-up period. This study suggested that for adolescents non-invasive testing may have a greater impact on their choice of a rapid method than the availability of same day test results. A high preference for rapid oral tests in comparison to invasive blood tests has also been demonstrated elsewhere (Pugatch et al., 2001; Peralta et al., 2001). Studies of rapid testing in specific settings have shown that paediatric emergency departments have been highly rated by adolescents aged 14-21 years, as a preferred location for rapid HIV testing. This supports the need for increased development of prevention and testing programs in this setting (Haines et al., 2011). It has been acknowledged that rapid testing should be followed by HIV prevention opportunities and rapid linkage to care (Peralta et al., 2001).

Adult populations

A high level of acceptance for rapid testing and a preference for rapid oral tests in comparison to invasive blood tests has been demonstrated in adult 'at risk' populations including MSM, high-risk heterosexual populations and injecting drug users (Speilberg et al., 2000; Greensides et al., 2003; Colfax et al., 2002; Sy et al., 1998, Chen et al., 2010). Research has shown that the majority of adults tested (95%) preferred results to be disclosed by telephone, again highlighting the importance of privacy issues in testing procedures (Speilberg et al., 2000). Positive implications of, rapid testing also include potential for, and increased monitoring and awareness of HIV related risk-behaviour (Speilberg et al., 2000). In MSM, injecting drug users and high risk heterosexuals attending a sexual health clinic (Greensides et al., 2003; Colfax et al., 2002), concerns have been raised about rapid testing in relation to associated costs, privacy issues, accuracy and reliability of results, access to post-test counselling and information, lack of access to testing, and lack of knowledge about testing centres and procedures (Greensides et al., 2003). It has been suggested that concerns regarding the accuracy of the rapid test might limit test acceptance and should be addressed during pre-test information procedures (Merchant et al., 2009).

Nevertheless, despite these concerns, a strong preference has been identified for non-invasive quick testing procedures, in particular, rapid oral testing methods (Chen et al., 2010). Although rapid testing procedures appear to be preferred in these populations, a large proportion of these individuals (almost half) remain unaware of the availability of home collection kits for HIV testing in areas where these are accessible (Greensides et al., 2003; Colfax et al., 2002). Many individuals 'at risk' have reported that they would test more frequently if testing was available for clinic or home use (Chen et al., 2010). In certain populations, such as MSM, those who prefer rapid testing may be significantly more likely to have some formal education, to have discussed testing with a sexual partner, to be aware of rapid testing, and to have had a previous test (Cohall et al., 2010).

Research has investigated the potential for offering rapid testing in commercial and community venues, although a significant number of barriers have been raised. Again, concerns have been raised about the lack of confidentiality and privacy for testing in social venues, and about the potential lack of post-test support for those who test positive (Prost et al., 2007).

Healthcare populations

Studies of HIV testing have mainly considered *patient* preferences, although recent work has investigated the attitudes of *healthcare* staff towards testing (Arbelaez et al., 2009; Sahoni et al., 2010). For example, it has been shown that hospital staff satisfaction and overall attitudes towards HIV testing program in an emergency department is high, and that healthcare staff attitudes do not represent a barrier to program implementation (Sahoni et al., 2010). Rapid advances in technology have also led to widening of training opportunities for rapid testing across geographically remote healthcare facilities (Knapp et al., 2011). Further, research is emerging which considers the role of various healthcare professionals rapid diagnostic testing for HIV in various regions of the world (e.g. oral health care workers; Patton et al., 2011). Whilst conducting rapid screening in the dental clinic setting has been identified as a viable option (Dietz et al., 2008; Patton et al., 2011), oral healthcare professionals have expressed a lack of confidence that graduating dentists have the skills and willingness to conduct HIV counselling and testing in dental practice; in fact lack of training in prevention counselling has been identified as a primary barrier (Patton et al., 2002). Additional challenges to rapid testing have been identified in a range of medical settings including insufficient staffing, inadequate privacy or space, associated administration, time limitations and competing priorities.

4. Conclusions

This is a rapidly advancing field and as such this chapter presents an overview of the key issues with selected evidence. In conclusion, it seems that rapid screening tests and/or alternative biological samples (such as oral fluid) are now thought to be effective in HIV prevention strategies by reaching a larger population through improved accessibility and general consent in approaches to screening, immediate referral of HIV positives for medical treatment and partner notification. Oral fluid testing has been implemented in a range of settings. The test appears to perform well in field settings, and can be considered a good alternative to blood samples, suitable for use in epidemiologic surveys aiming to estimate HIV prevalence in general populations and in high risk groups. There are several limitations in that oral fluid assays may be unlikely to detect those in early stages of HIV infection or with reduced viral load, and have shown altered accuracy in pregnancy; however, such limitations also apply to other rapid assays.

Research has suggested that in adults the most important factors in HIV testing are test accuracy, time to results and privacy of results. Studies have also suggested that patients express a preference for oral testing over venepuncture sampling since it is rapid and less invasive, although preferences may vary in different settings. Less invasive methods are preferred also in youth. Indeed, offering less invasive rapid testing to at-risk youth may assist clinicians in increasing the proportion of teens who agree to undergo testing and receive their test result. In general rapid testing is better accepted by patients in both developed and resource-limited settings. Point of care tests specifically assist in making testing accessible in areas with limited laboratory facilities. These tests have the potential for reducing the number of people who do not return to clinics to learn of their test result, and thus reduce the proportion of infected individuals who remain unaware of their diagnosis.

Overall, the majority of studies have demonstrated high sensitivity and specificity of oral fluid-based rapid HIV test in comparison with routinely utilized methods. With recent research showing comparable accuracy for a range of currently approved tests and specimen types, it may be characteristics such as convenience, time to result, shelf life, and cost that will be likely determining factors for selection of a rapid screening test for a specific application (Delaney et al., 2011). This suggests that rapid tests with well documented performance characteristics should be made available in public health and clinical settings.

Specifically, it seems that saliva specimens can be easily collected under difficult field conditions with minimal training and provide a valuable alternative to testing blood for HIV-seroprevalence studies. Salivary testing for HIV may therefore be a convenient and potentially accurate epidemiological tool, although should be used with caution since single test systems may be less appropriate to diagnose HIV infection in an individual without follow-up testing. There is a drive for continual improvement of test performance, such that is has been suggested that all initial positive findings should be repeated by second test method with a second confirmatory specimen found positive prior to informing the patient. This may serve to mitigate the emotional distress and unnecessary treatments associated with false positive HIV testing.

5. References

Andersson, S., da Silva, Z., Norrgren, H., Dias, F. & Biberfeld, G. (1997). Field evaluation of alternative testing strategies for diagnosis and differentiation of HIV-1 and HIV-2 infections in an HIV-1 and HIV-2-prevalent area, *AIDS*, 11 (15), 1815-1822.

Arbelaez, C., Wright, E., Losina, E. & et al. (2009). Emergency provider attitudes and barriers to universal HIV testing in the emergency department. *J Emerg Med*. Oct 13 [Epub ahead of print].

Balram, B. & Pai, N. (2011). Salivary and oral fluid based HIV antibody assays for rapid diagnosis of HIV infection. The 9th Annual Cochrane Canada Symposium, Early Exposure to Cochrane: accessible, credible & practical, 16-17 Feb 2011, Vancouver, BC.

Branson, B. (2000a). Rapid Tests for HIV Anti-body, *AIDS Reviews*, 2, 76-83.

Branson, B. (2000b). Assessing Diagnostic Technologies Marketed to Less Industralised Countries, *Journal of International Physicians in AIDS Care*, Feb 2000, 28-30.

Branson, B. (2003). Point of Care Rapid Tests for HIV Antibodies, *Journal of Laborqtory Medicine*, 27 (7/8), 288-295.

Branson, B., Handsfield, H., Lampe, M. & et al. (2006). Revised recommendations for HIV testing of adults, adolescents, and pregnant women in health-care settings. *MMWR Recomm Rep*, 55(RR-14), 1–17.

British HIV Association (2005). *Guidelines for the treatment of HIV-infected adults with antiretroviral therapy*. www.bhiva.org/cms1191541.asp.

Carne, C. (1988). *Testing and screening for HIV infection*. Health Education Authority: London.

Chen Y., Bilardi, J., Lee, D., Cummings, R., Bush, M. & Fairley, C. (2010). Australian men who have sex with men prefer rapid oral HIV testing over conventional blood testing for HIV. *Int J STD AIDS* 21(6):428-30.

Chin, B., Lee, S., Kim, G., Kee, M., Suh, S., & Kim, S. (2007). Early Identification of Seronegative Human Immunodeficiency Virus Type 1 Infection with Severe Presentation. *Journal of Clinical Microbiology*, 45, 1659-1662.

Chou, R., Huffman, L., Fu, R., Smits, A. & Korthuis, P. (2005). Screening for HIV: a review of the evidence for the U.S. Preventive Services Task Force, *Annals of Internal Medicine*, 143, 55-73.

Cohall, A., Dini, S., Nye, A., Dye, B., Neu, N. & Hyden, C. (2010). HIV testing preferences among young men of color who have sex with men. *Am J Public Health*. 100(10), 961-6. Epub 2010 Jan 14.

Colfax, G., Lehman, J., Bindman, A., Vittinghoff, E., Vranizan, K., & Fleming, P., et al. (2002). What happened to home HIV test collection kits? Intent to use kits, actual use, and barriers to use among persons at risk for HIV infection. *AIDS Care* 2 (14), 675-82.

Crepaz, N., Lyles, C., Wolitski, R., Passin, W., Rama, S., Herbst, J. & et al. (2006). Do prevention interventions reduce HIV risk behaviours among people living with HIV? A meta-analytic review of controlled trials [Editorial], *AIDS*, 20 (1), 143-157.

Debattista, J., Bryson, G., Roudenko, N., Dwyer, J., Kelly, M., Hogan, P., & Patten, J. (2007). Pilot of non-invasive (oral fluid) testing for HIV within a clinical setting. Sexual Health, 4 (2), 105-109.

Delaney, K., Branson, B., Uniyal, A., Kerndt, P., Keenan, P., Jafa, K., Gardner, A., Jamieson, D. & Bulterys, M. (2006). Performance of Oral Fluid HIV- 1/2 test: experience from four CDC studies, *AIDS*, 20, 1655-1660.

Department of Health (2001). *National Strategy for Sexual Health and HIV*, DoH, London.

Dietz, C., Ablah, E., Reznik, D. & Robbins, D. (2008). Patients' attitudes about rapid oral HIV screening in an urban, free dental clinic. *AIDS Patient Care STDS* 22(3):205-12.

Everett, D., Baisley, K., Changalucha, J., Vallely, A., Watson-Jones, D., Cook, C., Knight, L., Ross, D., Mugeye, K., McCormack, S., Lacey, C., Jentsch, U. & Hayes, R. (2009). Suitability of simple human immunodeficiency virus rapid tests in clinical trials in community-based clinic settings. *J Clin Microbiol* 47 (4), 1058-62. Epub 2009 Feb 25.

Franco-Paredes, C., Tellez, I., & del-Rio, C. (2006). Rapid HIV testing: A review of the literature and implications for the clinician. *Current HIV/AIDS Reports*, 3, 159-165.

Galvan, F., Brooks, R. & Leibowitz, A. (2004), Rapid HIV Testing: Issues in Implementation, *Aids Patient Care and STDS*, 18 (1), 15-18.

Goodman, E., Tipton, A., Hecht, L. & et al. (1994). Perseverance pays off: health care providers' impact on HIV testing decisions by adolescent females. *Pediatrics* 94 (6 Pt 1), 878–82.

Greensides, D., Berkelman, R., Lansky, A., & Sullivan, P. (2003). Alternative HIV Testing Methods Among Populations at High Risk for HIV Infection. *Public Health Reports*, 118, 531-539.

Greenwald, J., Burstein, G., Pincus, J. & Branson, B. (2006). A Review of Rapid HIV Antibody Tests, *Current Infectious Disease* Reports, 8, 125-131.

Haines, C., Uwazuoke, K., Zussman, B., Parrino, T., Laguerre, R. & Foster, J. (2011). Pediatric emergency department-based rapid HIV testing: adolescent attitudes and preferences. *Pediatr Emerg Care* 27 (1), 13-16.

Hamers, R., de Beer, I., Kaura, H., van Vugt, M., Caparos, L., & Rinke, de Wit T. (2008). Diagnostic accuracy of 2 oral fluid-based tests for HIV surveillance in Namibia. *Journal of Acquired Immune Deficiency Syndromes*, 48(1):116-8.

Hamill, M., Burgoine, M., Farrell, F., Hamelaar, J., Patel, G., Welchew, D. & Jaffe HW (2007). Time to move towards opt-out testing for HIV in the UK. *BMJ*, 334: 1352-4.

Hare, C., Pappalardo, B., Busch, M., Phelps, B., Alexander, S., Ramstead, C., Levy, J. & Hecht, F. (2004). Negative HIV antibody test results among individuals treated with antiretroviral therapy (ART) during acute/early infection. The XV International AIDS conference. pp. abstract No MoPeB3107.

Health Protection Agency (2007). Testing Times. HIV and other Sexually Transmitted Infections in the United Kingdom. London: Health Protection Agency, Centre for Infections. November 2007. Holt, M. (2009). *Rapid HIV testing: A literature review.* Australian Federation of AIDS Organisation Inc.

Ilegbodu, A., Frank, M., Poindexter, A., & et al. (1994). Characteristics of teens tested for HIV in a metropolitan area. *J Adolesc Health* 15 (6), 479–84.

Kane, B. (1999). Rapid testing for HIV: Why so fast. *Annals of Internal Medicine*, 133 (6), 481-483.

Kendrick, S., Kroc, K., Withum, D., Rydman, R., Branson, B. & Weinstein, R. (2005). Outcomes of Offering Rapid Point-of-Care HIV Testing in A Sexually Transmitted Disease Clinic, *J Acquir Immune Defic Syndr*, 38 (2), 142-146.

Knapp, H., Chan, K., Anaya, H., Goetz, M. (2011). Interactive Internet-Based Clinical Education: An Efficient and Cost-Savings Approach to Point-of-Care Test Training. *Telemed J E Health*. Apr 14. [Epub ahead of print]

Kurtzweil, P. (1999). Internet sales of bogus HIV test kits result in first-of-kind wire fraud conviction. *FDA Consum*, 33 (4), 34-5.

Lazebnik, R., Hermida, T., Szubski, R. & et al. (2001). The proportion and characteristics of adolescents who return for anonymous HIV test results. *Sex Transm Dis* 28 (7), 401–4.

Lee, B.E., Plitt, S., Fenton, J., Preiksaitis, J.K., Singh, A.E. Rapid HIV tests in acute care settings in an area of low HIV prevalence in Canada. *J Virol Methods* 172 (1-2), 66-71. Epub 2010 Dec 28.

Losina, E., Schackman, B., Sadownik, S., Gebo, K., Walensky, R. & et al. (2009). Racial and Sex Disparities in Life Expectancy Losses among HIV-Infected Persons in the

United States: Impact of Risk Behavior, Late Initiation, and Early Discontinuation of Antiretroviral Therapy. *Clin Infect Dis* 49, 1570–1578.

McCarthy, B., Wong, J., Munoz, A., & Sonnenberg, F. (1993). Who should be screened for HIV infection? A cost-effectiveness analysis. *Archives of Internal Medicine*, 153, 1107-1116.

Makuwa, M., Souquie`re ,S., Niangui, M., Rouquet, P., Apetrei, C. & et al. (2002). Reliability of rapid diagnostic tests for HIV variant infection. *J Virol Methods*, 103, 183–190.

Marks, G., Crepaz, N., Senterfitt, J. & Janssen, R. (2005). Meta-analysis of high-risk sexual behavior in persons aware and unaware they are infected with HIV in the United States: implications for HIV prevention programs, *Jounral of Acquired Immune Deficiency Syndrome*, 39, 446-453.

Mehta, S., Hall, J., Lyss, S. & et al. (2007). Adult and pediatric emergency department sexually transmitted disease and HIV screening: programmatic overview and outcomes. *Acad Emerg Med*, 14 (3), 250-8.

Merchant, R., Clark, M., Seage, G. 3rd, Mayer, K., Degruttola, V. & Becker, B. (2009). Emergency department patient perceptions and preferences on opt-in rapid HIV screening program components. *AIDS Care*, 21 (4), 490-500.

Mortimer, P., Parry, J. (1992). Letter to the Editor: Salivary testing for HIV infection. *BMJ*, 305, 1093.

Mullins, T., Braverman, P., Dorn, L, Kollar, L., & Kahn, J. (2010). Adolescent Preferences for Human Immunodeficiency Virus Testing Methods and Impact of Rapid Tests on Receipt of Results. *Journal of Adolescent Health*, 46, 162–168.

Mutale, W., Michelo, C., Jürgensen, M.& Fylkesnes, K. (2010). Home-based voluntary HIV counselling and testing found highly acceptable and to reduce inequalities. *BMC Public Health*, 10, 347.

Owens, D., Nease, R. & Harris, R. (1996). Cost-effectiveness of HIV screening in acute care settings. *Archives of Internal Medicine*, 156, 394-404.

Paltiel, D., Walensky, R., Schackman, B., Seage, G., Mercincavage, L., Weinstein, M., & Freedberg, K. (2006). Expanded HIB Screening in the United States: Effects on Clinical Outcomes, HIV Transmission and Costs, *Annals of Internal Medicine*, 145 (11), 797-806.

Pai, N., Tulsky, J., Cohan, D., Colford, J. & Reingold, A. (2007). Rapid point-of-care HIV testing in pregnant women: a systematic review and meta-analysis. *Trop Med Int Health*, 12 (2), 162-73.

Pascoe, S., Langhaug, L., Mudzori, J., Burke, E., Hayes, R. & Cowan, F. (2009). Field Evaluation of Diagnostic Accuracy of an Oral Fluid Rapid Test for HIV, Tested at Point-of-Service Sites in Rural Zimbabwe, *Aids, Patient Care and STDs.*, 23 (7), 571-6.

Patton, L., Ranganathan, K., Naidoo, S., Bhayat, A., Balasundaram, S., Adeyemi, O., Taiwo, O., Speicher, D. & Chandra, L. (2011). Oral Lesions, HIV Phenotypes, and Management of HIV-Related Disease: Workshop 4A. *Adv Dent Res*, 23 (1), 112-116.

Patton, L., Santos, V., McKaig, R., Shugars, D. & Strauss, R. (2002). Education in HIV risk screening, counseling, testing, and referral: survey of U.S. dental schools. *J Dent Educ*, 66 (10), 1169-77.

Pavie, J., Rachline, A., Loze, B., Niedbalski, L., Delaugerre, C., Laforgerie, E., Plantier, J., Rozenbaum, W., Chevret, S., Molina, J. &, Simon, F. (2010). Sensitivity of Five Rapid HIV Tests on Oral Fluid or Finger-Stick Whole Blood: A Real-Time Comparison in a Healthcare Setting. *PLoS ONE* , 5(7): e11581. doi:10.1371/journal.pone.0011581

Peeling, R. & Mabey, D. (2010). Point-of-care tests for diagnosing infections in the developing world. *Clin Microbiol Infect*, 6 (8), 1062-1069.

Peralta, L., Constantine, N., Griffin D., Martin, L., & Ghalib, K. (2001). Evaluation of youth preferences for rapid and innovative human immunodeficiency virus antibody tests. *Archives of Pediatric and Adolescent Medicine*, 155 (7), 761-762.

Pugatch, D., Levesque, B., Lally, M., Reinert, S., Filippone, W., Combs, C., Flanigan, T. & Brown, L. (2001). HIV testing among young adults and older adolescents in the setting of acute substance abuse treatment. *Journal of Acquired Immune Deficiency Syndrome*, 27, 135-42.

Prost, A., Chopin, M., McOwan, A., Elam, G., Dodds, J., Macdonald, N. & Imrie, J. (2007). "There is such a thing as asking for trouble": taking rapid HIV testing to gay venues is fraught with challenges. *Sex Transm Infect*, 83, 185–188.

Sohoni, A., Gordon, D., Vahidnia, F. & White, D. (2010). Emergency Department Staff Satisfaction With Rapid Human Immunodeficiency Virus Testing. *Academic Emergency Medicine* 17, 561–565.

Schopper, D., & Vercauteren, G. (1996). Testing for HIV at home: what are the issues? *AIDS*, 10, 1455-1465.

Sherrard, M. & Gatt, I. (1987). Human immunodeficiency virus (HIV) antibody testing. Guidance from an opinion provided for the British Medical Association. *Br Med J (Clin Res Ed)*. 295 (6603), 911-912.

Smith, P., Buzi, R. & Weinman, M. (2005). HIV testing and counseling among adolescents attending family planning clinics. *AIDS Care*, 17 (4), 451–456.

Spielberg, F., Critchlow, C., Vittinghoff, E., Coletti, A.S., Sheppard, H., Mayer, K., Metzgerg, D., Judson, F., Buchbinder S., Chesney, M., & Gross, M. (2000). Home collection for frequent HIV testing: acceptability of oral fluids, dried blood spots and telephone results. HIV Early Detection Study Group. *AIDS*, 14 (12), 1819-1828.

Spielberg, F., Branson, B., & Goldbaum, G., et al. (2005). Choosing HIV counseling and testing strategies for outreach settings: a randomized trial. *Journal of Acquired Immune Deficiency Syndrome*, 38, 348–355.

Stetler, H., Granade, T., Nunez, C., Meza, R., Terrell, S., Amador, L. & George, R. (1997). Field evaluation of rapid HIV serologic tests for screening and confirming HIV-1 infection in Honduras, *AIDS*, 11, 369–375.

Sy, F., Rhodes, S., Choi, S., Drociuk, D., Laurent, A., Naccash, R., & Kettinger, L. (1998). The acceptability of oral fluid testing for HIV antibodies. A pilot study in gay bars in a predominantly rural state. *Sexually Transmitted Diseases*, 25 (4), 211-215.

Tsu, R., Burm, M., Gilhooly, J. & et al (2002). Telephone vs. face-to-face notification of HIV results in high-risk youth. *J Adolesc Health* 30 (3), 154–60.

Tweed, E., Hale, A., Hurrelle, M., Smith, R., Delpech, V., Ruf, M., Klapper, P., Ramsay, M. & Brant, L. (2010) Monitoring HIV testing in diverse healthcare settings: results from a sentinel surveillance pilot study. *Sex Transm Infect* 86 (5), 360-4. Epub 2010 Apr 28.

UNAIDS (1997). HIV Testing Methods – UNAIDS technical update, UNAIDS, Geneva.

UNAIDS/WHO (2004). HIV Assays: Operational Characteristics (Phase 1) Simple/Rapid tests (Report 14) 2004.

Walensky, R., Freedberg, K., Weinstein, M. & Paltiel, A. (2007). Cost-effectiveness of HIV testing and treatment in the United States. *Clin Infect Dis*, 45 (Suppl 4), S248-54.

Wesolowski, L., MacKellar, D., Facente, S., Dowling, T., Ethridge, S., Zhu, J., Sullivan, P. & Post-marketing Surveillance Team (2006). Post-marketing surveillance of OraQuick whole blood and oral fluid rapid HIV testing. *AIDS*, 20 (12), 1661-1666.

11

Molecular Epidemiology of HIV-1 Infection in the Amazon Region

Antonio Carlos Rosário Vallinoto, Luiz Fernando Almeida Machado,
Marluísa de Oliveira Guimarães Ishak and Ricardo Ishak
Federal University of Para, Institute of Biological Sciences, Virus Laboratory,
Brazil

1. Introduction

No other group of infectious agents has received increased attention from scientists in recent years than that of retroviruses. This reflects not only their importance as pathogens of humans and animals, but also its great value in studying the interactions between pathogens and host.

The family *Retroviridae* comprises a large number of viruses that have the ability to insert its genome into the host cell and infect primarily vertebrates, despite having been described infections in other animals such as snails and insects.

Viruses pathogenic to humans which cause infections worldwide can be divided into two main groups: the transformants and the cytopathic. The first, induce changes in the control of cell division and can lead to tumors, such as Human T-lymphotropic virus (HTLV), belonging to the genus *Deltaretrovirus* and is linked to neurological and hematological. Cytopathic retroviruses are members of the *Lentivirus* genus, such as the Human immunodeficiency virus (HIV), and are related to severe immunodeficiency condictions.

The ubiquotous conditions, now known by the name of acquired immunodeficiency syndrome (AIDS) is caused by HIV and was first recognized in the summer of 1981. The spread of an emerging virus in all regions of the world, caused great losses both in terms of human lives as well as in the economic point of view.

HIV infection results in a profound disorder in the host immune system, which is characterized by a decrease in the number of lymphocytes with the CD4 glycoprotein on their surface, especially helper T lymphocytes (ATL), with subsequent reversal of the ratio of CD4+ or CD8+ T lymphocytes.

In Brazil, the HIV-1 dissemination reflects the grandeur and diversity sociogeographic of the country and its regional heterogeneity. The first cases of HIV/AIDS in Brazil, dates from 1982 and were originated the Southeast individual, which today still has the highest number of reported cases of the disease. Subtypes B, F, C and D, in addition to samples of virus recombinants and dual infections in different geographical areas. In the present chapter, we describe the molecular epidemiology of HIV-1 infection in the Brazilian Amazon region, emphasizing its impact in the city of Belem, Capital of the Para State, which is the main port of entry into the Amazon, highlighting the occurrence of the circulating subtypes and the genetic profile of the host which is associated with the infection.

Currently HIV-1 genetic heterogeneity is classified into four phylogenetic groups: M, N, O and P, which may reflect four interspecific transmission events from chimpanzees (Plantier et al., 2009). Group M (major) is the most frequently involves with human infectious worldwide and is composed of nine genetically distinct subtypes, named A, B, C, D, F, G, H, J and K, whose gene sequences differ approximately 20% (Taylor et al., 2008).

In Brazil, HIV-1 is characterized by the occurrence of several subtypes of the M group, and includes subtype B, the most prevalent in the majority of the regions, followed by subtypes F, C, and D, (Monteiro et al., 2009) although some cities present a distinct pattern of distribution of these subtypes (Vicente et al., 2000; Soares et al., 2003). This diversity of subtypes could represent more than one port of entry of HIV-1 in the country, with the emergence of the epidemic occurring, probably in the late 1970's or early 1980's (Morgado et al., 1998).

The circulating recombinant forms of HIV (CRFs) have an important role in regional and global epidemics of the virus, particularly in regions where multiple subtypes circulate simultaneously. Currently over 40 CRFs are recognized worldwide (http://www.hiv.lanl. gov), and five have been described in Brazil, designated as CRF28_BF, CRF29_BF, CRF39_BF, CRF40_BF e CRF31_BC (Sanabani et al., 2006; De Sá Filho et al., 2006, http://www.hiv.lanl.gov/content/sequence/HIV/CRFs/CRFs.html), where CRF_BC represents 11% of the HIV-1 viruses circulating in the Southern region of the country (Santos et al., 2006).

In addition to the CRF, a large number of unique recombinant forms (URFs) have been characterized worldwide (McCutchan, 2006). Notoriously, a recombination is a potentially important mechanism that significantly contributes to HIV genetic variability with serious implications for diagnosis, drug treatment and optimal vaccine development (Sanabani et al., 2010).

2. HIV-1 infection in the Brazilian Amazon region

The molecular epidemiology of HIV-1 strains circulating in the Northern region of Brazil is poorly known (Table 1). The State of Para has 43.3% of the cases. Until June 2006, there were 5919 infected individuals, in which 80.4% were men and 19.6% were women (Brasil, 2008). The prevalence of the infection in the State of Amapa is still low, although the region borders French Guiana and a great number of indigenous populations move freely between the two countries. The cities of Belem (State of Para), Manaus (State of Amazonas) and Macapa (State of Amapa) can be considered as the main entry of HIV-1 in northern Brazil. The city of Belem has one of the largest ports in the Brazilian Amazon and receives a great input of tourists throughout the year, while the city of Macapa is located next to several Indian tribes and borders countries such as Guyana, which generates a large population movement between two locations. The city of Belem shows the highest diversity of subtypes of HIV-1 in Brazil, having been identified the subtypes B, F, D, C and recombinant CRF02_AG subtype reflecting in this way, the same epidemiological profile found in almost all regions of Brazil (Sabino et al., 1996; Morgado et al., 1998; Ramos et al., 1999, Tanuri et al., 1999; Vicente et al., 2000) and from South America (Marquina et al., 1996; Navas et al., 1999; Avila et al., 2002; Castro et al., 2003).

The population group studied presented epidemiological characteristics which indicated that the heterosexual transmission of HIV-1 associated with sexual promiscuity, was the main way of virus dissemination. HIV-1 occurred mostly in the group of individuals who reported having only primary and secondary education, as well as those with a heterosexual behavior. There was no statistically correlation between sex, educational level, sexual orientation and risk behavior for HIV-1, with subtypes B and F infection.

Subtype C was identified in Belem and phylogenetic analysis supports the hypothesis that the virus was imported from the Southeast and Southern Brazil. Additionally, the recombinant CRF02_AG subtype, circulating in Belém-PA probably was reported for the first time in the Amazon region and reinforces the importance of epidemiological surveillance for the virus in the country.

In Belem four subtypes were described in relation to *env*: B (88.3%), F (8.3%), D (1.7%), and C (1.7%); subtype B was the only one found in Macapa. In relation to the *pro* segment, there were four distinct subtypes in Belem: B (88.3%), F (9.3%), D (1.2%), and CRF02_AG (1.2%). In Macapa, subtypes B (97.1%) and F (2.9%) were detected. Six strains were characterized as mosaics: two were B^{env}/F^{pro} (1.6%), two F^{env}/B^{pro} (1.6%), one C^{env}/B^{pro} (0.85%), and one B^{env}/D^{pro} (0.8%) (Machado et al., 2009).

When compared to the State of Amazonas, there is a higher concentration of cases of disease in Manaus (capital), which holds approximately 90% of cases (Fundação de Medicina Tropical do Amazonas, 2006). Manaus has greater human genetic diversity because of their indigenous origin and sociocultural strong influence of migration from the Northeast region of Brazil since the 1800's when colonization occurred more intensely because of the business cycles of the rubber extractive exploratory projects, settlement of forest areas its transformation into an industrial area (Carneiro Filho, 1998).

There is evidence that the HIV / AIDS in the city of Manaus evolved with different patterns of distribution and expansion, whose characteristics define its consolidation in the initially affected districts still in the emergency epidemic, spreading later to other spaces receptive City (Silva et al., 2009).

In Manaus, it was found almost equal proportions of HIV-1 strains belonging to subtype B (51.6%) and F (48.4%), a finding that differs from previous results from studies conducted in urban areas of southeastern Brazil (Vicente et al., 2000).

Region	State	Subtypes	Gene(s)	References
North	Pará	B, F, D e C	*env*	Machado *et al.*, 2009
	Pará	B, F, D, CRF02_AG	*pro*	Machado *et al.*, 2009
	Pará	B^{env}/F^{pro}, F^{env}/B^{pro}, C^{env}/B^{pro}, B^{env}/D^{pro}		Machado *et al.*, 2009
	Amapá	B	*env*	Machado *et al.*, 2009
	Amapá	B e F	*pro*	Machado *et al.*, 2009
	Amazonas	B, F e B/F	*env*	Vicente *et al.*, 2000

Table 1. Geographic distribution of subtypes of HIV-1 in northern Brazil.

3. Genetic background of HIV-1 infected subjects

The pathogenesis of human immunodeficiency virus 1 infection is very complex and of course influenced by both viral and host factors (Cohen et al., 1997). Studies have focused the attention about the role of *MBL* gene variants and its serum concentration on the progression of AIDS in HIV-1-infected subjects (Garred et al., 1997; Prohászka et al., 1997).

Mannose-binding lectin (MBL) is a liver-derived pluripotent serum lectin that has a role in the host's innate immune system (Turner, 2003) by binding with high affinity to mannose or other carbohydrate components existent in viruses, bacteria and yeast (Kuipers et al., 2003). However, MBL function is directly associated with its serum concentrations which are determined by the interplay between promoter and structural gene mutations (Madsen et al., 1995; Jüliger et al., 2000).

Three mutations have been described in the structural region of the molecule (codons 52, 54 and 57) from which are derived three allelic variants named *MBL*D*, *MBL*B* and *MBL*C*, respectively. On the other hand, the wild allele is called *MBL*A* (Madsen et al., 1994). The occurrence of these variants have been associated with MBL serum deficiency and consequently to susceptibility/resistance to infection by various pathogens, including HIV-1 (Drogari-Apiranthitou et al., 1997; Garred et al., 1997; Prohászka et al., 1997; Luty et al., 1998; Hibberd et al., 1999; Peterslund et al., 2001; Klabunde et al., 2002; Roy et al., 2002; Song et al., 2003).

It was investigated the association between *MBL* gene polymorphism and the susceptibility to HIV-1 infection (Vallinoto et al., 2006). The study of 145 HIV-1-infected subjects and 99 healthy controls showed the presence of alleles *MBL*A*, *MBL*B* and *MBL*D*, whose frequencies were 69%, 22% and 09% among patients and 71%, 13% and 16% among healthy controls, respectively. The presence of the variant *MBL*B* was associated with higher plasma viral load levels, suggesting the importance of the *MBL* gene polymorphism in the clinical evolution of HIV-1-infected patients.

The prevalence of mutations in the -550 (H/L) and -221 (X/Y) mannose-binding lectin (MBL) gene promoter regions and their impact on infection by human immunodeficiency virus 1 (HIV-1) was investigated in a population of 128 HIV-1 seropositive and 97 seronegative patients (Vallinoto et al, 2008). The allele identification was performed through the sequence-specific primer polymerase chain reaction method, using primer sequences specific to each polymorphism. The evolution of the infection was evaluated through CD4+ T-lymphocyte counts and plasma viral load. The allele and haplotype frequencies among HIV-1-infected patients and seronegative healthy control patients did not show significant differences. CD4+ T-lymphocyte counts showed lower levels among seropositive patients carrying haplotypes LY, LX and HX, as compared to those carrying the HY haplotype. Mean plasma viral load was higher among seropositive patients with haplotypes LY, LX and HX than among those carrying the HY haplotype. When promoter and exon 1 mutations were matched, it was possible to identify a significantly higher viral load among HIV-1 infected individuals carrying haplotypes correlated to low serum levels of MBL. The current study shows that haplotypes related to medium and low MBL serum levels might directly influence the evolution of viral progression in patients. Therefore, it is suggested that the identification of haplotypes within the promoter region of the MBL gene among HIV-1 infected persons should be further evaluated as a prognostic tool for AIDS progression.

4. References

Avila, M.M., Pando, M.A., Carrion, G., Peralta, L.M., Salomon, H., Carrillo, M.G., Sanchez, J., Maulen, S., Hierholzer, J., Marinello, M., Negrete, M., Russell, K.L. & Carr, J.K. (2002). Two HIV-1 epidemics in Argentina: different genetic subtypes associated with different risk groups. *Journal of Acquired Immune Deficiency Syndrome*. Apr 1, 29(4):422-426, ISSN:1525-4135

Brasil. Ministério da Saúde. *Boletim Epidemiológico* (2008). AIDS, 12: 1–57, http://portal.saude.gov.br/portal/svs/visualizar_texto.cfm?idtxt=21168.

Carneiro Filho, A (1998). Manaus: fortaleza extrativismo-cidade, uma história da dinâmica urbana. *In*: Espaço e Doença Um Olhar Sobre o Amazonas. Rojas, L.B.I., Toledo, L.M. I.6.1-I.6.5, Fundação Oswaldo Cruz, Rio de Janeiro,.

Castro, E., Echeverría, G., Deibis, L., González de Salmen, B., Dos Santos Moreira, A., Guimarães, M.L., Bastos, F.I. & Morgado, M.G. (2003). Molecular epidemiology of HIV-1 in Venezuela: high prevalence of HIV-1 subtype B and identification of a B/F recombinant infection. *Journal of Acquired Immune Deficiency Syndrome*. Mar 1, 32(3): 338-344, ISSN:1525-4135

Cohen, O.J., Kinter, A. & Fauci, A.S. (1997). Host factors in the pathogenesis of HIV disease. *Immunology Reviews*, 159: 31-48, ISSN:0105-2896.

De Sa Filho, D.J., Sucupira, M.C., Caseiro, M.M., Sabino, E.C., Diaz, R.S. & Janini, L.M. (2006). Identification of two HIV type 1 circulating recombinant forms in Brazil. *AIDS Research and Human Retroviruses*, 22:1-13, ISSN: 0889-2229

Drogari-Apiranthitou, M., Fijen, C.A.P., Thiel, S., Platonov, A., Jensen, L., Dankert, J. & Kuijper, E.J. (1997). The effect of mannan-binding lectin on opsonophagocytosis of *Neisseria meningitides*. *Immunopharmacology*, 38: 93-99, ISSN:0162-3109.

Fundação de Medicina Tropical do Amazonas (2006). Coordenação Estadual do Programa de DST/Aids do Amazonas. Boletim Epidemiológico 1: 1-20.

Garred, P., Richter, C., Andersen, A.B., Madsen, H.O., Mtoni, I., Svejgaard, A. & Shao, J. (1997). Mannan-binding lectin in the sub-Saharan HIV and tuberculosis epidemics. *Scandinavian Journal of Immunology.*, 46: 204–208, ISSN:0300-9475

Hibberd, M.L., Sumiya, M., Summerfield, J.A., Booy, R. & Levin, M. (1999). Association of variants of the gene for mannose-binding lectin with susceptibility to meningococcal disease. *Lancet*, 353: 1049-1053, ISSN:0099-5355

Jüliger, S., Luckner, D., Mordmüller, B., May, J., Weierich, A., Lell, B., Luty, A., Kremsner & Kun, F.J., 2000. Promoter variants of the human mannose-binding lectin gene show different binding. *Biochemical and biophysical research communications*, 275: 617-622, ISSN:0006-291X

Klabunde, J., Berger, J., Jensenius, J.C., Klinkert, M.Q., Zelck, U.E., Kremsner, P.G. & Kun, J.F. (2000). Schistosoma mansoni: adhesion of mannan-binding lectin to surface glycoproteins of cercariae and adult worms. *Experimental Parasitology*, 95: 231–239, ISSN:0014-4894

Kuipers, S., Aerts, P.C. & Van Dijk, H. (2003). Differential microorganism-induced mannose-binding lectin activation. *FEMS Immunology and Medical Microbiology*, 36: 33-39, ISSN:0928-8244

Luty, A.J., Kun, J.F. & Kremsner, P.G. (1998). Mannose-binding lectin plasma levels and gene polymorphisms in *Plasmodium falciparum* malaria. *Journal of Infectious Diseases*, 178: 1221-1224, ISSN:0022-1899

Machado, L.F., Ishak, M.O., Vallinoto, A.C., Lemos, J.A., Azevedo, V.N., Moreira, M.R., Souza, M.I., Fernandes, L.M., Souza, L.L. & Ishak, R (2009). Molecular epidemiology of HIV type 1 in northern Brazil: identification of subtypes C and D and the introduction of CRF02_AG in the Amazon region of Brazil. *AIDS Research and Human Retroviruses*, 25(10): 961-966, ISSN: 0889-2229

Madsen, H.O., Garred, P., Kurtzhals, J.A., Lamm, L.U., Ryder, L.P., Thiel, S. & Svejgaard, A. (1994). A new frequent allele is the missing link in the structural polymorphism of the human mannan-binding protein. *Immunogenetics*, 40: 37–44, ISSN:0093-7711

Madsen, H.O., Garred, P., Thiel, S., Kurtzhals, J.A.L.,Lamm, L.U., Ryder, L.P. & Svejgaard, A. (1995). Interplay between promoter and structural gene variants control basal serum level of Mannan-Binding Protein. *Journal of Immunology*, 155: 3013-3020, ISSN:0022-1767

Marquina, S., Leitner, T., Rabinovich, R.D., Benetucci, J., Libonatti, O. & Albert, J. (1996). Coexistence of subtypes B, F, and as B/F env recombinant of HIV type 1 in Buenos Aires Argentina. *AIDS Research and Human Retroviruses*. Nov 20, 12(17):1651-1654, ISSN: 0889-2229.

McCutchan, F.E. (2006). Global epidemiology of HIV. *Journal of Medical Virology.*, 78(Suppl 1): S7-S12, ISSN:0146-6615

Monteiro, J.P., Alcantara, L.C., de Oliveira, T., Oliveira, A.M., Melo, M.A., Brites, C. & Galvão-Castro, B. (2009). Genetic variability of human immunodeficiency virus-1 in Bahia state, Northeast, Brazil: High diversity of HIV genotypes. *Journal of Medical Virology*, 81(3): 391–399, ISSN:0146-6615

Morgado, M.G., Guimarães, M.L., Gripp, C.B., Costa, C.I., Neves Jr, I., Veloso, V.G., Linhares-Carvalho, M.I., Castello-Branco, L.R., Bastos, F.I., Kuiken, C., Castilho, E.A., Galvão-Castro, B. & Bongertz, V (1998). Molecular epidemiology of HIV-1 in Brazil: high prevalence of HIV-1 subtype B and identification of an HIV-1 subtype D infection in the city of Rio de Janeiro, Brazil. Evandro Chagas Hospital AIDS Clinical Research Group. *Journal of Acquired Immune Deficiency Syndrome*, Aug 15, 18(5): 488-494, ISSN:1525-4135

Navas, M.C., Letourneur, F., Gomas, E., Boshell, J. & Saragosti, S (1999). Analysis of the V3 loop sequences from 12 HIV type 1-infected patients from Colombia, South America. *AIDS Research and Human Retroviruses*, Aug 10, 15(12): 1141-1144, ISSN: 0889-2229

Peterslund, N.A., Koch, C., Jensenius, J.C. & Thiel, S. (2001). Deficiency of mannan-binding lectin (MBL), association with severe infections after chemotherapy. *Lancet*, 358: 637-638, ISSN:0099-5355

Plantier, J.C., Leoz, M., Dickerson, J.E., De Oliveira, F., Cordonnier, F., Lemée, V., Damond, F., Robertson, D.L., Simon, F (2009). A new human immunodeficiency virus derived from gorillas. *Nature Medicine*, Aug, 15(8): 871-872, ISSN:1078-8956

Prohaszka, Z., Thiel, S., Ujhelyi, E., Szlavik, J., Banhegyi, D., Fust, G. (1997). Mannan-binding lectin serum concentrations in HIV-infected patients are influenced by the stage of disease. *Immunology Letters*, 58: 171-175, ISSN:0165-2478

Ramos, A., Tanuri, A., Schechter, M., Rayfield, M.A., Hu, D.J., Cabral, M.C., Bandea, C.I., Baggs, J. & Pieniazek, D (1999). Dual and recombinant infections: an integral part of the HIV-1 epidemic in Brazil. *Emerging Infectious Diseases*, 5(1): 65-74, ISSN:1080-6040

Roy, S., Knox, K., Segal, S., Griffiths, D., Moore, C.E., Welsh, K.I., Smarason, A., Day, N.P., Mcpheat, W.L., Crook, D.W. & Hill, A.V.S. (2002). MBL genotype and risk of invasive pneumococcal disease: a case-control study. *Lancet*, 359: 1569-1573, ISSN:0165-2478.

Sabino, E.C., Diaz, R.S., Brigido, L.F., Learn, G.H., Mullins, J.I., Reingold, A.L., Duarte, A.J., Mayer, A. & Busch, M.P. (1996). Distribution of HIV-1 subtypes seen in an AIDS clinic in Sao Paulo City, Brazil. *AIDS*, 10(13): 1579-84, ISSN:0953-0096

Sanabani, S., Kleine Neto, W., Kalmar, E.M., Diaz, R.S., Janini, L.M. & Sabino, E.C. (2006). Analysis of the near full length genomes of HIV-1 subtypes B, F and BF recombinant from a cohort of 14 patients in Sao Paulo, Brazil. *Infection, Genetics and Evolution*, 6:368-377, ISSN:1567-1348

Sanabani, S.S., Pastena, E.R., Neto, W.K., Martinez, V.P. & Sabino, E.C. (2010). Characterization and frequency of a newly identified HIV-1 BF1 intersubtype circulating recombinant form in São Paulo, Brazil. *Virology Journal*, 16, 7:74, ISSN:1743-422X

Santos, A.F., Sousa, T.M., Soares, E.A., Sanabani, S., Martinez, A.M., Sprinz, E., Silveira, J., Sabino, E.C., Tanuri, A. & Soares, M.A (2006). Characterization of a new circulating recombinant form comprising HIV-1 subtypes C and B in southern Brazil. *AIDS*, 20: 2011-2019, ISSN:0953-0096

Silva, L.C., Santos, E.M., Silva, Neto, A.L., Miranda, A.E., Talhari, S. & Toledo, L.M. (2009). Pattern of HIV/AIDS infection in Manaus, State of Amazonas, between 1986 and 2000. *Revista da Sociedade Brasileria de Medicina Tropical*, Sep-Oct,42(5): 543-50, ISSN:0037-8682

Soares, E.A., Santos, R.P., Pellegrini, J.A., Sprinz, E., Tanuri, A. & Soares, M.A. (2003). Epidemiologic and molecular characterization of human immunodeficiency virus type 1 in southern Brazil. *Journal of Acquired Immune Deficiency Syndrome*, 34: 520–526, ISSN:1525-4135

Song, L.H., Binh, V.Q., Duy, D.N., Jüliger, S., Bock, T.C., Luty, A.J.F., Kremsner, P.G. & Kun, J.F.J. (2003). Mannose-binding lectin gene polymorphisms and hepatitis B virus infection in Vietnamese patients. *Mutation Research*, 522: 119-125, ISSN:0027-5107

Tanuri A, Vicente AC, Otsuki K, Ramos CA, Ferreira OC Jr, Schechter M, Janini LM, Pieniazek D & Rayfield M.A. (1999). Genetic variation and susceptibilities to protease inhibitors among subtype B and F isolates in Brazil. *Antimicrobial Agents Chemotherapy*, 43(2): 253-258, ISSN:0066-4804

Taylor, B.S., Sobieszczyk, M.E., McCutchan, F.E., Hammer, S.M. (2008). The challenge of HIV-1 subtype diversity. *The New England Journal of Medicine*, Apr 10, 358(15): 1590-1602, ISSN:0028-4793

Turner, M.W. (2003). The role of mannose-binding lectin in health and disease. *Molecular Immunology*, 40: 423-429, ISSN:0161-5890

Vallinoto, A.C., Menezes-Costa, M.R., Alves, A.E., Machado, L.F., Azevedo, V.N., Souza, L.L., Ishak, M.O.G. & Ishak, R. (2006). Mannose-binding lectin gene polymorphism and its impact on human immunodeficiency virus 1 infection. *Molecular Immunology*, 43: 1358-1362, ISSN:0161-5890

Vallinoto, A.C.R., Muto, N.A., Alves, A.E.M., Machado, L.F.A., Azevedo, V.N., Souza, L.L.B., Ishak, M.O.G. & Ishak, R. (2008). Characterization of the polymorphisms in the mannose-binding lectin gene promoter among human immunodeficiency virus 1 infected subjects. *Mem Inst Oswaldo Cruz*, 103: 645–649, ISSN:1678-8060

Vicente, A.C., Otsuki, K., Silva, N.B., Castilho, M.C., Barros, F.S., Pieniazek, D., et al. (2000). The HIV epidemic in the Amazon Basin is driven by prototypic and recombinant HIV-1 subtypes B and F. *Journal of Acquired Immune Deficiency Syndrome*, 23: 327–331, ISSN:1525-4135.

12

Cannabinoids – Influence on the Immune System and Their Potential Use in Supplementary Therapy of HIV/AIDS

Alicja Szulakowska and Halina Milnerowicz
Department of Biomedical and Environmental Analyses, Faculty of Pharmacy,
Silesian Piasts University of Medicine in Wroclaw
Poland

1. Introduction

Cannabis sativa (Fig. 1.) has been valued for its medicinal as well as its psychotropic properties dating back to ancient times. In nineteenth century W.B. O'Shaughnessy used marijuana for pain relief and Jean-Jacques Moreau de Tours – French psychiatrist, said, that cannabis is very helpful in therapy of psychiatric disorders (Booth, 2004). Main constituents of *Cannabis sativa* were discovered in 1960's and named after the plant – cannabinoids. The identification of the chemical structure of *cannabis* components and the possibility of obtaining its pure constituents were related to a significant increase in scientific interest in this plant. This interest was renewed in the 1990's with the description of cannabinoid receptors and the identification of an endogenous cannabinoid system in the brain (Zuardi, 2006).

The most notable of the cannabinoids are: tetrahydrocannabinol (THC) – the most psychoactive substance found in the cannabis plant and cannabidiol – constituent which has displayed sedative effects. Both constituents can be found in the brown resin secreted by the hair which covers female plants (Truta et al., 2002). Cannabinoids bind to the cannabinoid receptors (CB receptors), change metabolism of the cells, moderate neurotransmission and hormones extraction, what affect main functions of the human body (Demuth et al., 2006, ElSohly et al., 2005).

The cannabinoid receptor family currently includes two types: CB1, characterized mostly in neuronal cells and brain, and CB2, characterized in immune cells (lymphocytes and macrophages) and tissues (spleen and tonsils) (Demuth et al., 2006). Both receptors are proteins and consist of seven transmembrane–spanning domains (Fig. 2.)(Joy et al., 1999). The CB1 molecule is larger than CB2. However, both receptor molecules are alike in four of the seven regions embedded in the cell membrane (known as the transmembrane regions). The intracellular loops of the two receptor subtypes are quite different, which might affect the cellular response to the ligand (Szulakowska&Milnerowicz, 2007). Human body also produces substances that activate CB receptors, they are known as endocannabinoids. The studies have revealed a broad role of endocannabinoids and cannabinoid receptors in a variety of physiological processes as neuromodulation, pain and appetite sensation, motor learning (Saito et al., 2010).

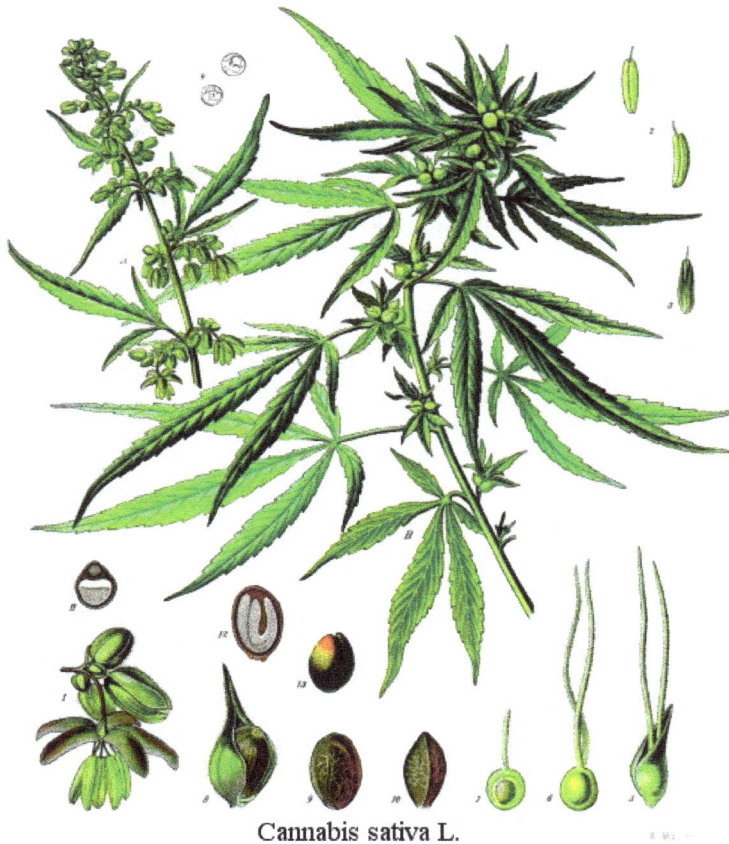

Cannabis sativa L.

Fig. 1. *Cannabis sativa* (Kohler, 1887).

2. Cannabinoids and the immune system

The study of marijuana cannabinoid biology has led to many important discoveries in immunology; not only existence of a new physiological system - the endocannabinoid system, but also its role in the regulation of the immune system. Studies examining the effect of cannabinoids on immunity have shown that many cellular and cytokine mechanisms are suppressed by these agents (Klein&Cabral, 2006).

2.1 Cellular effects

Scientists have already suggested in 1970s that cannabinoids can change the number and function of T cells. Various functions from cytotoxic T cell killing to antibody production by B cells have been examined. Nong and Co. have studied the T-cell rosetting capacity of lymphocytes in CD4 and CD8 subsets – it was impaired in peripheral blood cells from marijuana users. Scientists examined also the effects on the number of lymphocytes in CD4 and CD8 subsets. The percentage of CD4 T cells was increased in peripheral blood cells from marijuana smokers, with a mean CD4/CD8 ratio of 1.95 as opposed to 1.27 in controls (Nong et al., 2002; Massi et al., 2006). Finally, Klein and Co. proved that cannabinoids affect cytotoxic T lymphocytes (CTL) – after incubation with THC, the cytolytic activity of CTL was depressed by about 60% (Klein et al., 1991). It also appeared that cannabinoids can disrupt proliferation and cytolytic activity in natural killer cells (NK), which plays very important role in host defences against tumors and microbes (Massi et al., 2006).

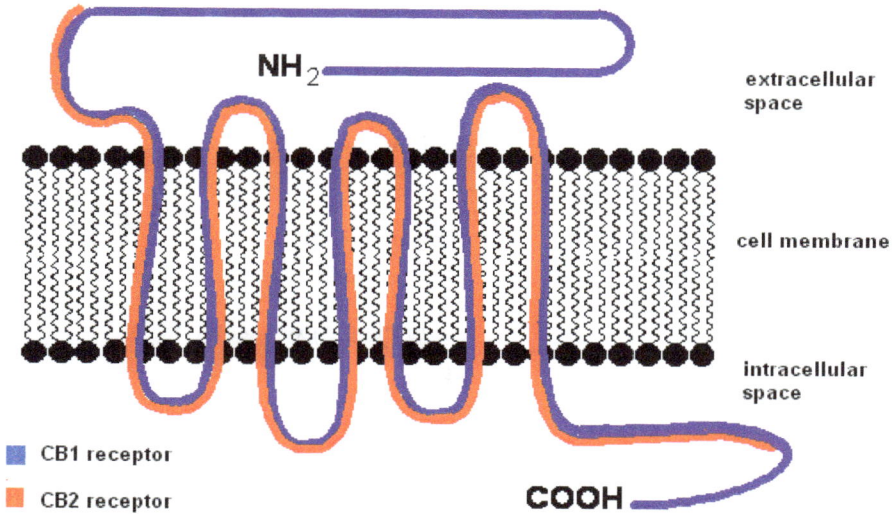

Fig. 2. Cannabinoid receptors CB1 and CB2 (Joy et al., 1999).

Functions of macrophages are also impaired by cannabinoids through either a receptor- or non-receptor-mediated mechanism. Studies with pulmonary alveolar macrophages showed that cannabinoids significantly lowered the level of tumor necrosis factor α (TNFα) in the bronchoalveolar lavage (Klein et al., 1991). Scientists proved that cannabinoids influenced the ability of macrophages to process antigens necessary for the activation of CD4+ T lymphocytes (McCoy et al., 1999), reduced chemotaxis (Sacerdote et al., 2000) and affect the production of arachidonic acid metabolites in macrophage cultures (Berdyshev et al., 2000). The influence of cannabinoids on NO production is still unclear (Massi et al., 2006).

2.2 Cytokines and hormones
Cannabinoids can modulate the action of cytokines mostly by affecting immune cells, for example macrophages or Th cells, their immunomodulatory properties are complex, what was shown in the Table 1.
Scientists proved that cannabinoids can modulate immune response also by affecting hormones release. For example administration of THC, may increase level of adrenocorticotropic hormone and corticosterone, what is causing downstream release of immunoregulatory molecules as cortizol and sex hormones and inhibition of immune response (Massi et al., 2006; Tanasescu&Constantinescu, 2010; Baker et al., 2007).

Name of the cytokine	Cannabinoid infulence	General result	References
IFNγ	Decreased level	Anti-inflammatory action	(Zheng et al., 1992, 1996)
TNFα	Decreased level	Anti-inflammatory action	(Zheng et al., 1992, 1996)
Il-1	Decreased level	Anti-inflammatory action	(Kozela et al., 2010)
Il-2	Decreased level	Anti-inflammatory action	(Zhu et al., 1993)
Il-4	Increased level	Action unclear	(Klein et al., 2000)
Il-6	Decreased level	Anti-inflammatory action	(Kozela et al., 2010)
Il-10	Decreased level	Action unclear	(Sacerdote et al., 2005)
Il-12	Decreased level (THC)/increased level (CBD)	Anti-inflammatory action (THC)/ Anti-inflammatory action	Massi et al., 2006; Klein et al., 2000; Sacerdote et al., 2005)

Table 1. Cannabinoid influence on cytokines profile

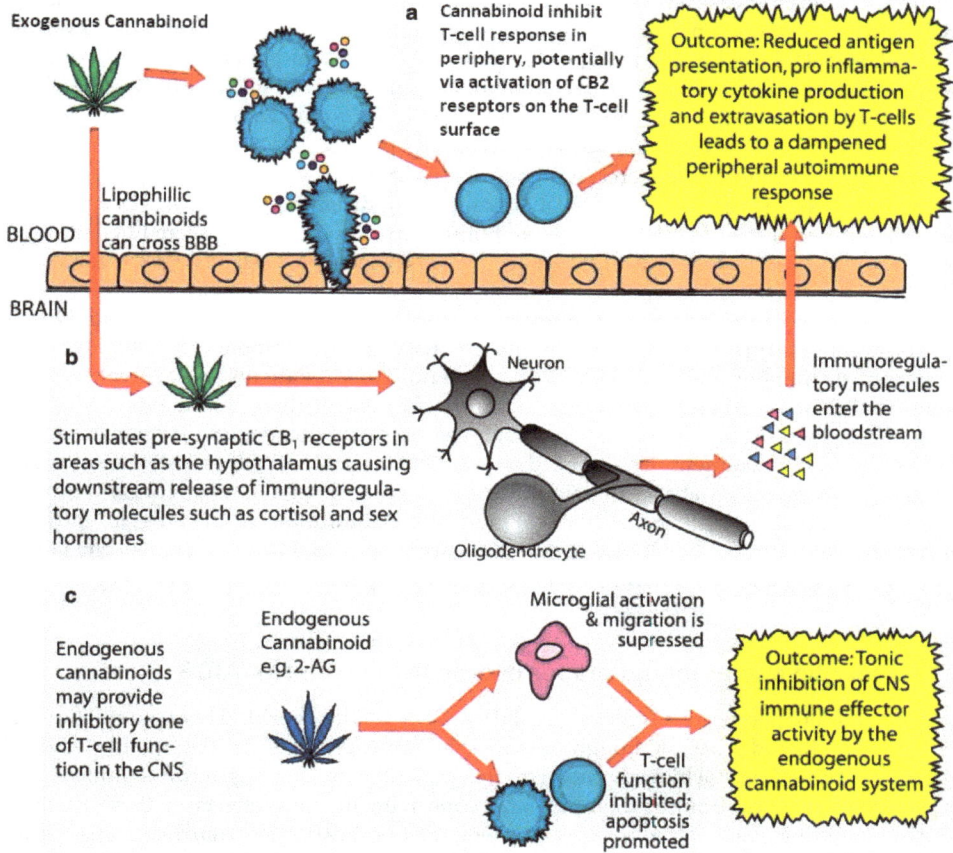

Exogenous Cannabinoid

a Cannabinoid inhibit T-cell response in periphery, potentially via activation of CB2 reseptors on the T-cell surface

Outcome: Reduced antigen presentation, pro inflammatory cytokine production and extravasation by T-cells leads to a dampened peripheral autoimmune response

Lipophillic cannbinoids can cross BBB

BLOOD

BRAIN

b Stimulates pre-synaptic CB₁ receptors in areas such as the hypothalamus causing downstream release of immunoregulatory molecules such as cortisol and sex hormones

Neuron

Oligodendrocyte

Axon

Immunoregulatory molecules enter the bloodstream

c Endogenous cannabinoids may provide inhibitory tone of T-cell function in the CNS

Endogenous Cannabinoid e.g. 2-AG

Microglial activation & migration is supressed

T-cell function inhibited; apoptosis promoted

Outcome: Tonic inhibition of CNS immune effector activity by the endogenous cannabinoid system

Fig. 3. Immune regulation by cannabinoids. Exogenously administered cannabinoids (a, b) or endocannabinoids (c) may inhibit the action of the immune response in either the periphery (a, b) or the central nervous system (CNS; c) via either a direct (a, c) or indirect (b) action on leukocytes (from Baker et al., 2007).

Cannabinoids can modulate immune reactions in the periphery but also in the brain, influence T cell subset balance and cytokine expression. Generally, they alter many functions of the immune response, what was shown in the Fig. 3. (Baker et al., 2007).

3. Immunological consequences of cannabinoids use by HIV/AIDS patients

Anti-inflammatory potential action of cannabinoids tends to be evident from the studies discussed in the previous paragraph. Cannabinoids do induce apoptosis in immune cells and alleviate inflammatory responses (Rieder et al., 2010). Even though the progressive failure of the immune system is a cause of AIDS disease, no conclusive data have been obtained as to potential risk associated with HIV infection and the use of cannabinoids. In 2003 Abrams and co. examined short-term effects of cannabinoids in patients with HIV-1 infection. Scientists measured HIV RNA level and CD4+ and CD8+ cell subsets, during 21 days of oral and smoked marijuana administration among 67 patients with HIV-1 infection. At days 0 and 21, HIV RNA was undetectable in 50% to 55% of patients in each group, the mean changes were decreases in both cannabinoid groups: marijuana group and dronabinol group. The unadjusted mean increases in CD4+ cell counts were greater for patients receiving cannabinoids than for patients receiving placebo. CD8+ cell counts were on average 20% greater for patients receiving marijuana than for patients receiving placebo and marginally greater (average 10%) for patients receiving dronabinol than for those receiving placebo. Authors concluded that smoked and oral cannabinoids did not seem to be unsafe in patients with HIV infection with respect to HIV RNA levels, CD4+ and CD8+ cell counts (Abrams et al., 2003).

Kosel and co. decided to examine effects of cannabinoids on the pharmacokinetics of indinavir and nelfinavir – protease inhibitors used as a component of highly active antiretroviral therapy to treat HIV infection and AIDS. Patients on stable regimens containing indinavir or nelfinavir were randomized to one of three treatments: 3.95% THC marijuana cigarettes, dronabinol 2.5 mg capsules or placebo capsules administered three times daily. The treatment lasted 14 days. Authors concluded that their results after marijuana treatment (statistically significant decrease in maximum concentration of nelfinavir - C(max)) by -17.4% (P=0.46) and the magnitude of changes in indinavir concentration - C(max) by -14.1% (P=0.039)), are likely to have no short-term clinical consequence. The use of cannabinoids is unlikely to impact antiretroviral efficacy (Kosel et al., 2002).

4. Therapeutic use of marijuana for people living with HIV/AIDS

Over 40 million people are affected by HIV/AIDS in the world. There is still no cure available for this disease, although remarkable improvements in the quality and life expectancy have been achieved. Most of the patients are on long-term treatment with combinations of antiretroviral therapies and cope with the side effects of these therapies (nausea, vomiting, pain, reduced appetite, weight loss, headaches, diarrhea, constipation, anxiety and depression) (Woolridge et al., 2005). Recently, therapeutic use of marijuana has emerged as an important issue for people living with HIV/AIDS. Fogarty et al. reported that people with HIV/AIDS who use marijuana indicate improved moods, sensory experiences, creativity, increased socialising, elation and changes in appetite (Fogarty et al., 2007; Woolridge et al., 2005). In 2005 Woolridge et al. surveyed 143 HIV positive people who reported using marijuana to manage side effects of long-term anti-retroviral treatment. Results were shown in the table below (Table 2.) (Woolridge et al., 2005).

The ability of cannabinoid to treat pain, nausea, appetite loss, muscle spasm and a wide variety of other symptoms causes that more and more HIV/AIDS patients reach for marijuana as an alternative remedy. The actual numbers of HIV/AIDS patients that use marijuana to treat HIV related symptoms is a difficult number to quantify, but some researchers report that this number is quite significant (Cannon, 2010).

In 1998/1999, in Canada approximately 15% of 977 responders were using marijuana for medical purposes (Braitstein et al., 2001). In California in 2001 – 33.3% of the 442 responders reported the use of marijuana (Cannon, 2010). Regarding this data, in 2007 scientists examined people living with HIV/AIDS in Australia. The results show that among 408 participants, 59.8% reported some use of marijuana in the past six months. 244 (55.7% of those) reported recreational use only of marijuana and 44.3% admitted mixed use of marijuana for therapeutic and recreational purposes (Fogarty et al., 2007). In 2007/2008 in South Africa only 3.7% of 618 admitted that was using marijuana in the past six month, mostly for stress relief (85.7%) and to a lesser extent for recreational purposes (relaxation) (23.5%) and pain relief (17.6%) (Peltzer et al., 2008). These results from different places in the world show that substantial proportion of people living with HIV/AIDS use marijuana for therapeutic purposes, despite considerable legal barriers, suggesting that cannabis represents another option in their health management (Fogarty et al., 2007). The small percentage of South Africans with HIV/AIDS using marijuana for therapeutic purposes may be caused by poverty (marijuana is more expensive than other alternative, supplementary methods like micronutrients, religious healing) and limited access to information about alternative therapy (Peltzer et al., 2008).

Symptom	Number of complaints	Much better [%]	Little better [%]	No change [%]	Little worse [%]	Much worse [%]
Lack of appetite	111	79	18	2	0	1
Pain in muscle	65	63	31	6	0	0
Nausea	62	56	37	3	2	2
Anxiety	98	64	49	3	2	2
Nerve pain	53	51	40	9	0	0
Depression	94	56	30	9	4	1
Tingling	46	37	48	9	7	0
Numbness	42	36	36	24	5	0
Weight loss	62	45	24	31	0	0
Headaches	46	35	30	33	2	0
Tremor	24	37	29	21	13	0
Constipation	24	21	29	46	4	0
Tiredness	60	17	33	33	15	2
Diarrhea	48	13	23	56	6	2
Vision dimness	22	9	27	55	9	0
Weakness	48	10	21	54	15	0
Memory loss	38	13	5	34	34	13
Slurred speech	9	11	0	78	11	0

Table 2. Effect of marijuana on Complaint of Symptoms in 143 HIV Patients (from Woolridge et al., 2005).

4.1 Pain management

Neuropathic pain and muscular pain is reported by people living with HIV/AIDS. Patients describe pain as "aching", "burning" and "painful numbness" of legs and hands mostly (Cannon, 2010). Despite management with opioids and other pain modifying therapies, neuropathic pain continues to reduce the quality of life among 30% or more of HIV-infected individuals. Scientists suppose that pain perception is modulated by cannabinoid receptors in the central and peripheral nervous system (Ellis et al., 2009) via endocannabinoids, an endogenous system of retrograde neuromodulatory messengers that work in tandem with endogenous opioids (McCarberg, 2007).

Cannabinoids have been shown to inhibit the experience of pain in both – animal and human studies. It was demonstrated in 2007 in a study conducted by Abrams et al. He decided to determine the effect of smoked cannabis on the neuropathic pain of HIV-associated sensory neuropathy and an experimental pain model. Scientists asked fifty patients to smoke either cannabis or identical placebo cigarettes with the cannabinoids extracted three times daily for 5 days. Reduction in pain intensity was measured. It occurred that smoked cannabis reduced daily pain by 34% with placebo. Greater than 30% reduction of pain was reported by 52% in the cannabis group and by 24% in the placebo group. The first cannabis cigarette reduced chronic pain by a median of 72% vs 15% with placebo (Abrams et al., 2007). Similar trial was conducted by American scientists in 2009. Ellis et al. examined 127 HIV-associated distal sensory predominant polyneuropathy and measured change in pain intensity by the Descriptor Differential Scale (DDS) from a pretreatment baseline to the end of each treatment week. Treatments were placebo and delta-9-tetrahydrocannabinol, smoked four times daily for 5 consecutive days during each of 2 treatment weeks, separated by a 2-week washout. Among all the patients, pain relief was greater with cannabis than placebo and the proportions of subjects achieving at least 30% pain relief with cannabis vs placebo were 0.46 and 0.18. Results were shown in Fig. 4. (Ellis et al., 2009). This study's findings are equivalent to those achieved by Abrams et al. in 2007 and consistent with other recent research supporting the short-term efficacy of cannabis for neuropathic pain (Ellis et al., 2009; Abrams et al., 2007).

Results of other studies show that cannabis can treat not only the neuropathic pain but also muscular and chronic pain. Woolridge study demonstrated that 94% of participants reported positive results for muscular pain management using marijuana (Cannon, 2010; Woolridge et al., 2005). Finally, as it was mentioned in the previous paragraph, 30% reduction in chronic pain was reported by 52% of the smoked cannabis group (Cannon, 2010; Abrams et al., 2007).

Scientists suppose that analgetic properties of cannabinoids are effect of additional receptor and non-receptor mechanisms of their activity. Synergy between opioids and cannabinoids may produce opioid-sparing effects, as well as extend the duration of analgesia and reduce opioid tolerance and dependence, what is very important in long-term palliative treatment (McCarberg, 2007; Karst&Wippermann, 2009).

4.2 Management of wasting syndrome

Wasting is big problem for people living with HIV/AIDS and is linked to disease progression and death. It is defined as the involuntary loss of more than 10% of normal body weight in addition to at least 30 days of diarrhea, fever and generalized weakness. It is caused by several factors:

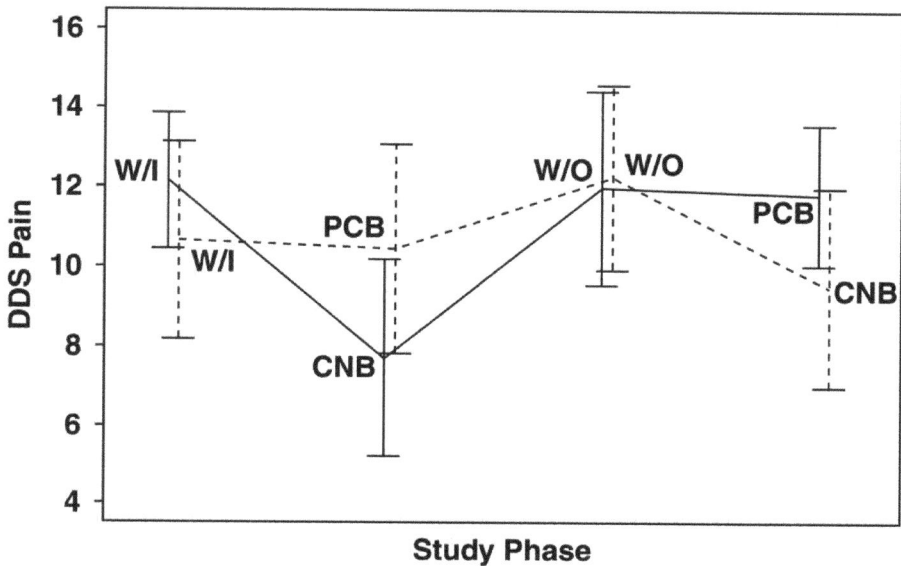

Fig. 4. DDS pain severity scores for participants in the cannabis (CNB) and placebo (PCB) arms before study treatment (W/I), during each of the 2 treatment weeks (1, 2) and during the Washout (W/O) between treatment weeks (from Ellis et al., 2009).

- Low food intake – low appetite is common among HIV/AIDS patients and is mostly caused by anti-retroviral drugs (their side effects such as nausea, changes in the sense of taste, or tingling around the mouth also decrease appetite). Moreover, opportunistic infections in the mouth, throat or stomach may also reduce food intake.
- Poor nutrient absorption – opportunistic infections of the gastrointestinal tract can interfere with the absorption of nutrients. Moreover, HIV may directly affect the intestinal lining and reduce nutrient absorption; diarrhea may affect nutrient absorption indirectly – it flushes the system of needed nutrients and calories.
- Altered metabolism – HIV/AIDS affects food processing and protein building. It is probably caused by the increased activity of the immune system. People need more calories just to maintain their body weight (Cannon, 2010; The Body, 2011).

5. Antiemetic action

Scientists suppose that emesis (the side effect of anti-retroviral therapy) is caused by the stimulation of receptors in the central nervous system or the gastrointestinal tract. This stimulation appears to be caused by the drug used in treatment itself or a metabolite of the drug. The high concentration of cannabinoid receptors in the nucleus of the solitary tract, suggest that exogenous cannabinoids bind to receptors and prevent them from binding with drugs and metabolites (Szulakowska&Milnerowicz, 2007). Recent findings suggest that the mechanism of anti-emetic action of cannabinoids is more complex – CB1 agonist suppresses vomiting, which is reversed by CB1 antagonism, and CB1 inverse agonism promotes vomiting. Parker et al. proved that cannabinoid agonists –THC suppress nausea. It occurred that cannabidiol (CBD) can also be used in the supplementary therapy of HIV/AIDS. The antiemetic effects of CBD may be mediated by indirect activation of somatodendritic 5-HT (1A) receptors in the dorsal raphe nucleus; activation of these autoreceptors reduces the release of 5-HT in terminal forebrain regions and inhibit nausea and emesis (Parker et al., 2010).

In 2001 Tramer et al. decided to search systematically for randomised controlled comparisons of the antiemetic efficacy of cannabinoids with any antiemetic or placebo (control) in chemotherapy, radiotherapy, surgery or HIV/AIDS. Scientist analyzed data from 30 randomised controlled trials published between 1975 and 1997 (1366 patients). Across all the trials, cannabinoids were more effective than active comparators and placebo. Results were shown in the Table 3. (Tramer et al., 2001).

	Cannabinoids % (number of patients)	Control % (number of patients)
Control of nausea and vomiting		
Complete control of nausea *vs* placebo	70 (81/116)	57 (66/115)
Complete control of vomiting *vs* placebo	66 (76/116)	36 (41/115)
Complete control of nausea *vs* active comparator	59 (122/207)	43 (93/215)
Complete control of vomiting *vs* active comparator	57 (111/194)	45 (90/201)
Patients' rating		
Cannabinoids *vs* placebo	76 (153/202)	13 (27/202)
Cannabinoids *vs* active comparator	61 (371/604)	26 (156/608)

Table 3. Control of nausea and vomiting and patients' preference for treatment in trials of cannabinoids against active antiemetic or control treatment (Tramer et al., 2001).

6. Appetite stimulation

Cannabinoids can also stimulate appetite and food intake. This property is connected with the presence of functional cannabinoid type 1 receptors in the digestive system, especially the liver. Hepatocytes express CB1 receptors, the activation of which increase the expression of lipogenic genes and *de novo* fatty acid synthesis, which contributes to the development of diet-induced obesity. Cannabinoids can also stimulate AMP-activated protein kinase in the hypothalamus, whereas they inhibit it in the liver and adipose tissues (Osei-Hyiaman, 2007). Moreover, scientists proved that CBs can activate fatty acid synthase (FAS), whereas the inhibition of FAS is a result of profound anorexia. These finding thus suggest that the same molecular pathway is involved in both central appetitive and the peripheral anabolic effects of cannabinoids (Szulakowska&Milnerowicz, 2007; Osei-Hyiaman et al., 2005).

In 2007 Haney et al. decided to check tolerability and efficacy of smoked marijuana and oral dronabinol in HIV-positive marijuana smokers. This placebo-controlled within-subjects study evaluated marijuana and dronabinol across a range of eating topography and mood. Scientists administered 4 times daily for 4 days each dronabinol and marijuana, but only one drug was active per day. Administration of drugs was separated by four days of placebo washout. Results were shown in the Fig. 5. In comparison to placebo, marijuana and dronabinol increased daily caloric intake and body weight. It is probably caused by the increased number of eating occasions – marijuana and dronabinol increased the number of eating occasions but didn't alter the number of calories intake. Moreover, marijuana and dronabinol produced significant shifts in the distribution of macronutrient administration by enhancing the proportion of calories derived from fat. The final effect of increased caloric intake and macronutrients administration was weight gain – 1.2 kg after 4 days of dronabinol and 1.1 kg after 4 days of marijuana (Haney et al., 2007).

6.1 Mood control

Scientists consider that prevalence of psychiatric disorders (mostly depression) is really high among the people living with HIV/AIDS. In 2001 in the USA nearly half of the population screened positive for a psychiatric disorder (36% major depression, 26.5% dysthymia, 15.8% generalized anxiety disorder, 10.5% panic attack)(Bing et al., 2001). Psychiatric disorders may be triggered by side effects of medications or the effects of HIV on the brain. Research show that depression can limit the energy needed to keep focused on staying health and may accelerate HIV's progression to AIDS (The Body, 2002).

Clinical data suggests that cannabinoids can strongly modulate mood of the people living with HIV/AIDS. Marijuana and dronabinol can help to overcome psychiatric disorders like anxiety, depression and sleeping disorders. In 2004 Prentiss et al. reported that 60.3% of 133 people living with HIV/AIDS and coping with psychological disorders recently used marijuana to alleviate the symptoms. Only few of them (9.1%) reported smoking marijuana/using dronabinol ineffective (Prentiss et al., 2004). Moreover, Haney et al. showed also that cannabinoids from marijuana or dronabinol can improve mood without producing disruptions in psychomotor functioning and add benefit of improving rating of sleep (Haney et al., 2007). In general, people living with HIV/AIDS reported that using marijuana cause reduction in stress, relief from anxiety and improve sleep (Cannon, 2010; Fogarty et al., 2007).

Scientists suppose that anti-depressive properties of THC and CBD are probably effect of involvement of these cannabinoids in the modulation of serotonergic signaling by their capacity to increase the availability of circulating tryptophan (precursor necessary for the biosynthesis of the 5-HT). The compensation of tryptophan degradation might be an important mechanism, by which THC and CBD may improve mood disturbances – mainly cause by alteration of serotonergic activity) (Jenny et al., 2010).

7. Medical marijuana use – Legal issues

Scientists from all over the world have explored the use of medical marijuana. Many of them have clearly reported that cannabinoids have therapeutic benefits (Cannon, 2010). According to this information, many countries, including Canada, Australia, The Netherlands and Switzerland, have legalized marijuana for medical purposes. The process of legislation of medical marijuana began in the United States in 2005. Today medical marijuana is legal at least in thirteen states (Active State Medical Marijuana Programs, 2011). Table 4. shows a summary of the main features of medical marijuana programs in different countries (Cannon, 2010).

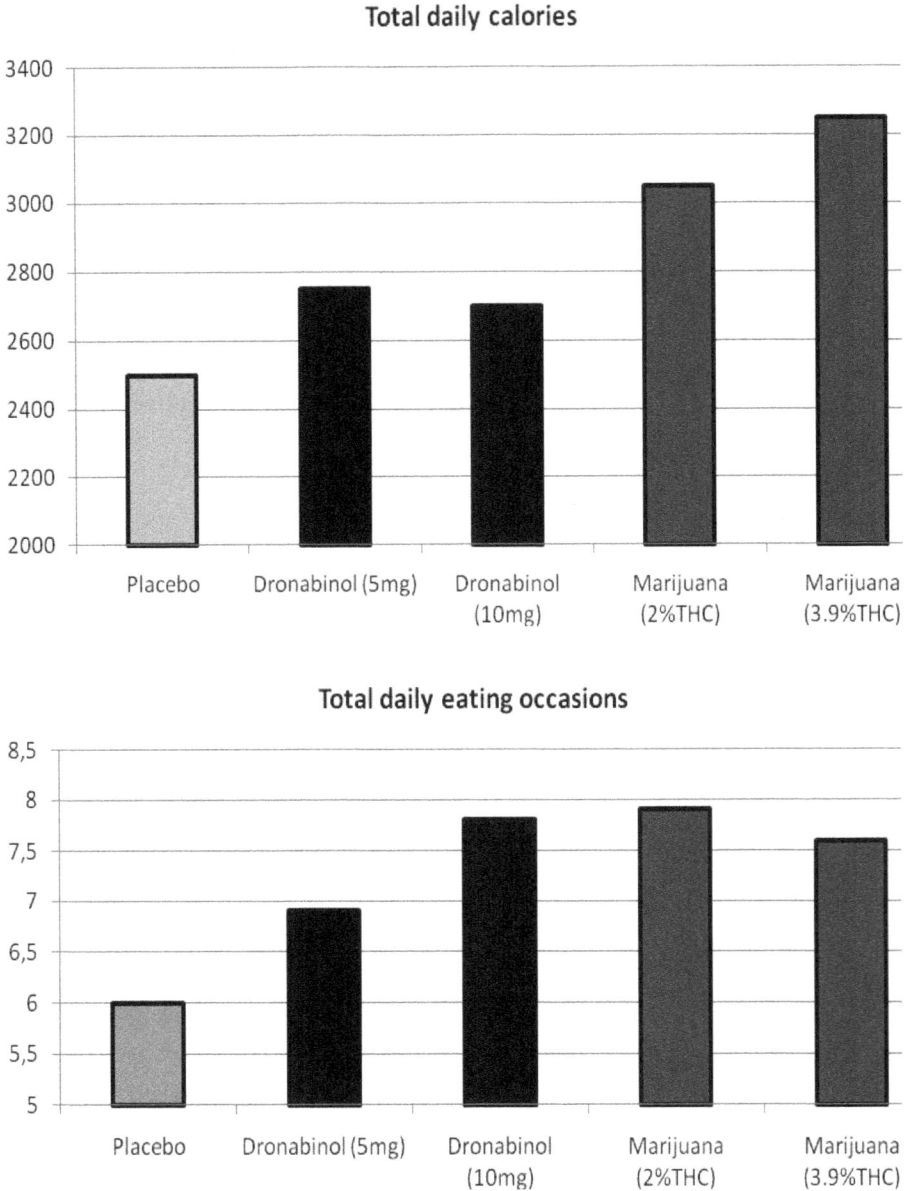

Fig. 5. Mean total daily caloric intake and total number of eating occasions as a function of marijuana (MJ) and dronabinol (Dronab) dose (Haney et al., 2007).

Country	Legal issues	Eligible health conditions	Access
United States of America	Legal for medical purposes in 13 states	HIV/AIDS Cancer Arthritis Anorexia Chronic pain Spasticity Glaucoma Migraine	Patients must receive a prescription from a physician
Canada	Legal for medical purposes	HIV/AIDS Cancer Multiple Sclerosis Spinal cord injury/disease Severe arthritis Epilepsy Part of a palliative care treatment program	Patients must become licensed by the Medical Marijuana Resource Centre to access marijuana
The Netherlands	Illegal – exception for personal use	HIV/AIDS Cancer Multiple Sclerosis Tourette's Syndrome Chronic pain Spasticity	Patients must voluntarily apply through the Department of Public Health to join the program and be issued with an identification car

Table 4. A summary of the main features of the medical marijuana programs in different countries (Cannon, 2010).

8. Conclusion

There is constant debate whether cannabis should be considered therapeutic for HIV/AIDS patients. According to the literature, management of HIV-associated symptoms is one of the most common applications ascribed to medical marijuana (Prentiss et al., 2004). More and more studies have characterized the extent of cannabis use for medical benefit to address HIV-related symptoms like nausea (Parker et al., 2010), lack of appetite (Tramer et al., 2001), emesis (Parker et al., 2010), pain (McCarberg, 2007), depression (Bing et al., 2001), anxiety Haney et al., 2007) and weight loss (Fogarty et al., 2007). However, it has to be mentioned, that use of cannabinoids can have side effects. Several scientists have warned about the negative effects of marijuana use on the cardiovascular, respiratory and nervous system (Cannon, 2010; Corless et al., 2009), and psychological dysfunction including loss of memory (Seamon et al., 2007) and pointed out the necessity for further investigation of the effects of cannabinoids. Moreover, recent legislative efforts to support legalization of medical marijuana suggest the need for more precise understanding of the typical patterns and determinants of marijuana use, and better characterization of the epidemiology of cannabis use for relief of symptoms commonly associated with HIV/AIDS (Cannon, 2010; Abrams et al., 2007).

9. References

Abrams, D.I.; Hilton, J.F.; Leiser, R.J.; et al. (2003). Short-Term Effects of Cannabinoids in Patients with HIV-1 Infection. A Randomized, Placebo-Controlled Clinical Trial, *Ann Intern Med*, 139, 258-266.

Abrams, D.I.; Jay, C.A.; Shade, S.B.;Vizoso, H.; Reda, H.; Press, S.; Kelly, M.E.; Rowbotham, M.C.; Petersen, K.L. (2007). Cannabis in painful HIV-associated sensory neuropathy. A randomized placebo-controlled trial, *Neurology*, 68, 7, 515-521.

Active State Medical Marijuana Programs, *NORML*, http://www.norml.org/index.cfm?Group_ID=3391#Maryland (downloaded April 20, 2011).

Baker, D.; Jackson, S.J.; Pryce, G. (2007). Cannabinoid control of neuroinflammation related to multiple sclerosis, *British Journal of Pharmacology*, 152, 649–654.

Berdyshev, E.V. (2000). Cannabinoid receptors and the regulation of im-mune response. *Chem Phys Lip*, 108, 169-190.

Bing, E.G.; Burnam, M.A.; Longshore D. et al. (2001). The estimated prevalence of psychiatric disorders, drug use and drug dependence among people with HIV disease in the United States: results from the HIV Cost and Services Utilization Study. *Archives of General Psychiatry*, 58, 721-728.

The Body: The Complete HIV/AIDS Resource, (2002). Depression and HIV: Fact Sheet 2-5005, *The Body: The Complete HIV/AIDS Resource*, viewed 10 March 2011, http://www.thebody.com/content/art6295.html#sup1

The Body: The Complete HIV/AIDS Resource, (2007). Wasting Syndrome: Fact Sheet 519, *The Body: The Complete HIV/AIDS Resource*, viewed 10 March 2011, http://www.thebody.com/content/art6127.html

Both, M. (2004). *Cannabis: A history*, Thomas Dunne Books

Braitstein, P.; Kendall, T.; Chan, K.; Wood, E.; Montaner, J.S.; O'Shaughnessy, M.V.; Hogg, R.S. (2001). Mary-Jane and her patients: sociodemographic and clinical characteristics of HIV-positive individuals using medical marijuana and antiretroviral agents, *AIDS*, 15, 4, 532-533.

Cannon, R. (2010). The medicinal use of marijuana for people living with HIV/AIDS in South Australia, *AIDS Council of South Australia information paper No. 2*, ISBN 978-0-9808084-3-8.

Corless, I.; Lindgren, T.; Holzemer, W.; Robinson, L.; Moezzi, S.; Kirksey, K.; Coleman, C.; Tsai, Y.F.; Sanzerro, L.; Hamilton, M.J.; Sefcik, E.F.; Canaval, G.E.; Rivero Mendez, M.; Kemppainen, J.K.; Bunch, E.H.; Nicholas, P.; Nokes, K.M.; Dole, P.; Reynolds, N. (2009). Marijuana Effectiveness as an HIV Self-Care Strategy, *Clinical Nursing Research*, 18, 2, 172-193.

Demuth, D.G.; Molleman, A. (2006). Cannabinoid signaling, *Life Sci*, 78, 549–563.

Ellis,R.J.; Toperoff,W.; Vaida,F.; van den Brande,G.; Gonzales,J.; Gouaux,B.; Bentley,H.; Atkinson, J.H. (2009). Smoked Medicinal Cannabis for Neuropathic Pain in HIV: A Randomized, Crossover Clinical Trial, *Neuropsychopharmacology*, 2009, 34, 3, 672-680.

ElSohly, M.A.; Slade, D. (2005). Chemical constituents of marijuana: The complex mixture of natural cannabinoids, *Life Sci*, 78, 539-548.

Fogarty, A.; Rawstorne, P.; Prestage, G.; Crawford, J.; Grierson J.; Kippax, S. (2007). Marijuana as therapy for people living with HIV/AIDS: social and health aspects, *AIDS Care*, 19, 2, 295-301.

Haney, M.; Gunderson, E.W.; Rabkin, J.; Hart, C.L.; Vosburg, S.K.; Comer, S.D.; Foltin, R.W. (2007). Dronabinol and Marijuana in HIV-positiive Marijuana Smokers. Caloric intakie, Mood, and Sleep, *J Acquir Immune Defic Syndr*, 45, 5, 545-554.

Jenny, M.; Schrocksnadel, S.; Uberall, F.; Fuchs, D. (2010). The Potential Role of Cannabinoids in Modulating Serotonergic Signaling by Their Influence on Tryptophan Metabolism, *Pharmaceuticals*, 3, 2647-2660.

Joy, J.E.; Watson S.J.Jr.; Benson J.A.Jr. (1999). *Marijuana and Medicine:Assessing the Science Base*, National Academy Press, Washington D. C., 1999

Karst, M.; Wippermann, S. (2009). Cannabinoids against pain. Efficacy and strategies to reduce psychoactivity: a clinical perspective, *Expert Opin Investig Drugs*, 18, 2, 125-133.

Klein, T.W; Kawakami, Y; Newton, C; Friedman, H. (1991). Marijuana com-ponents suppress induction and cytolytic function of murine cyto-toxic T cells in vitro and in vivo, *J Toxicol Environ Health* , 32, 465-477.

Klein, T.W; Newton A; Nakachi, N; Friedman, H. (2000). Delta 9-tetrahydrocannabinol treatment suppresses immunity and early IFN-gamma, IL-12, and IL-12 receptor beta 2 responses to Legionella pneumophila infection, *J Immunol*, 164, 12, 6461-6.

Klein, T.W.; Cabral, C.A. (2006). Cannabinoid-induced immune suppression and modulation of antigen-presenting cells, *J Neuroimmune Pharmacol*, 1,1, 50-64.

Kohler, F.E. (1887). Medizinal Pflantzen. http://upload.wikimedia.org/wikipedia/commons/1/19/Koeh-026.jpg (downloaded March 11, 2011)

Kosel, B.W.; Aweeka, F.T.; Benowitz, N.L.; Shade, S.B.; Hilton, J.F.; Lizak, P.S.; Abrams, D.I. (2002). The effects of cannabinoids on the pharmacokinetics of indinavir and nelfinavir, *AIDS*, 16, 4, 543-50.

Kozela, E; Pietr, M; Juknat, A; Rimmerman, N; Levy, R; Vogel, Z. (2010) Cannabinoids Δ9-Tetrahydrocannabinol and Cannabidiol Differentially Inhibit the Lipopolysaccharide-activated NF-κB and Interferon-β/STAT Proinflammatory Pathways in BV-2 Microglial Cells, *J Biol Chem*, 285, 3, 1616–1626.

Massi, P; Vaccani, A; Parolaro, D. (2006). Cannabinoids, immune system and cytokine network, *Curr Pharm Des*, 12, 24, 3135-46.

McCarberg, B.H. (2007). Cannabinoids: their role in pain and palliation, *J Pain Palliat Care Pharmacother*, 21, 3, 19-28.

McCoy, K.L; Matveyeva, M; Carlisle, S.J; Cabral, G.A. (1999). Cannabinoidinhibition of the processing of intact lysozyme by macrophages:evidence for CB2 receptor participation, *J Pharmacol Exp Ther*, 289, 1620-1625.

Nong, L; Newton, C; Cheng, Q; Friedman, H; Roth, M.D; Klein, T.W. (2002). Altered cannabinoid receptor mRNA expression in peripheralblood mononuclear cells from marijuana smokers, *J Neuroimmunol*, 127, 169-176.

Osei–Hyiaman, D.; DePetrillo, M.; Pacher, P.; Liu, J.; Radaeva, S.; Bátkai, S.; Harvey–White, J.; Mackie, K.; Offertáler, L.; Wang, L.; Kunos, G. (2005). Endocannabinoid activation at hepatic CB1 receptors stimulates fatty acid synthesis and contributes to diet–induced obesity, *J Clin Invest*, 115, 5, 1298–1305.

Osei–Hyiaman, D. (2007). Endocannabinoid system in cancer cachexia. Nutrition in wasting disease, *Curr Opin Clin Nutr Metab Care*, 10, 4, 443–448.

Parker, L.A.; Rock, E.; Limebeer, C. (2010). Regulation of nausea and vomiting by cannabinoids, *Br J Pharmacol*, "Accepted article", doi: 10.1111/j.1476-5381.2010.01176.x

Peltzer, K.; Friend-du Preez, N.; Ramlagan,S.; Fomundam, H. (2008). Use of traditional complementary and alternative medicine for HIV patients in KwaZulu-Natal, South Africa, *BMC Public Health*, 8, 255.

Prentiss, D.; Power, R.; Balmas, G.; Tzuang, G.; Israelski, D.M. (2004). Patterns of marijuana use among patients with HIV/AIDS followed in the public health care setting, *J Acquir Immune Defic Syndr*, 35, 1, 38-45.

Rieder, S.A.; Chauhan, S.; Singh, U.; Nagarkatti, M.; Nagarkatti, P. (2010). Cannabinoid-induced apoptosis in immune cells as a pathway to immunosuppression, *Immunobiology*, 215, 8, 598–605.

Sacerdote, P; Massi, P; Panerai, A.E; Parolaro, D. (2000). In vivo and in vitro treatment with the synthetic cannabinoid CP-55,940 decreases the in vitro migration of macrophages in the rat: involvement of bothCB1 and CB2 receptors, *J Neuroimmunol*, 109, 155-163.

Sacerdote, P; Martucci, C; Vaccani, A; Bariselli, F; Panerai, A.E; Colombo, A; Parolaro, D; Massi, P. (2005). The nonpsychoactive component of marijuana cannabidiol modulates chemotaxis and IL-10 and IL-12 production of murine macrophages both in vivo and in vitro., *J Neuroimmunol*, 159, 1-2, 97-105.

Saito, V.M.; Wotjak, C.T.; Moreira, F.A. (2010). Pharmacological exploitation of the endocannabinoid system: new perspectives for the treatment of depression and anxiety disorders?, *Rev. Bras. Psiquiatr*, 32, 1, 7-14.

Seamon, M.; Fass, J.; Maniscalco-Feichtl, M.; Abu-Shraie, N.A. (2007). Medical Marijuana and the developing role of the pharmacist, *American Journal of Health-System Pharmacy*, 64, 1037-1044.

Szulakowska, A.; Milnerowicz H. (2007). Cannabis sativa in the light of scientific research, *Adv Clin Exp Med*, 16, 6, 807-815.

Tanasescu, R; Constantinescu, C.S. (2010). Cannabinoids and the immune system: an overview, *Immunobiology*, 215, 8, 588-97.

Tramèr, M.R.; Carroll, D.; Campbell, F.A.; Reynolds, D.J.M.; Moore, R.A.; McQuay, H.J. (2001). Cannabinoids for control of chemotherapy induced nausea and vomiting: quantitative systematic review, *BMJ*, 323, 7303, 16.

Truta, E.; Gille, E.; Toth, E.; Maniu, M. (2002). Biochemical differences in Cannabis sativa L. depending on sexual phenotype, *J Appl Genet*, 43, 4, 451–462.

Woolridge, E.; Barton, S.; Samuel, J.; Osorio, J.; Dougherty, A.; Holdcroft, A.; (2005). Cannabis use in HIV for pain and other symptoms,*Journal of Pain and Symptom Management*, 29, 4, 358-367.

Zheng, Z.M; Specter, S; Friedman, H. (1992). Inhibition by delta-9-tetra-hydrocannabinol of tumor necrosis factor alpha production bymouse and human macrophages, *Int J Immunopharmacol*, 14, 1445-1452.

Zheng, Z.M;Specter, S.C. (1996). Δ9-Tetrahydrocannabinol suppresses tumornecrosis factor alpha maturation and secretion but not its transcrip-tion in mouse macrophages, *Int J Immunopharmacol*, 18, 53-68.

Zhu, W; Igarashi, T; Qi, Z.T; Newton, C; Widen, R.E; Friedman, H.(1993) Delta-9-tetrahydrocannabinol (THC) decreases the number of high and intermediate affinity IL-2 receptors of the IL-2 dependentcell line NKB61A2, *Int J Immunopharm*, 15, 401-408.

Zuardi, A. (2006). History of cannabis as a medicine: a review, *Rev Bras Psiquiatr*, 28,2, 153-157.

13

HAART and Causes of Death in Perinatally HIV-1-Infected Children

Claudia Palladino[1], Jose María Bellón[2], Francisco J. Climent[3],
María del Palacio Tamarit[1], Isabel de José[4] and
Mª Ángeles Muñoz-Fernández[1]
[1]Laboratorio de Inmuno-Biología Molecular, Hospital General Universitario
"Gregorio Marañón"
[2]Unidad de Investigación, Fundación de Investigación Biomédica Hospital
"Gregorio Marañón"
[3]Servicio Infecciosas, Hospital "Ramón y Cajal"
[4]Servicio Infecciosas Infantil, Hospital Universitario "La Paz", Madrid,
Spain

1. Introduction

Children represent a population at higher risk of Human Immunodeficiency Virus type 1 (HIV-1) infection and AIDS-related death. Approximately 2.5 million (1.6–3.4) children are infected at present, accounting for 370,000 [230,000–510,000] new infections and 260,000 [150,000–360,000] deaths (Gray et al., 2001). About 90% of children living with HIV-1 are in sub-Saharan Africa. The paediatric HIV-1 epidemic is fuelled by HIV-1 infection in women of childbearing age. In fact, mother-to-child (perinatal) HIV-1 transmission during pregnancy, birth or breastfeeding accounts for the vast majority of HIV-1 cases in children. An estimated 2.4 million infected women give birth annually. This results in the birth of approximately 1,000 HIV-1–infected babies per day, of which 80% occur in resource-limited countries where there are no effective programs for prevention of mother-to-child transmission (MTCT) of HIV-1 . Almost two decades ago, the introduction of antiretroviral chemoprophylaxis to prevent MTCT of HIV-1 was an important milestone in paediatric HIV-1. The use of antiretroviral drugs and elective caesarean section have reduced the incidence of MTCT in industrialised countries to <2% since 1997 (The European Collaborative Study [ECS], 2005; Connor et al., 1994). However, such interventions to prevent MTCT of HIV-1 are still not widely accessible or available in most resource-limited countries where the rate of transmission is estimated at 12–40% (De Cock et al., 2000). Concerning the diagnosis and treatment of HIV-1, significant improvements have been made over the last few years, yet much more needs to be done. The first evidence of the efficacy of antiretroviral therapy (ART) in HIV-1–infected children was published 20 years ago (Pizzo et al., 1988). Since then, the introduction of highly active antiretroviral therapy (HAART) into medical care for HIV-1–infected children and adolescents has increased life expectancy and resulted in AIDS incidence decline in both industrialised countries and resource-limited settings (Judd et al., 2007; Patel et al., 2008; Puthanakit et al., 2007; Reddi et al., 2007). Some studies have also described the immunovirological impact of HAART (Fraaij et al., 2005; Scherpbier et al., 2006; Walker et al., 2004). Nevertheless, in developing countries early diagnosis is a major challenge and ART is often started late. The clinical impact of early treatment has been recognised (Faye et al., 2004; Violari et al., 2007); in fact, in the absence of treatment, 50% of infants die before their second birthday (Newell et al., 2004). Moreover, lack of resources restricts drug supply. Despite the number of children receiving ART increased from about 75,000 in 2005 to 360,000 in 2009, these represent en estimated ART coverage of 28% [21-43%] of all children less than 15 years who need ART in resource-limited settings (WHO, 2010). On the contrary, in industrialised countries antiretroviral drugs are widely available. In addition, new therapeutic options have been developed for the paediatric population in recent years, such as the protease inhibitor darunavir approved for children aged ≥ 6 years and adolescents (Blanche et al., 2009), or are under evaluation in ongoing clinical trials, including the second generation non-nucleoside reverse transcriptase inhibitor etravirine (ClinicalTrials.gov 2008b, 2009a), the new protease inhibitor tipranavir (Salazar et al., 2008), and the new families of antiretrovirals, such as the CCR5 antagonists and integrase inhibitors (ClinicalTrials.gov 2007, 2008a, 2009b).

2. Impact of antiretroviral therapy

Given that HIV-1 infection has turned into a chronic condition and that exposure to antiretrovirals is likely to be life-long, continuous assessment of the impact of HAART on progression of perinatal HIV-1 infection remains an important public health issue to improve health care strategies. Here, we report the evaluation of HAART effectiveness on the incidence of AIDS and death, and the trends in the underlying causes of death at population level over almost three decades in Madrid (Spain). In Western Europe, Spain continues to be one of the countries with the highest AIDS incidence rate and prevalence. Within Spain, the *Comunidad Autónoma de Madrid* is the area most affected by the infection, with a total of 18,866 AIDS cases up to 2010 (24% of the national cases) (Centro Nacional de Epidemiología [CNE], 2010). The high HIV-1 prevalence had a direct impact on the spread of the infection within the infant population and although the risk of perinatal transmission of HIV-1 has decreased below 2% in recent years, paediatric HIV-1 cases are still being diagnosed (Palladino et al., 2008). In the *Comunidad Autónoma de Madrid*, a total of 237 cumulative AIDS cases due to vertical transmission were reported to the National AIDS Registry from 1981 to 2010 (CNE, 2010). The introduction of HAART in late 1996 and its universal and free availability (Ministerio de sanidad y Consumo, 1998) offered the opportunity to control HIV-1 disease progression in the paediatric population (2005; Resino et al., 2006b). The aim of this study was to describe the mortality and AIDS rates and changes in underlying causes of death in HIV-1–infected paediatric patients. Moreover, risk factors associated with shorter first-line HAART duration among antiretroviral-naïve patients who began HAART after 1996 were examined.

2.1 Study population and methods

The HIV Paediatric Cohort of the *Comunidad Autónoma de Madrid* was established in 1995 as an open cohort of paediatric patients infected by HIV-1 through MTCT, for whom it was assumed that HIV-1 transmission occurred on the date of birth (de Martino et al., 2000). The cohort has included all HIV-1–infected patients identified in a multicenter network of nine referral paediatric hospitals from January 1982 (birth date of the first MTCT–infected child in Madrid). Children infected before 1995 were enrolled retrospectively, while those infected after 1995 were enrolled prospectively. Complete ascertainment of all records was carefully sought. Informed consent was obtained from mothers of all patients. The Institutional Ethics Committee approved the study. HIV-1 testing during pregnancy was offered to all women until 1998, when routine testing was introduced for all pregnant women. Patients were actively followed up every 3–6 months (Centers for Disease Control and Prevention [CDC] 1998). At the beginning of the study, the diagnosis of HIV-1 infection was based on the results of a serologic test for HIV-1 antibody, which was performed routinely for children born to seropositive women. When the result of the serologic test was positive, the infection was confirmed by paediatricians and/or through hospital summaries. Later, the diagnosis was done by positive results of HIV-1 PCR DNA and peripheral blood mononuclear cells viral culture assays on two separate samples (Resino et al., 2006a). The clinical classification and definition of AIDS-related events were based on international guidelines (CDC 1994). Children in the A or B clinical category who became older than 13 years were not categorised as having AIDS by CD4+ cell count criteria when they had <200 cells/ml (CDC 1992).

Deaths were reported by paediatricians. The underlying cause of death (the disease/injury which initiated the morbid event leading to death) was confirmed by reviewing medical histories or autopsy certificates and interviewing paediatricians. Patients were cross-checked with the National Death Index to validate their causes of death classified as: "AIDS-defining" when attributable to a disease in the C clinical category (CDC 1992, 1994); "HIV-related" when attributable to a category A or B disease (CDC 1992, 1994) or to ARV adverse events; "non-HIV-related": all other causes. To report the underlying cause of death, when multiple concurrent causes contributed to death, patients were included as many times as the number of illnesses diagnosed. The study period comprised a pre-HAART era (1982-1996) and a post-HAART era (1997-2009), and was divided into six calendar periods (CP) on the basis of the changing HIV-1 therapy management. CP1 (1982-1989): it was chose as the reference period, when ART was not routinely available; CP2 (1990–1993): the standard of care was zidovudine monotherapy; CP3 (1994–1996): children were receiving dual-nucleoside regimen; CP4 (1997–1998): when HAART, a combination of three or more drugs, was introduced; CP5 (1999–2004): early-HAART period; CP6 (2005–2009): late-HAART period. Information on socio-demographic characteristics, mother's transmission category, clinical and immunovirological data and the antiretroviral therapy were recorded. Any change in two or more antiretroviral drugs that lasted ≥14 days, excluding dosage changes, in the presence of detectable HIV-1 RNA, was considered to indicate the start of a new regimen.

2.1.1 Statistical analysis

AIDS and mortality rates were calculated as the number of new AIDS and death cases per hundred person-years (p-y) of follow-up. Individuals were followed from the date of enrolment (i.e., date of HIV-1 diagnosis or first blood test) until the date of development of the event of interest (AIDS or death) or December 31, 2009 (administrative censoring date), whichever occurred first. The risk of progression to AIDS and death over time was estimated by survival analyses using Kaplan-Meier curves and Cox proportional hazards models. Time was calculated from the birth date so that comparisons across different calendar periods were based on individuals who were infected for the same length of time. All models were stratified by hospital and adjusted for potential confounders (gender, mother's transmission category and immunological category). Fisher exact test, χ^2 or Mann-Whitney U test were used to derive P-values. Poisson regression was used to compare mortality and infection rates between our cohort and the age-similar general population living in the *Comunidad Autónoma de Madrid*. The median duration of initial HAART regimen was determined by Kaplan-Meier analysis. Univariate proportional hazards regressions were used to identify factors associated with a shorter initial regimen. The variables examined included demographics, socio-economic characteristics, baseline laboratory values (CD4+ cell count, HIV-1 RNA, haemoglobin), clinical status and adherence to initial HAART regimen. Then, multivariate regression analysis was performed including all factors for which the results of univariate analysis were statistically significant ($P<0.05$, 2-sided). Analyses were performed with SPSS 16 and Epidat 3.1.

3. Results

Overall, 484 children who acquired HIV-1 from their mothers between 1982 and 2009 were enrolled and followed for 5298.2 person-years (11.6 years; interquartile range (IQR): 5.2-16.7). HIV-1 infection occurred mainly in 1992 [IQR: 1988-1995]; 270 (56%) patients were girls and 299 (62%) had a mother who acquired the virus through injection drug use. Table 1 provides the characteristics of the children at the end of each calendar period (CP). The cohort had the highest number of enrolled children between 1994 and 1996; in the last period (2005-2009) there were 279 children included, of whom 13 were born in this period. The sex ratio remained stable over time (CP1: 1.0; CP6: 1.4), while the median age (CP1: 2.6 [1.0-4.4]; CP6: 14.8 [11.6-17.5]; $P<0.001$) and the proportion of immigrants (CP1: 3.1; CP6: 15.5; $P<0.0001$) increased. An increase of the median CD4+ cell percentage at the end of each calendar period was observed (CP2: 22.5 [11.9-32.1]; CP4: 26.5 [18.2-33.7]; CP6: 33.4 [28.0-39.7]) and a concomitant decrease of HIV-1 RNA since 1997 (median $\log_{10}$ copies/ml CP4: 4.31 [3.80-4.91]; CP6: 2.60 [1.70-3.55]). The proportion of children with <400 copies/ml was 9% (13/151) in CP3, 20% (39/196) in CP4, 60% (150/248) in CP5, and 80% (160/199) in CP6. Two adolescents died in CP2 achieving undetectable HIV-1 RNA at death. The CD8+ cell percentage remained stable (CP2: 42.0 [29.0-52.0]; CP4: 43.7 [35.6-52.5]; CP6: 38.9 [31.7-45.7]). The changes over time in antiretroviral therapy management are described in Fig. 1. Monotherapy was used in the early 1990s and dual-nucleoside therapy in mid-1990s. An increasing proportion of children receiving HAART from 1997 onward was observed; by 2005, up to 80% of the children were on HAART.

3.1 Time to AIDS or death

Information on 471 children, of whom 285 (61%) developed an AIDS-defining disease, was available for the progression to AIDS analyses. The AIDS incidence rate increased over time until 1989 (32.6 per 100 p-y), it arose again during the first half of the 1990s (13.2 in 1991; 18.8 in 1995) and waned off thereafter (3.2 in 1999; 0.0 in 2009) (Fig. 2). The cumulative incidence curves showed a reduction in the proportion of patients developing AIDS after 1997 compared to the period 1982-1989 (Fig. 3A). Multivariate Cox analysis showed a more pronounced decline in the last period (CP6) (AHR: 0.07; 95%CI: 0.04-0.16) than in the CP5 (AHR: 0.23; 95%CI: 0.15-0.37) (Table 2). A total of 159/484 (33%) deaths occurred. The death incidence rate was 7.4 per 100 p-y at risk in 1986, it peaked in 1995 (10.1 per 100 p-y) and declined thereafter (0.7 in 1999; 0.0 in 2009) (Fig. 2). The incidence of death decreased since 1997 compared to the period 1982-1989 (Fig. 3B, Table 2). Multivariate analysis showed more marked improvements in survival in the CP6 (AHR: 0.16; 95%CI: 0.05-0.50) than in the CP5 (AHR: 0.25; 95%CI: 0.11-0.56).

Characteristics	Period					
	CP1 (80-89)	CP2 (90-93)	CP3 (94-96)	CP4 (97-98)	CP5 (99-04)	CP6 (05-09)
N. of HIV-1–infected patients	168	280	317	282	315	279
Age, years (median, IQR)	2.6 (1.0 – 4.4)	4.0 (1.8 – 6.6)	5.0 (2.6 – 8.0)	6.7 (3.8 – 9.6)	11.1 (7.8 – 14.0)	14.8 (11.6–17.5)
Date of birth, n. of patients						
1980-1989	168	144	115	85	79	47
1990-1993	–	136	115	93	90	85
1994-1996	–	–	87	73	68	63
1997-1998	–	–	–	31	29	27
1999-2004	–	–	–	–	49	44
2005-2009	–	–	–	–	–	13
Sex ratio, n. of girls	1.00	1.19	1.23	1.27	1.32	1.41
Geographic origin, n. (%)						
Spain	156 (92.9)	264 (94.3)	298 (94.0)	256 (90.8)	271 (86.0)	235 (84.0)
Central America	0 (0)	3 (1.1)	4 (1.3)	8 (2.8)	10 (3.2)	9 (3.2)
South America	3 (1.8)	4 (1.4)	6 (1.9)	6 (2.1)	8 (2.5)	8 (2.9)
North Africa	0 (0)	0 (0)	1 (0.3)	1 (0.4)	1 (0.3)	2 (0.7)
Sub-Sahara Africa	0 (0)	3 (1.1)	5 (1.6)	8 (2.8)	19 (6.0)	20 (7.2)
Other	2 (1.2)	2 (0.7)	2 (0.6)	3 (1.1)	5 (1.6)	4 (1.4)
Unknown/Unavailable	7 (4.2)	4 (1.4)	1 (0.3)	–	1 (0.3)	1 (0.4)
Maternal transmission, n. (%)						
Injecting drug use	119 (70.8)	189 (67.5)	196 (61.8)	168 (59.6)	185 (58.7)	154 (55.2)
Heterosexual	29 (17.3)	56 (20.0)	69 (21.8)	69 (24.5)	78 (24.8)	74 (26.5)
IDU / Heterosexual	13 (7.7)	23 (8.2)	29 (9.1)	24 (8.5)	23 (7.3)	19 (6.8)
Transfusion	3 (1.8)	3 (1.1)	7 (2.2)	6 (2.1)	6 (1.9)	6 (2.2)
Unknown/Unavailable	4 (2.4)	9 (3.2)	16 (5.0)	15 (5.3)	23 (7.3)	26 (9.3)
Clinical category C, n. (%)	69 (41.3)	106 (38.3)	137 (44.1)	102 (37.4)	124 (40.8)	102 (37.5)
Death, n. (%)	21 (12.5)	49 (17.5)	63 (19.9)	12 (4.3)	10 (3.2)	4 (1.4)

Table 1. Demographic and clinical characteristics of the HIV-1–infected patients enrolled in the HIV Paediatric Cohort of the *Comunidad Autónoma de Madrid* at the end of each calendar period (CP). IQR: interquartile range; clinical classification was based on the 1994 revised CDC guidelines. IDU: injecting drug use.

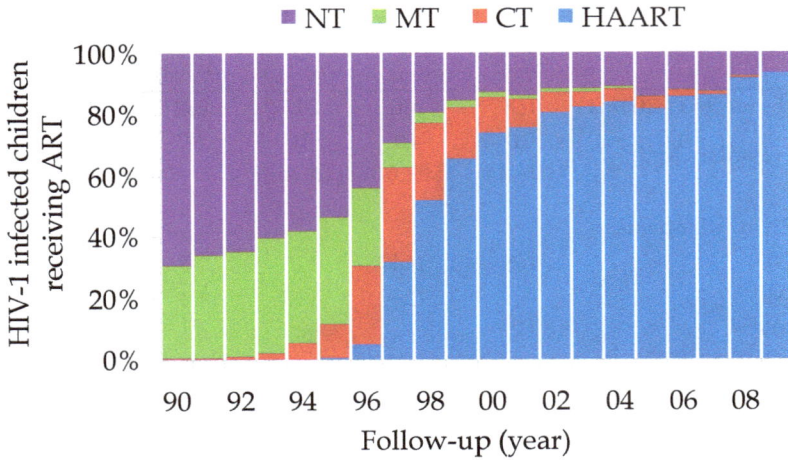

Fig. 1. Use of antiretroviral therapy among HIV-1 vertically infected children enrolled in the HIV Paediatric Cohort of the *Comunidad Autónoma de Madrid*. NT: not treated; MT: monotherapy; combined/dual-nucleoside therapy; HAART: highly active antiretroviral therapy.

	AIDS		
Calendar period	N.	N. of cases	Adjusted HR (95% CI)
1982 – 1989	167	69	1.00
1990 – 1993	232	61	0.49 (0.33 - 0.69)
1994 – 1996	255	81	0.64 (0.44 - 0.91)
1997 – 1998	199	28	0.39 (0.25 - 0.63)
1999 – 2004	216	37	0.23 (0.15 - 0.37)
2005 – 2009	178	9	0.07 (0.04 - 0.16)
	Death		
Calendar period	N.	N. of cases	Adjusted HR (95% CI)
1982 – 1989	168	21	1.00
1990 – 1993	280	49	1.33 (0.77 - 2.28)
1994 – 1996	317	63	1.71 (1.00 - 2.94)
1997 – 1998	282	12	0.54 (0.25 - 1.14)
1999 – 2004	315	10	0.25 (0.11 - 0.56)
2005 – 2009	279	4	0.16 (0.05 - 0.50)

Table 2. Effect of calendar period on the risk of AIDS and death. Note: Adjusted hazard ratios were derived from a standard Cox proportional hazard model that included calendar period (external time-dependent covariate), gender, mother's transmission category, immunological category and it is stratified by hospital.

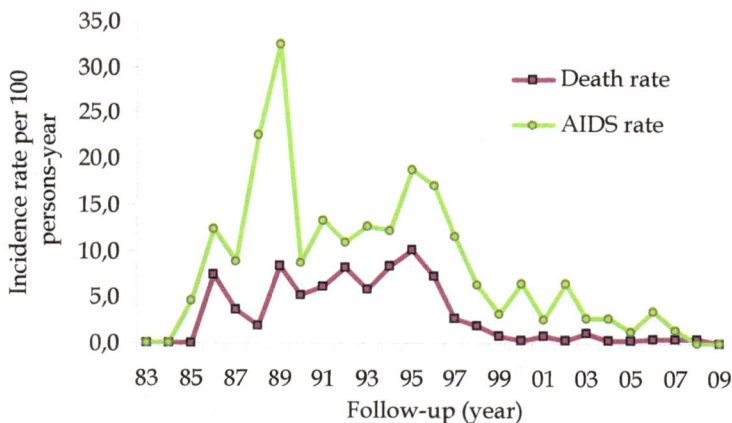

Years	AIDS			Death		
	p-y	N.	Rate	p-y	N.	Rate
1982	2	0	0,0	2	0	0,0
1983	10	0	0,0	10	0	0,0
1984	24	0	0,0	24	0	0,0
1985	44	2	4,6	45	0	0,0
1986	65	8	12,4	68	5	7,4
1987	79	7	8,9	84	3	3,6
1988	89	20	22,6	105	2	1,9
1989	98	32	32,6	133	11	8,3
1990	103	9	8,7	154	8	5,2
1991	121	16	13,2	177	11	6,2
1992	147	16	10,9	206	17	8,3
1993	158	20	12,7	221	13	5,9
1994	173	21	12,2	239	20	8,4
1995	170	32	18,8	248	25	10,1
1996	164	28	17,1	248	18	7,3
1997	156	18	11,5	256	7	2,7
1998	158	10	6,3	263	5	1,9
1999	155	5	3,2	269	2	0,7
2000	155	10	6,5	275	1	0,4
2001	155	4	2,6	278	2	0,7
2002	155	10	6,5	283	1	0,4
2003	152	4	2,6	276	3	1,1
2004	151	4	2,6	271	1	0,4
2005	150	2	1,3	263	1	0,4
2006	142	5	3,5	244	1	0,4
2007	136	2	1,5	233	1	0,4
2008	132	0	0,0	217	1	0,5
2009	128	0	0,0	209	0	0,0

Fig. 2. Annual AIDS and mortality incidence rates per 100 person-years (p-y) in the HIV Paediatric Cohort of the *Comunidad Autónoma de Madrid*.

In the population aged 0-19 years of the *Comunidad Autónoma de Madrid*, the mortality decreased from 4.2 deaths per 10,000 inhabitants in 1996 to 3.5 in 2007. In spite of the mortality decline in our cohort, it still was 10.4-fold (95%CI: 5.8-18.8; $P<0.001$) higher than in age-similar general population after 1999. Since 1999, the HIV-1–infected infants had a higher mortality rate than children/adolescents (IRR: 6.9; 95%CI: 2.3-20.3; $P<0.001$), as in the general population (IRR: 18.9; 95%CI: 17.9-19.9; $P<0.001$). A lower decrease of mortality among HIV-1–infected infants (IRR: 2.6; 95%CI: 0.9-7.4; $P=0.069$) between pre-HAART and post-HAART era than among older patients (IRR: 12.5; 95%CI: 7.6-20.4; $P<0.001$) was observed. On the contrary, mortality decreased equally in infants (IRR: 1.8; 95%CI: 1.8-1.9; $P<0.001$) and children/adolescents (IRR: 1.5; 95%CI: 1.5-1.6; $P<0.001$) in the general population.

3.2 Causes of death

Overall, 169 causes of death were documented for 151/159 (95%) patients (Table3). The 81% (137/169) were AIDS-defining, 12% (20/169) HIV-related and 7% (12/169) non-HIV-related. Multiple causes of death were reported in 16/151 (11%) patients, 3.2 (0.6–6.3) years old at death, of which 7 were infants: 13/129 (10%) died in pre-HAART era and 3/22 (14%) in post-HAART era. Concomitant pathologies were diagnosed in 101/151 (67%) patients (Table 4). The majority (83%) of the subjects died in the post-HAART era had a low/medium socio-economic status. From 1999 to 2007, the risk of death from infections was 115.9 times (95% CI: 42.0–265.8; $P<0.001$) higher in our cohort than in the *Comunidad Autónoma de Madrid*. It was not possible to evaluate the risk of death from other causes than infections due to the low number of events.

AIDS-defining causes were 82% (118/144) in pre-HAART and 76% (19/25) in post-HAART era. The most frequent contributing events were opportunistic infections (58%, 79/137) (Table 4), wasting syndrome (19%, 26/137) and lymphoid interstitial pneumonia (12%, 16/137). The largest components of opportunistic infections were bacterial (20%, 28/137), fungal (mainly *Pneumocystis jiroveci*; 15%, 20/137), and mycobacterial infections (mainly *Mycobacterium tuberculosis*; 10%, 14/137). These three etiologic pathogens were associated with the only cases of death occurred in 2005-2007. No statistically significant changes over time were observed in the proportions of the causes of death. HIV-related causes were 11% (16/144) in pre-HAART and 16% (4/25) in post-HAART era. Overall, the leading causes of death were infections (75%, 15/20), mainly bacterial (65%, 13/20), and bleeding (15%, 3/20). The causes of death reported in post-HAART era were: bacterial infection, pulmonary bleeding caused by thrombocytopenia, pulmonary arterial hypertension and lactic acidosis (1 case each). Non-HIV-related causes were 7% (10/144) in pre-HAART and 8% (2/25) in post-HAART era. Infections were the main cause of death (75%, 9/12), mainly viral infections (67%, 8/12), followed by cancer (17%, 2/12) and hepatic pathology (8%, 1/12). The only causes of death reported in post-HAART era were cancer and hepatic failure (1 case each).

3.3 Duration of HAART regimen

Of 484 patients included in the HIV Paediatric Cohort of the *Comunidad Autónoma de Madrid*, 105 (22%) were naïve to antiretrovirals when HAART began as of January 1997. It was possible to analyse the duration of the first HAART regimen in 82 of them. Half of the patients were girls (42; 51%) and had a median age at HAART initiation of 3.6 years (0.6-7.3).

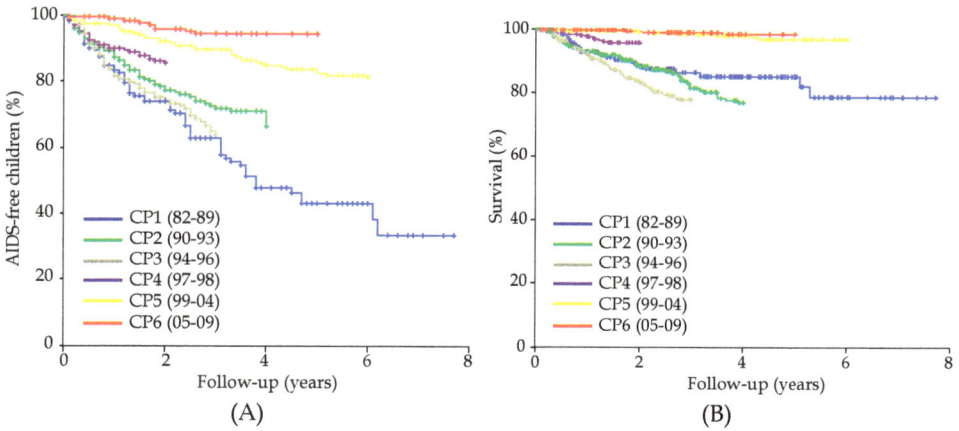

Fig. 3. Kaplan-Meier curves for HIV-1–infected children enrolled in the HIV Paediatric Cohort of the *Comunidad Autónoma de Madrid* without AIDS (A) and for survival (B) in different calendar periods.

Cause of death	Pre-HAART (1982-1996) N=144 (85.2%)	Post-HAART (1997-2009) N=25 (14.8%)
Cancer	6 (4.2)	3 (12.0)
NHL	5 (3.5)	2 (8.0)
HL	1 (0.7)	--
Others	--	1 (4.0)
Infections	90 (62.5)	13 (52.0)
Bacterial infections	34 (23.6)	7 (28.0)
Pneumonia	20 (13.9)	3 (12.0)
Sepsis	14 (9.7)	3 (12.0)
Meningitis	--	1 (4.0)
Fungal infections	17 (11.8)	3 (12.0)
Pneumonia	13 (9.0)	3 (12.0)
Esophageal	4 (2.8)	--
Mycobacterial infections	13 (9.0)	3 (12.0)
Nontuberculous	8 (5.6)	2 (8.0)
Tuberculosis	5 (3.5)	1 (4.0)
Viral infections	15 (10.4)	--
Pneumonia	5 (3.5)	
Sepsis	6 (4.2)	
AGE	3 (2.1)	
PML	1 (0.7)	
Parasitic infections	11 (7.6)	--
Cryptosporidiasis	9 (6.3)	
Toxoplasmosis	1 (0.7)	
Leishmaniasis	1 (0.7)	
Other causes	48 (33.3)	9 (36.0)
Wasting	22 (15.3)	4 (16.0)
Pulmonary	15 (10.4)	2 (8.0)
Encephalopathy	9 (6.3)	--
Hepatic	--	1 (4.0)
Bleeding	2 (1.4)	1 (4.0)
Lactic acidosis	--	1 (4.0)

Table 3. All causes of death for HIV-1–infected children enrolled in the HIV Paediatric Cohort of the *Comunidad Autónoma de Madrid* stratified by pre-HAART era and post-HAART era. Pulmonary cause of death includes lymphoid interstitial pneumonia cases and 1 case of pulmonary hypertension. AGE: acute gastroenteritis; HL: Hodgkin's lymphoma; NHL: non-Hodgkin's lymphoma; PML: progressive multifocal leukoencephalopathy (JC virus). Percentage may not total 100 because of rounding.

	Pre-HAART (1982-1996)	Post-HAART (1997-2009)
Opportunistic infection	N=67/129 (51.9%)	N=12/22 (54.5%)
Recurrent bacterial infection	22 (32.8)	6 (50.0)
Pneumocystis jiroveci	13 (19.4)	3 (25.0)
Cryptosporidiosis	9 (13.4)	0
Nontuberculous mycobacteria	6 (9.0)	2 (16.7)
Mycobacterium tuberculosis	5 (7.5)	1 (8.3)
Candidasis	4 (6.0)	0
Cytomegalovirus	6 (9.0)	0
Toxoplasmosis	1 (1.5)	0
JC virus	1 (1.5)	0
Comorbidity*	N= 87/129 (64.9%)	N=14/22 (60.9%)
Wasting	52 (38.8)	11 (47.8)
Encephalopathy	50 (37.3)	7 (30.4)
Hepatic	17 (12.7)	2 (8.7)
Miocardiophaty	20 (14.9)	2 (8.7)
Hematologic alterations	15 (11.2)	3 (13.0)
Candidiasis	10 (7.5)	--
Hypertension	3 (2.2)	--
Nephropathology	3 (2.2)	--
Giardiasis	1 (0.7)	--
HSV	1 (0.7)	--

Table 4. Prevalence of opportunistic infections and comorbidity in the deceased patients of the HIV Paediatric Cohort of the *Comunidad Autónoma de Madrid*, stratified by pre-HAART and post-HAART era. HSV: Herpes simplex virus. *Note: Patients can be counted more than once.

The majority originated from Spain (58; 71%) and 19 (23%) were adopted or lived in institutions. The socio-economic status was medium-high for 28 (56%) out of 50 patients and low for 22 (44%). At baseline, the median CD4+ cell count was 707 (19%) cells/ml (212-1,443) and HIV-1 RNA was 100,000 (5.0 $\log_{10}$) copies/ml. The median duration of the first HAART regimen was 40.5 months (20.9-80.2). Fifty (61%) subjects were still on the same regimen at the end of the follow-up (Fig. 4, circle chart), being the median HAART duration in this group of 64.5 months (28.6-95.1). The rest of the study group (32/82; 39%) switched to a second regimen after 25.9 months (12.4-39.2) of first regimen. The median first-line HAART duration was significantly different between the two groups ($P<0.0001$). Among the 32 patients who experienced first-line HAART discontinuation, up to 6 switches to successive regimens were observed and had a median duration of 25.9 months (20.7-29.2) (Fig. 4, bar chart). The cumulative incidence curves for time to initial HAART regimen discontinuation showed a longer median HAART duration for the 65/82 (79%) children who started the therapy after 6 months of age compared with the 17 (21%) infants who started at or before 6 months (*P*=0.033) (Fig 5A). In addition, this analysis showed a longer median HAART duration for the 31 (60%) out of 52 subjects with good/perfect adherence compared with the 21 (40%) subjects with poor/intermediate adherence (*P*<0.0001) (Fig. 5B). Initial HAART regimen discontinuation remained associated to younger ages (AHR: 4.56; 95%CI: 1.76–11.86; *P*=0.002) and poor adherence (AHR: 5.02; 95%CI: 2.02–12.47; *P*=0.001) in the multivariate analysis performed for 52 patients (Table 5). The most frequently prescribed first-line regimen was based on protease inhibitors, while one-quarter of the patients received therapy based on non-nucleoside reverse-transcriptase inhibitors (Fig. 6). Two nucleosides backbone therapy remains the cornerstone for all patients but one who had 3 nucleosides. For patients who discontinued the first-regimen, there was a difference, approaching statistical significance, between the duration of the PI-based therapy (30.0 months [13.1-40.5]) and the NNRTI-based therapy (15.2 [5.5-23.2]; *P*=0.054).

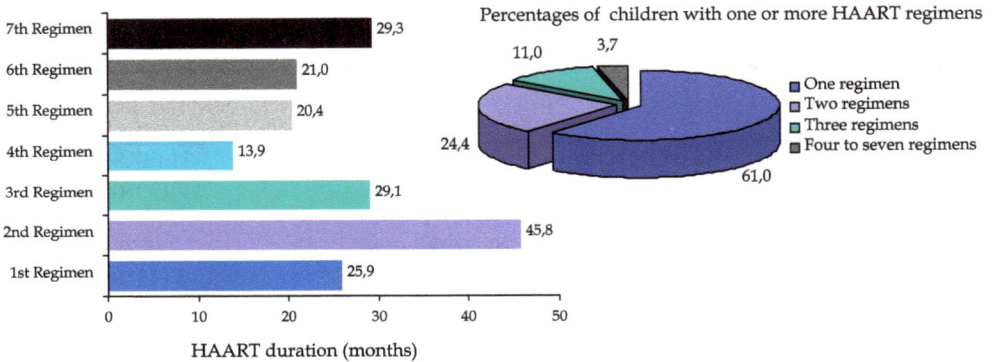

Fig. 4. Relative proportion of patients according to the number of HAART regimens among the 82 antiretroviral-naïve patients who start HAART since 1997 (circle chart); months of HAART regimen duration among the 32 patients with regimen switch (bat chart).

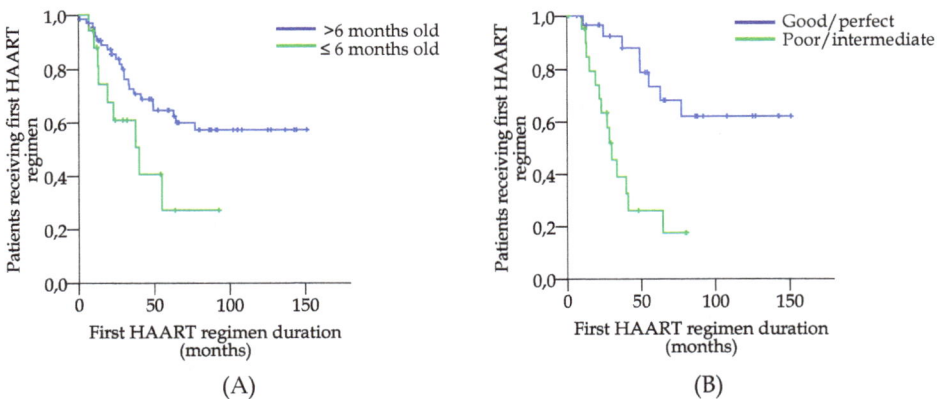

Fig. 5. Kaplan-Meier curves for time to discontinuation of first HAART regimen according to the age of HAART initiation (A) and to adherence to first HAART regimen (B).

| | First HAART regimen discontinuation | | |
	N.	N. of cases (%)	Adjusted HR (95% CI)
Age at HAART initiation			
> 6 months	40	14 (35.0)	1.00
≤ 6 months	12	8 (66.7)	4.56 (1.76 – 11.86)
Adherence to first HAART regimen			
Good/perfect	31	8 (25.8)	1.00
Poor/intermediate	21	14 (66.7)	5.02 (2.02 – 12.47)

Table 5. Effect of age at HAART initiation and adherence on the risk of first HAART regimen discontinuation. Note: Adjusted hazard ratios were derived from a standard Cox proportional hazard model.

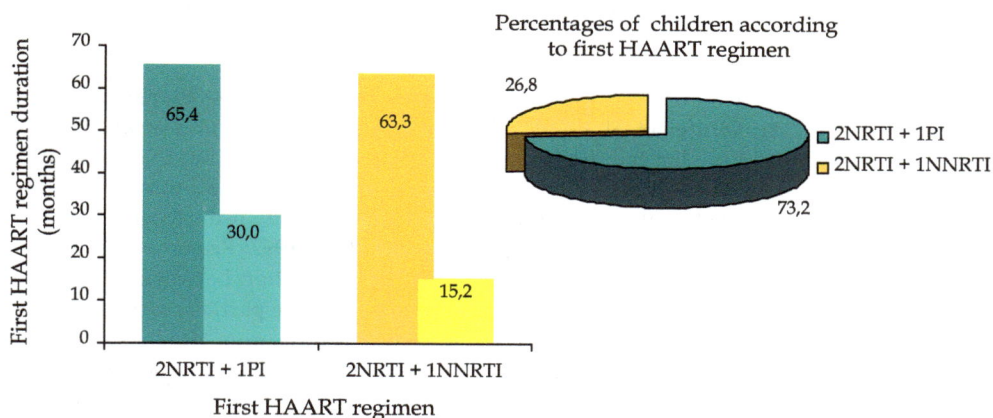

Fig. 6. Relative proportion of initial HAART regimen types among the 82 antiretroviral-naïve patients who started HAART since 1997 (circle chart); months of HAART regimen duration in patients who did not suspended the first HAART regimen (dark coloured bars) and who suspended the first regimen (light coloured bars). NRTI: nucleoside reverse-transcriptase inhibitor; NNRTI: non-nucleoside reverse-transcriptase inhibitor; PI: protease inhibitor.

4. Discussion

The results of this multicenter study on 484 patients infected by HIV-1 through perinatal transmission from the region of Madrid, show that the immunovirological response observed after the introduction of HAART has improved steadily since 1997. Also, an increase in clinical outcome with calendar period was observed. The marked reduction in progression to AIDS and death (by 93% and 84%, respectively) in recent years compared to 1982-1989 suggests a relationship between clinical outcome and HAART, which became widely available from 1997 onward. However, in the latter period, a low but stable mortality rate was recorded, in accordance with those recently reported by others (Brady et al., 2010; Judd et al., 2007).

Remarkably, mortality continued to be more than ten-fold higher in our cohort than in age-similar general population after 1996 and mainly affected patients of low/medium socio-economic status (Palladino et al., 2008). In addition, HIV-1-infected infants were still at higher risk for death compared with older paediatric patients, being this pattern mirrored in the general paediatric population and maybe attributable to the immature of the immune system (Gortmaker et al., 2001). Finally, the mortality trend had a strikingly lower decrease among infants than among children aged ≥ 1 year in our cohort, where it decreased equally in both groups in the general population. These findings highlight the HIV-1-infected infants as a major target for healthcare policy. We observed very high AIDS and mortality incidence rates during the first years of follow-up. These data on mortality are consistent with historical European series (ECS, (1994). and with data on HIV-1 progression in children living in setting where they do not receive medical care (Brahmbhatt et al., 2006; Marinda et al., 2007). In fact, zidovudine monotherapy administration to paediatric patients started only in 1988 (Pizzo et al., 1988) and in our cohort the majority of the children were still untreated in this year. Moreover, the high HIV-1 prevalence among the female population fuelled by the so called "epidemic of heroin" had a direct impact on the spread of the infection in infants.

Our study shows that monotherapy exerted some benefit in the management of symptomatic children (Butler et al., 1991; McKinney et al., 1991; Resino et al., 2006b). Nevertheless, it had a time-limited effect due to ongoing viral replication that inevitably leads to the emergence of resistant HIV-1 quasispecies, which was also promoted by the lack of drug dosage adjustments for children at that time. The dual-nucleoside therapy proved to be more effective than monotherapy (Englund et al., 1997; Resino et al., 2006b). However, in our setting its effect on mortality or AIDS prevention between 1994- 1996 was similar to that exerted by monotherapy. This finding might be partially attributable to the regimen switch to dual-drug therapy (mainly zidovudine plus didanosine) after several years of zidovudine treatment in many children, when zidovudine was not more completely active. Thus, even with perfect adherence, dual-drug therapy was only partially suppressive being administered as functional monotherapy and due to cross-resistance within the nucleoside analogue class. In addition, during this period more than 40% of the children were still untreated and more than 35% were on monotherapy. Previous studies reported the effectiveness of HAART on the risk of death in the setting of large paediatric cohorts, but these had limited follow-up and lacked assessment of the progression to AIDS (de Martino et al., 2000; Gortmaker et al., 2001). In 2000, the Italian Register for HIV Infection in Children (de Martino et al., 2000) observed a reduction in the mortality rate of 71% in individuals undergoing triple-combination therapy compared with untreated patients, while Gortmaker and colleagues found a 67% reduction comparing HAART with other therapy (Gortmaker et al., 2001). Important reductions of 76% have also been reported recently by a 10-year follow-up survey (Patel et al., 2008). Our analyses found a stronger reduction (84%), but it is not directly comparable with previous published data due to the longer follow-up and to the difference in the performed analyses. In fact, we dealt with the trend of the risk of death in different calendar periods considered as an external time-dependent covariate. The high prevalence of comorbidities, along with multiple causes of death, resulted in increasing complexity of the management of patients with HIV/AIDS.

In terms of specific causes of death, AIDS–defining events were the most represented, with proportions higher than that recently observed in adults (Martinez et al., 2007; Palella et al., 2006). This finding might be directly linked to a late HIV-1 diagnosis at the beginning of the epidemic and to the persistence of opportunistic infections, that were the leading AIDS–defining causes of death (Brady et al., 2010; Selik & Lindegren 2003), although less represented since HAART advent (Currier et al., 1998; Kaplan et al., 2001). As in previous studies, bacterial infections were the largest component of opportunistic infections (Gona et al., 2006; Langston et al., 2001). Although specific information for their aetiology was mainly unavailable, we supposed that pneumococcus (*Streptococcus pneumoniae*) might has been the prominent microbial on the basis of recent reports (Cotton et al., 2008; Gortmaker et al., 2001; Kapogiannis et al., 2008). In addition, the pneumococcal conjugate vaccine available since 2000 (Black et al., 2000) and recommended for all HIV-infected children, has a lower efficacy in these patients than in HIV-uninfected children (Bliss et al., 2008). Some bacterial infections occurred with normal CD4$^+$ cell percentage ($\geq 25\%$), consistently with previous report (Gona et al., 2006), maybe because the HIV-1 infection does not allow the correct development of primary immune function leading to the production of polyclonal, non-specific immunoglobulin increasing the risk of infections with encapsulated bacteria (Brady et al., 2010; Cotton et al., 2008; Gortmaker et al., 2001; Kapogiannis et al., 2008). The population-based analysis yielded consistent results with studies of HIV–infected patients (Kapogiannis et al., 2008; Martinez et al., 2007), highlighting a higher incidence of infections in our cohort than in the general population of similar age from the same region. Along with host immune factors (Janoff et al., 1992), antimicrobial resistance (Cotton et al., 2008; Jaspan et al., 2008), comorbidity and co-infections might have contributed to the high risk of death from opportunistic infections. The introduction of both *Pneumocystis* pneumonia prophylaxis (CDC 1995; Simonds et al., 1995) and HAART in our cohort has been accompanied by substantial reductions in mortality caused by *Pneumocystis* pneumonia (Gona et al., 2006; Kaplan et al., 2000), which have continued to occur in post-HAART era only in infants born to women with late HIV-1 diagnosis or unmonitored pregnancy, causing failure to implement *Pneumocystis* pneumonia prophylaxis (Gibb et al., 2003; Simpson et al., 2000). The cases of *M. avium* complex infection in our cohort have decreased over time (Gona et al., 2006). The cases reported in CP2 were diagnosed in children 6-11 years old, probably as a complication of advanced immunologic deterioration and the difficulty to realize a complete adherence to HAART and *M. avium* complex chemoprophylaxis. On the other hand, our data have shown an increase in the median age at death over time that might reflect improved management and prolongation in the time to development of a first bacteremia (Kapogiannis et al., 2008). More prolonged survival might allow chronic underlying comorbid conditions to become more clinically relevant in the next future. The proportion of HIV–related causes of deaths (12%) increased over time even if not statistically significant. Interestingly, the case of lactic acidosis was related to HAART regimen (stavudine + didanosine + efavirenz) that caused mitochondrial toxicity, whose rate is known to be increased by stavudine + didanosine co-administration (Blanco et al., 2003; Cote et al., 2002). Among non-HIV–related causes of death, the 7% of all the underlying causes, the fulminant hepatic failure occurred in 2008 was HCV-associated. We did not observe the increase of conditions, including diabetes mellitus, cancer, cardiovascular, liver and renal diseases that have become frequent in HIV-1–infected adults (Crum et al., 2006;

Lewden et al., 2008; Novoa et al., 2008; Palella et al., 2006; Sackoff et al., 2006; Smit et al., 2006). The lack of increase of non-HIV–related causes of death might be due to the long duration pathogenesis of these diseases as well as to their rarity, which might have limited power to identify such evolution.

The duration of initial HAART regimens for antiretroviral-naïve children has not been reported. On the contrary, several studies have assessed this public health issue in HIV-1-infected adults (Chen et al., 2003; Miller et al., 1999; Palella Jr et al., 2002; Phillips et al., 2001). The median duration of the first regimen observed in our study population was more than 3 years, the double of the duration described by Cheng and colleagues (2003) in a group of 405 antiretroviral-naïve adults and longer than that observed by Palella et al. (2002) who enrolled patients with previous antiretroviral experience. Notably, our study had a longer follow-up which could in part explain this difference. Among the therapy-naïve paediatric patients enrolled in the HIV Paediatric Cohort of the *Comunidad Autónoma de Madrid*, poor adherence has been identified as primary risk factor for initial HAART regimens discontinuation and short duration. This result is in agreement with the association between adherence and response to antiretroviral therapy reported for paediatric patients, being incomplete adherence the primary cause of treatment failure (Chiappini et al., 2006; Gray et al., 2001; Hainaut et al., 2003; Resino et al., 2003). In addiction, the age at HAART initiation was found to be another independent risk factor for first HAART regimen discontinuation. The impact of HAART on the morbidity and mortality in Spanish HIV-1 vertically infected children has been discussed elsewhere (Resino et al., 2006b; Sanchez et al., 2003). However, an assessment of underlying causes of mortality and a population effectiveness analysis have never been performed in the context of an observational paediatric cohort in Spain. A number of limitations of this study should be noted. First, temporal changes in the spectrum of causes of deaths were not statistically significant; whether this result has been due to the limited number of deaths occurred after 1996 should be cautiously taken into account. Second, a survivor bias due to the partially retrospective enrolment might have caused mortality underestimation in infants at the beginning of the epidemic. Nevertheless our cohort remains more than representative of the HIV-1 epidemic in one of the Spanish regions most affected by the disease over almost three decades.

5. Conclusion

Despite the population effectiveness of HAART in reducing HIV-1-associated mortality, new challenges could arise for national surveillance systems as prolonged survival and long-term antiretroviral exposure might contribute to additional and different causes of death in perinatally infected patients in the future.

6. Acknowledgments

The authors thank patients for their participation and the HIV HGM BioBank belonging to the Spanish AIDS Research Network (RED RIS) and Red Nacional de BioBancos, and The cohort of the Spanish Paediatric HIV Research Network CoRISpe cohort node 1.

This study was partially supported by grants from Red Temática de Investigación Cooperativa Sanitaria ISCIII (RETIC RD06/0006/0035), Fundación para la Investigación y Prevención del SIDA en España (FIPSE 240800/09 and 380910/10), Paediatric European

Network for Treatment of AIDS (PENTA), Fundación Caja Navarra, Fondo de Investigación Sanitaria (FIS INTRASALUD PI09/02029). The Spanish MICINN through the Juan de la Cierva program (JCI-2009–05650) (to C.P.).

7. References

Black, S., Shinefield, H., Fireman, B., Lewis, E., Ray, P., Hansen, J. R., Elvin, L., Ensor, K. M., Hackell, J., Siber, G., Malinoski, F., Madore, D., Chang, I., Kohberger, R., Watson, W., Austrian, R., & Edwards, K. (2000). Efficacy, safety and immunogenicity of heptavalent pneumococcal conjugate vaccine in children. Northern California Kaiser Permanente Vaccine Study Center Group. *Pediatr Infect Dis J*, Vol. 19, No. 3, (Mar 2000), pp. 187-195, 0891-3668 (Print) 0891-3668 (Linking)

Blanche, S., Bologna, R., Cahn, P., Rugina, S., Flynn, P., Fortuny, C., Vis, P., Sekar, V., van Baelen, B., Dierynck, I., & Spinosa-Guzman, S. (2009). Pharmacokinetics, safety and efficacy of darunavir/ritonavir in treatment-experienced children and adolescents. *AIDS*, Vol. 23, No. 15, (Sep 2009), pp. 2005-13, 1473-5571 (Electronic)   0269-9370 (Linking)

Blanco, F., Garcia-Benayas, T., Jose de la Cruz, J., Gonzalez-Lahoz, J., & Soriano, V. (2003). First-line therapy and mitochondrial damage: different nucleosides, different findings. *HIV Clin Trials*, Vol. 4, No. 1, (Jan-Feb 2003), pp. 11-19, 1528-4336 (Print) 1528-4336 (Linking)

Bliss, S. J., O'Brien, K. L., Janoff, E. N., Cotton, M. F., Musoke, P., Coovadia, H., & Levine, O. S. (2008). The evidence for using conjugate vaccines to protect HIV-infected children against pneumococcal disease. *Lancet Infect Dis*, Vol. 8, No. 1, (Jan 2008), pp. 67-80, 1473-3099 (Print) 1473-3099 (Linking)

Brady, M. T., Oleske, J. M., Williams, P. L., Elgie, C., Mofenson, L. M., Dankner, W. M., & Van Dyke, R. B. (2010). Declines in mortality rates and changes in causes of death in HIV-1-infected children during the HAART era. *J Acquir Immune Defic Syndr*, Vol. 53, No. 1, (Jan 2010), pp. 86-94, 1944-7884 (Electronic) 1525-4135 (Linking)

Brahmbhatt, H., Kigozi, G., Wabwire-Mangen, F., Serwadda, D., Lutalo, T., Nalugoda, F., Sewankambo, N., Kiduggavu, M., Wawer, M., & Gray, R. (2006). Mortality in HIV-infected and uninfected children of HIV-infected and uninfected mothers in rural Uganda. *J Acquir Immune Defic Syndr*, Vol. 41, No. 4, (Apr 2006), pp. 504-508, 1525-4135 (Print) 1525-4135 (Linking)

Butler, K. M., Husson, R. N., Balis, F. M., Brouwers, P., Eddy, J., el-Amin, D., Gress, J., Hawkins, M., Jarosinski, P., Moss, H., & et al. (1991). Dideoxyinosine in children with symptomatic human immunodeficiency virus infection. *N Engl J Med*, Vol. 324, No. 3, (Jan 1991), pp. 137-44, 0028-4793 (Print)

Centers for Disease Control and Prevention. (Dec 1992). Revised classification system for HIV-1 infection and expanded surveillance case definition for AIDS among adolescents and adults. *Morbidity and Mortality Recomm Rep*, Vol. 41, No. RR-17, pp. 1-19, 17.02.2011, Available from:
    <http://www.cdc.gov/mmwr/preview/mmwrhtml/ 00018871.htm>

Centers for Disease Control and Prevention. (Sep 1994). Revised classification system for human immunodeficiency virus infection in children less than 13 years of age. *Morbidity and Mortality Weekly Report CDC Surveill Summ*, Vol. 43, No. RR-12, pp. 1-10, 17.02.2011, Available from:

<http://www.cdc.gov/mmwr/preview/mmwrhtml/ 00032890.htm>
Centers for Disease Control and Prevention. (Apr 1995). Revised guidelines for prophylaxis against Pneumocystis carinii pneumonia for children infected with or perinatally exposed to human immunodeficiency virus. *Morbidity and Mortality Weekly Report*, Vol. 44, No. RR-4, pp. 1-11, 17.02.2011, Available from: <http://www.cdc.gov/mmwr/PDF/rr/rr4404.pdf>

Centers for Disease Control and Prevention. (Apr 1998). Guidelines for use of antiretroviral agents in pediatric HIV infection. *Morbidity and Mortality Weekly Report*, Vol. 47, No. RR-4, pp. 1-31, 17.02.2011, Available from <http://www.cdc.gov/mmwr/preview/mmwrhtml/00053104.htm>

Centro Nacional de Epidemiología. Instituto de Salud Carlos III. (Jun 2010) Vigilancia epidemiológica del SIDA en España, 28.10.2010, Available from: <http://cne.isciii.es. Accessed January 15, 2011>

Chen, R. Y., Westfall, A. O., Mugavero, M. J., Cloud, G. A., Raper, J. L., Chatham, A. G., Acosta, E. P., Taylor, K. H., Carter, J., & Saag, M. S. (2003). Duration of highly active antiretroviral therapy regimens. *Clin Infect Dis*, Vol. 37, No. 5, (Sep 2003), pp. 714-722, 1537-6591 (Electronic) 1058-4838 (Linking)

Chiappini, E., Galli, L., Tovo, P. A., Gabiano, C., Gattinara, G. C., Guarino, A., Badolato, R., Giaquinto, C., Lisi, C., & de Martino, M. (2006). Virologic, immunologic, and clinical benefits from early combined antiretroviral therapy in infants with perinatal HIV-1 infection. *AIDS*, Vol. 20, No. 2, (Jan 2006), pp. 207-215, 0269-9370 (Print) 0269-9370 (Linking)

ClinicalTrials.gov. (2007). Safety and Effectiveness of Raltegravir (MK-0518) in Treatment-Experienced, HIV-Infected Children and Adolescents. NCT00485264. 25.01.2011, Available from: <http://clinicaltrials.gov/ct2/show/NCT00485264?term=NCT00485264&rank=1>

ClinicalTrials.gov. (2008a). An Open Label Pharmacokinetic, Safety And Efficacy Study Of Maraviroc In Combination With Background Therapy For The Treatment Of HIV-1 Infected, CCR5 -Tropic Children. NCT00791700. 28.02.2011, Available from: <http://clinicaltrials.gov/ct2/show/study/NCT00791700>

ClinicalTrials.gov. (2008b). Safety and Antiviral Activity of Etravirine (TMC125) in Treatment-Experienced, HIV Infected Children and Adolescents. NCT00665847. 25.01.2011, Available from: <http://clinicaltrials.gov/ct2/show/results/NCT00665847>

ClinicalTrials.gov. (2009a). Continued Access to Etravirine (ETR) in Treatment Experienced HIV-1 Infected Children and Adolescents. NCT00980538. Available from: <http://clinicaltrials.gov/ct2/show/NCT00980538>

ClinicalTrials.gov. (2009b). Pharmacokinetic Effects of New Antiretroviral Drugs on Children, Adolescents and Young Adults. NCT00977756. 25.01.2011, Available from: <http://clinicaltrials.gov/ct2/show/NCT00977756>

Connor, E. M., Sperling, R. S., Gelber, R., Kiselev, P., Scott, G., O'Sullivan, M. J., VanDyke, R., Bey, M., Shearer, W., Jacobson, R. L., & et al. (1994). Reduction of maternal-infant transmission of human immunodeficiency virus type 1 with zidovudine treatment. Pediatric AIDS Clinical Trials Group Protocol 076 Study Group. *N Engl J Med*, Vol. 331, No. 18, (Nov 1994), pp. 1173-80, 0028-4793 (Print) 0028-4793 (Linking)

Cote, H. C., Brumme, Z. L., Craib, K. J., Alexander, C. S., Wynhoven, B., Ting, L., Wong, H., Harris, M., Harrigan, P. R., O'Shaughnessy, M. V., & Montaner, J. S. (2002). Changes in mitochondrial DNA as a marker of nucleoside toxicity in HIV-infected patients. *N Engl J Med*, Vol. 346, No. 11, (Mar 2002), pp. 811-820, 1533-4406 (Electronic) 0028-4793 (Linking)

Cotton, M. F., Wasserman, E., Smit, J., Whitelaw, A., & Zar, H. J. (2008). High incidence of antimicrobial resistant organisms including extended spectrum beta-lactamase producing Enterobacteriaceae and methicillin-resistant Staphylococcus aureus in nasopharyngeal and blood isolates of HIV-infected children from Cape Town, South Africa. *BMC Infect Dis*, Vol. 8, (Apr 2008), pp. 40, 1471-2334 (Electronic) 1471-2334 (Linking)

Crum, N. F., Riffenburgh, R. H., Wegner, S., Agan, B. K., Tasker, S. A., Spooner, K. M., Armstrong, A. W., Fraser, S., & Wallace, M. R. (2006). Comparisons of causes of death and mortality rates among HIV-infected persons: analysis of the pre-, early, and late HAART (highly active antiretroviral therapy) eras. *J Acquir Immune Defic Syndr*, Vol. 41, No. 2, (Feb 2006), pp. 194-200, 1525-4135 (Print) 1525-4135 (Linking)

Currier, J. S., Williams, P. L., Grimes, J. M., Squires, K. S., Fischl, M. A., & Hammer, S. M. (1998). Incidence rates and risk factors for opportunistic infections in a phase III trial comparing indinavir + ZDV + 3TC to ZDV + 3TC. *Proceedings of the 5th Conference on Retroviruses and Opportunistic Infections*, Chicago, Illinois, USA, Feb 1-5, 1998

De Cock, K. M., Fowler, M. G., Mercier, E., de Vincenzi, I., Saba, J., Hoff, E., Alnwick, D. J., Rogers, M., & Shaffer, N. (2000). Prevention of mother-to-child HIV transmission in resource-poor countries: translating research into policy and practice. *JAMA*, Vol. 283, No. 9, (Mar 2000), pp. 1175-1182, 0098-7484 (Print) 0098-7484 (Linking)

de Martino, M., Tovo, P. A., Balducci, M., Galli, L., Gabiano, C., Rezza, G., & Pezzotti, P. (2000). Reduction in mortality with availability of antiretroviral therapy for children with perinatal HIV-1 infection. Italian Register for HIV Infection in Children and the Italian National AIDS Registry. *JAMA*, Vol. 284, No. 2, (Jul 2000), pp. 190-197, 0098-7484 (Print) 0098-7484 (Linking)

Englund, J. A., Baker, C. J., Raskino, C., McKinney, R. E., Petrie, B., Fowler, M. G., Pearson, D., Gershon, A., McSherry, G. D., Abrams, E. J., Schliozberg, J., & Sullivan, J. L. (1997). Zidovudine, didanosine, or both as the initial treatment for symptomatic HIV-infected children. AIDS Clinical Trials Group (ACTG) Study 152 Team. *N Engl J Med*, Vol. 336, No. 24, (Jun 1997), pp. 1704-1712,

Faye, A., Le Chenadec, J., Dollfus, C., Thuret, I., Douard, D., Firtion, G., Lachassinne, E., Levine, M., Nicolas, J., Monpoux, F., Tricoire, J., Rouzioux, C., Tardieu, M., Mayaux, M. J., & Blanche, S. (2004). Early versus deferred antiretroviral multidrug therapy in infants infected with HIV type 1. *Clin Infect Dis*, Vol. 39, No. 11, (Dec 2004), pp. 1692-1698, 1537-6591 (Electronic) 1058-4838 (Linking)

Fraaij, P. L., Verweel, G., van Rossum, A. M., van Lochem, E. G., Schutten, M., Weemaes, C. M., Hartwig, N. G., Burger, D. M., & de Groot, R. (2005). Sustained viral suppression and immune recovery in HIV type 1-infected children after 4 years of highly active antiretroviral therapy. *Clin Infect Dis*, Vol. 40, No. 4, (Feb 2005), pp. 604-608, 1058-4838 (Print)

Gibb, D. M., Duong, T., Tookey, P. A., Sharland, M., Tudor-Williams, G., Novelli, V., Butler, K., Riordan, A., Farrelly, L., Masters, J., Peckham, C. S., & Dunn, D. T. (2003). Decline in mortality, AIDS, and hospital admissions in perinatally HIV-1 infected children in the United Kingdom and Ireland. *BMJ*, Vol. 327, No. 7422, (Nov 2003), pp. 1019

Gona, P., Van Dyke, R. B., Williams, P. L., Dankner, W. M., Chernoff, M. C., Nachman, S. A., & Seage, G. R., 3rd. (2006). Incidence of opportunistic and other infections in HIV-infected children in the HAART era. *JAMA*, Vol. 296, No. 3, (Jul 2006), pp. 292-300, 1538-3598 (Electronic) 0098-7484 (Linking)

Gortmaker, S. L., Hughes, M., Cervia, J., Brady, M., Johnson, G. M., Seage, G. R., 3rd, Song, L. Y., Dankner, W. M., & Oleske, J. M. (2001). Effect of combination therapy including protease inhibitors on mortality among children and adolescents infected with HIV-1. *N Engl J Med*, Vol. 345, No. 21, (Nov 2001), pp. 1522-1528,

Gray, L., Newell, M. L., Thorne, C., Peckham, C., & Levy, J. (2001). Fluctuations in symptoms in human immunodeficiency virus-infected children: the first 10 years of life. *Pediatrics*, Vol. 108, No. 1, (Jul 2001), pp. 116-122, 1098-4275 (Electronic) 0031-4005 (Linking)

Hainaut, M., Ducarme, M., Schandene, L., Peltier, C. A., Marissens, D., Zissis, G., Mascart, F., & Levy, J. (2003). Age-related immune reconstitution during highly active antiretroviral therapy in human immunodeficiency virus type 1-infected children. *Pediatr Infect Dis J*, Vol. 22, No. 1, (Jan 2003), pp. 62-69, 0891-3668 (Print) 0891-3668 (Linking)

Janoff, E. N., Breiman, R. F., Daley, C. L., & Hopewell, P. C. (1992). Pneumococcal disease during HIV infection. Epidemiologic, clinical, and immunologic perspectives. *Ann Intern Med*, Vol. 117, No. 4, (Aug 1992), pp. 314-324, 0003-4819 (Print) 0003-4819 (Linking)

Jaspan, H. B., Huang, L. C., Cotton, M. F., Whitelaw, A., & Myer, L. (2008). Bacterial disease and antimicrobial susceptibility patterns in HIV-infected, hospitalized children: a retrospective cohort study. *PLoS One*, Vol. 3, No. 9, (Set 2008), pp. e3260, 1932-6203 (Electronic) 1932-6203 (Linking)

Joint United Nations Programme on HIV/AIDS. (July 2010). UNAIDS Outlook Report, Geneva, Switzerland: UNAIDS, p. 7, 20.01.2011, Available from: <http://data.unaids.org/pub/Outlook/2010/20100713_outlook_report_web_en.p df>

Judd, A., Doerholt, K., Tookey, P. A., Sharland, M., Riordan, A., Menson, E., Novelli, V., Lyall, E. G., Masters, J., Tudor-Williams, G., Duong, T., & Gibb, D. M. (2007). Morbidity, mortality, and response to treatment by children in the United Kingdom and Ireland with perinatally acquired HIV infection during 1996-2006: planning for teenage and adult care. *Clin Infect Dis*, Vol. 45, No. 7, (Oct 2007), pp. 918-924

Kaplan, J. E., Hanson, D., Dworkin, M. S., Frederick, T., Bertolli, J., Lindegren, M. L., Holmberg, S., & Jones, J. L. (2000). Epidemiology of human immunodeficiency virus-associated opportunistic infections in the United States in the era of highly active antiretroviral therapy. *Clin Infect Dis*, Vol. 30 Suppl 1, No., (Apr 2000), pp. S5-14, 1058-4838 (Print) 1058-4838 (Linking)

Kaplan, J. E., Sepkowitz, K., Masur, H., Sirisanthana, T., Russo, M., & Chapman, L. (2001). Opportunistic infections in persons with HIV or other immunocompromising conditions. *Emerg Infect Dis*, Vol. 7, No. 3 Suppl, (Aug 2001), pp. 541, 1080-6040 (Print) 1080-6040 (Linking)

Kapogiannis, B. G., Soe, M. M., Nesheim, S. R., Sullivan, K. M., Abrams, E., Farley, J., Palumbo, P., Koenig, L. J., & Bulterys, M. (2008). Trends in bacteremia in the pre- and post-highly active antiretroviral therapy era among HIV-infected children in the US Perinatal AIDS Collaborative Transmission Study (1986-2004). *Pediatrics*, Vol. 121, No. 5, (May 2008), pp. e1229-1239, 1098-4275 (Electronic) 0031-4005 (Linking)

Langston, C., Cooper, E. R., Goldfarb, J., Easley, K. A., Husak, S., Sunkle, S., Starc, T. J., & Colin, A. A. (2001). Human immunodeficiency virus-related mortality in infants and children: data from the pediatric pulmonary and cardiovascular complications of vertically transmitted HIV (P(2)C(2)) Study. *Pediatrics*, Vol. 107, No. 2, (Feb 2001), pp. 328-338, 1098-4275 (Electronic) 0031-4005 (Linking)

Lewden, C., May, T., Rosenthal, E., Burty, C., Bonnet, F., Costagliola, D., Jougla, E., Semaille, C., Morlat, P., Salmon, D., Cacoub, P., & Chene, G. (2008). Changes in causes of death among adults infected by HIV between 2000 and 2005: The "Mortalite 2000 and 2005" surveys (ANRS EN19 and Mortavic). *J Acquir Immune Defic Syndr*, Vol. 48, No. 5, (Aug 2008), pp. 590-598, 1525-4135 (Print) 1525-4135 (Linking)

Marinda, E., Humphrey, J. H., Iliff, P. J., Mutasa, K., Nathoo, K. J., Piwoz, E. G., Moulton, L. H., Salama, P., & Ward, B. J. (2007). Child mortality according to maternal and infant HIV status in Zimbabwe. *Pediatr Infect Dis J*, Vol. 26, No. 6, (Jun 2007), pp. 519-526

Martinez, E., Milinkovic, A., Buira, E., de Lazzari, E., Leon, A., Larrousse, M., Lonca, M., Laguno, M., Blanco, J. L., Mallolas, J., Garcia, F., Miro, J. M., & Gatell, J. M. (2007). Incidence and causes of death in HIV-infected persons receiving highly active antiretroviral therapy compared with estimates for the general population of similar age and from the same geographical area. *HIV Med*, Vol. 8, No. 4, (May 2007), pp. 251-258, 1464-2662 (Print) 1464-2662 (Linking)

McKinney, R. E., Jr., Maha, M. A., Connor, E. M., Feinberg, J., Scott, G. B., Wulfsohn, M., McIntosh, K., Borkowsky, W., Modlin, J. F., Weintrub, P., & et al. (1991). A multicenter trial of oral zidovudine in children with advanced human immunodeficiency virus disease. The Protocol 043 Study Group. *N Engl J Med*, Vol. 324, No. 15, (Apr 11 1991), pp. 1018-1025

Miller, V., Staszewski, S., Sabin, C., Carlebach, A., Rottmann, C., Weidmann, E., Rabenau, H., Hill, A., Lepri, A. C., & Phillips, A. N. (1999). CD4 lymphocyte count as a predictor of the duration of highly active antiretroviral therapy-induced suppression of human immunodeficiency virus load. *J Infect Dis*, Vol. 180, No. 2, (Aug 1999), pp. 530-533, 0022-1899 (Print) 0022-1899 (Linking)

Ministerio de sanidad y Consumo. (Nov 1998). Encuesta hospitalaria sobre la utilización de recursos y características de los pacientes VIH/SIDA, 17.02.2011, Available from: <www.msc.es/sida/epidemiologia>

Newell, M. L., Coovadia, H., Cortina-Borja, M., Rollins, N., Gaillard, P., & Dabis, F. (2004). Mortality of infected and uninfected infants born to HIV-infected mothers in Africa: a pooled analysis. *Lancet*, Vol. 364, No. 9441, (Oct 2004), pp. 1236-1243, 1474-547X (Electronic) 0140-6736 (Linking)

Novoa, A. M., de Olalla, P. G., Clos, R., Orcau, A., Rodriguez-Sanz, M., & Cayla, J. A. (2008). Increase in the non-HIV-related deaths among AIDS cases in the HAART era. *Curr HIV Res*, Vol. 6, No. 1, (Jan 2008), pp. 77-81, 1873-4251 (Electronic) 1570-162X (Linking)

Palella, F. J., Jr., Baker, R. K., Moorman, A. C., Chmiel, J. S., Wood, K. C., Brooks, J. T., & Holmberg, S. D. (2006). Mortality in the highly active antiretroviral therapy era: changing causes of death and disease in the HIV outpatient study. *J Acquir Immune Defic Syndr*, Vol. 43, No. 1, (Sep 2006), pp. 27-34, 1525-4135 (Print) 1525-4135 (Linking)

Palella Jr, F. J., Chmiel, J. S., Moorman, A. C., & Holmberg, S. D. (2002). Durability and predictors of success of highly active antiretroviral therapy for ambulatory HIV-infected patients. *AIDS*, Vol. 16, No. 12, (Aug 2002), pp. 1617-1626, 0269-9370 (Print) 0269-9370 (Linking)

Palladino, C., Bellon, J. M., Perez-Hoyos, S., Resino, R., Guillen, S., Garcia, D., Gurbindo, M. D., Ramos, J. T., de Jose, M. I., Mellado, M. J., & Munoz-Fernandez, M. A. (2008). Spatial pattern of HIV-1 mother-to-child-transmission in Madrid (Spain) from 1980 till now: demographic and socioeconomic factors. *AIDS*, Vol. 22, No. 16, (Oct 2008), pp. 2199-2205, 1473-5571 (Electronic) 0269-9370 (Linking)

Patel, K., Hernan, M. A., Williams, P. L., Seeger, J. D., McIntosh, K., Van Dyke, R. B., & Seage, G. R., 3rd. (2008). Long-term effectiveness of highly active antiretroviral therapy on the survival of children and adolescents with HIV infection: a 10-year follow-up study. *Clin Infect Dis*, Vol. 46, No. 4, (Feb 2008), pp. 507-515

Phillips, A. N., Miller, V., Sabin, C., Cozzi Lepri, A., Klauke, S., Bickel, M., Doerr, H. W., Hill, A., & Staszewski, S. (2001). Durability of HIV-1 viral suppression over 3.3 years with multi-drug antiretroviral therapy in previously drug-naive individuals. *AIDS*, Vol. 15, No. 18, (Dec 2001), pp. 2379-2384, 0269-9370 (Print) 0269-9370 (Linking)

Pizzo, P. A., Eddy, J., Falloon, J., Balis, F. M., Murphy, R. F., Moss, H., Wolters, P., Brouwers, P., Jarosinski, P., Rubin, M., Broder, S., Yarchoan, R., Brunetti, A., Maha, M., Nusinoff-Lehrman, S., & Poplack, D. G. (1988). Effect of continuous intravenous infusion of zidovudine (AZT) in children with symptomatic HIV infection. *N Engl J Med*, Vol. 319, No. 14, (Oct 1988), pp. 889-896, 0028-4793 (Print) 0028-4793 (Linking)

Puthanakit, T., Aurpibul, L., Oberdorfer, P., Akarathum, N., Kanjananit, S., Wannarit, P., Sirisanthana, T., & Sirisanthana, V. (2007). Hospitalization and mortality among HIV-infected children after receiving highly active antiretroviral therapy. *Clin Infect Dis*, Vol. 44, No. 4, (Feb 2007), pp. 599-604, 1537-6591 (Electronic)

Reddi, A., Leeper, S. C., Grobler, A. C., Geddes, R., France, K. H., Dorse, G. L., Vlok, W. J., Mntambo, M., Thomas, M., Nixon, K., Holst, H. L., Karim, Q. A., Rollins, N. C., Coovadia, H. M., & Giddy, J. (2007). Preliminary outcomes of a paediatric highly active antiretroviral therapy cohort from KwaZulu-Natal, South Africa. *BMC Pediatr*, Vol. 7, (Mar 2007), pp. 13-25, 1471-2431 (Electronic)

Resino, S., Bellon, J. M., Gurbindo, D., Leon, J. A., & Munoz-Fernandez, M. A. (2003). Recovery of T-cell subsets after antiretroviral therapy in HIV-infected children. *Eur J Clin Invest*, Vol. 33, No. 7, (Jul 2003), pp. 619-627, 0014-2972 (Print) 0014-2972 (Linking)

Resino, S., Alvaro-Meca, A., de Jose, M. I., Martin-Fontelos, P., Gutierrez, M. D., Leon, J. A., Ramos, J. T., Ciria, L., & Munoz-Fernandez, M. A. (2006a). Low immunologic response to highly active antiretroviral therapy in naive vertically human immunodeficiency virus type 1-infected children with severe immunodeficiency. *Pediatr Infect Dis J*, Vol. 25, No. 4, (Apr 2006a), pp. 365-368, 0891-3668 (Print)

Resino, S., Resino, R., Bellon, J. M., Micheloud, D., Gutierrez, M. D., de Jose, M. I., Ramos, J. T., Fontelos, P. M., Ciria, L., & Munoz-Fernandez, M. A. (2006b). Clinical outcomes improve with highly active antiretroviral therapy in vertically HIV type-1-infected children. *Clin Infect Dis*, Vol. 43, No. 2, (Jul 2006b), pp. 243-252, 1058-4838 (Print)

Sackoff, J. E., Hanna, D. B., Pfeiffer, M. R., & Torian, L. V. (2006). Causes of death among persons with AIDS in the era of highly active antiretroviral therapy: New York City. *Ann Intern Med*, Vol. 145, No. 6, (Sep 2006), pp. 397-406, 1539-3704 (Electronic) 0003-4819 (Linking)

Salazar, J. C., Cahn, P., Yogev, R., Negra, M. D., Castelli-Gattinara, G., Fortuny, C., Flynn, P. M., Giaquinto, C., Ruan, P. K., Smith, M. E., Mikl, J., & Jelaska, A. (2008). Efficacy, safety and tolerability of tipranavir coadministered with ritonavir in HIV-1-infected children and adolescents. *AIDS*, Vol. 22, No. 14, (Sep 2008), pp. 1789-1798, 1473-5571 (Electronic) 0269-9370 (Linking)

Sanchez, J. M., Ramos Amador, J. T., Fernandez de Miguel, S., Gonzalez Tomee, M. I., Rojo Conejo, P., Ferrnado Vivas, P., Clemente Vivas, J., Ruiz Contreras, J., & Nogales Espert, A. (2003). Impact of highly active antiretroviral therapy on the morbidity and mortality in Spanish human immunodeficiency virus-infected children. *Pediatr Infect Dis J*, Vol. 22, No. 10, (Oct 2003), pp. 863-867, 0891-3668 (Print)

Scherpbier, H. J., Bekker, V., van Leth, F., Jurriaans, S., Lange, J. M., & Kuijpers, T. W. (2006). Long-term experience with combination antiretroviral therapy that contains nelfinavir for up to 7 years in a pediatric cohort. *Pediatrics*, Vol. 117, No. 3, (Mar 2006), pp. e528-536, 1098-4275 (Electronic) 0031-4005 (Linking)

Selik, R. M., & Lindegren, M. L. (2003). Changes in deaths reported with human immunodeficiency virus infection among United States children less than thirteen years old, 1987 through 1999. *Pediatr Infect Dis J*, Vol. 22, No. 7, (Jul 2003), pp. 635-641, 0891-3668 (Print) 0891-3668 (Linking)

Simonds, R. J., Lindegren, M. L., Thomas, P., Hanson, D., Caldwell, B., Scott, G., & Rogers, M. (1995). Prophylaxis against Pneumocystis carinii pneumonia among children with perinatally acquired human immunodeficiency virus infection in the United States. Pneumocystis carinii Pneumonia Prophylaxis Evaluation Working Group. *N Engl J Med*, Vol. 332, No. 12, (Mar 1995), pp. 786-790, 0028-4793 (Print) 0028-4793 (Linking)

Simpson, B. J., Shapiro, E. D., & Andiman, W. A. (2000). Prospective cohort study of children born to human immunodeficiency virus-infected mothers, 1985 through 1997: trends in the risk of vertical transmission, mortality and acquired immunodeficiency syndrome indicator diseases in the era before highly active antiretroviral therapy. *Pediatr Infect Dis J*, Vol. 19, No. 7, (Jul 2000), pp. 618-624, 0891-3668 (Print) 0891-3668 (Linking)

Smit, C., Geskus, R., Walker, S., Sabin, C., Coutinho, R., Porter, K., & Prins, M. (2006). Effective therapy has altered the spectrum of cause-specific mortality following HIV seroconversion. *AIDS*, Vol. 20, No. 5, (Mar 2006), pp. 741-749, 0269-9370 (Print) 0269-9370 (Linking)

The European Collaborative Study. Mother-to-child transmission of HIV infection in the era of highly active antiretroviral therapy. *Clin Infect Dis*, Vol. 40, No. 3, (Feb 2005), pp. 458-465, 1537-6591 (Electronic) 1058-4838 (Linking)

The European Collaborative Study (1994). Natural history of vertically acquired human immunodeficiency virus-1 infection. *Pediatrics*, Vol. 94, No. 6 Pt 1, (Dec 1994), pp. 815-819, 0031-4005 (Print) 0031-4005 (Linking)

Violari, A., Cotton, M., Gibb, D., Babiker, A., Steyn, J., Jean-Phillip, P., J., M., & Team., o. b. o. t. C. S. (2007). Antiretroviral therapy initiated before 12 weeks of age reduces early mortality in young HIV-infected infants: evidence from the Children with HIV Early Antiretroviral Therapy (CHER) Study. Fourth Internationa AIDS Society Conference, Sydney, Australia, July 22–25, 2007, 17.02.2011, Available from; <http://www.ias2007.org/pag/Abstracts.aspx?AID=5557>

Walker, A. S., Doerholt, K., Sharland, M., & Gibb, D. M. (2004). Response to highly active antiretroviral therapy varies with age: the UK and Ireland Collaborative HIV Paediatric Study. *AIDS*, Vol. 18, No. 14, (Sep 2004), pp. 1915-1924, 0269-9370 (Print) 0269-9370 (Linking)

WHO/UNAIDS/UNICEF. (Sep 2010). Towards Universal Access: Scaling up Priority HIV/AIDS Interventions in the Health Sector: Progress Report 2010. Geneva, Switzerland: World Health Organization, pp. 1-146, 20.01.2011, Available from: <http://www.who.int/hiv/pub/2010progressreport/en/>

14

Small Livestock, Food Security, Nutrition Security and HIV/AIDS Mitigation

John Cassius Moreki[1] and Richard Dikeme[2]
[1]Department of Animal Science and Production, Botswana College of Agriculture
[2]Botswana Network of People Living with HIV and AIDS,
Botswana

1. Introduction

Livestock contribute to people's livelihoods in many ways, and their contributions tend to be particularly important for poorer people. These include source of cash income, liquid asset, inputs to crop production (draught power and manure), diversification of risk/ buffer to crop production, cultural value (livestock may be sacrificed at the time of a certain festival) and source of food (Conroy, 2005). Sale of livestock and their products can be a valuable source of income. For example, animals, especially small livestock (i.e., goats, sheep, poultry and rabbits) can be sold to meet immediate family needs such as food, clothing, medical expenses, school fees etc.

Livestock play an important role in supporting the social and economic safety nets of households and communities. They are central to people's livelihoods, food security and nutrition; they act as a "bank" to be called upon in times of stress or need (either sold, traded, or slaughtered). Also, livestock are central in many of the major events of life, i.e. birth ceremonies, weddings and funerals. However, it appears that little is known about how traditional community institutions, particularly around livestock production (e.g. women's poultry groups, grazing support and dairy cooperatives) are holding up under the stress induced by HIV and AIDS and related chronic illnesses (FAO, 2003). The study of Mutenje et al. (2008) in the Muzarabani and Bindura districts of Mashonaland Central Province in Zimbabwe found that livestock, particularly poultry and smallstock (sheep and goats), play a significant role in smoothing income fluctuations due to HIV and AIDS. The workers reported that about 90% of HIV and AIDS-afflicted households, headed mainly by women or children, used poultry and goats as consumption-smoothing strategies when faced with negative income shocks.

Africa is the hardest hit continent in the world in terms of HIV epidemic (Topouzis, 1999; FAO, 2005). The HIV and AIDS pandemic in sub-Saharan Africa is widely recognised as development disaster threatening poverty reduction, economic growth and not merely a health issue (Mohiddin & Johnson, 2006). HIV and AIDS affects households' nutrition by decreasing food consumption and impairing nutrient absorption (Hanze et al., 2005). According to FAO (2005), people that live with HIV and AIDS (PLWHA) have special nutritional needs to assist them to remain active and productive workers and to ward off the opportunistic infections that accompany the disease and in prolonging their lives. The PLWHA need good nutrition to stay as healthy as possible. However, good nutrition cannot cure AIDS or prevent HIV infection, but it can delay the progression from HIV to full-blown AIDS and related diseases, and improve the quality of life of PLWHA. Slater & Wiggins (2005) argued that households may sell off large livestock, such as cattle, and use smaller stock units, such as goats and chickens, that can be reared closer to the homestead, and that can be sold off in small quantities to release cash for purchase of medicines for the sick or basic needs where regular sources of income are lost. Small livestock, especially village chickens (also referred to as family chickens) are the most significant livestock species in terms of levels of ownership, supply of protein, and the potential for earning cash income. It has been demonstrated in Botswana, Lesotho and Zambia that livestock, especially village poultry can play an important role in mitigating the impacts of HIV and AIDS on household and community food security and nutrition, as well as, economic empowerment of the vulnerable groups.

As women are the main carers of sick people, chickens can play an important role in providing them with additional resources to perform the important task of caring for people living with HIV and AIDS (Alders et al., 2007a, 2007b). In Mozambique, Alders et al. (2009) reported that village chickens play an important role in households where there is lack of able-bodied workers, such as those affected by HIV and AIDS or those family members living with disabilities. In households headed by widows, children or grandparents, chickens represent the easiest species to raise for sale and home consumption, providing high quality protein and micronutrients, which play an important role in the nutrition of HIV and AIDS patients. Furthermore, village poultry production also provides women and children with experience in small-scale business management and improved knowledge about human nutrition (Alders et al., 2009).

Among the small livestock species reared by individuals and communities in the rural villages, village poultry predominates; hence the emphasis of this chapter is on village poultry. Livestock, especially poultry species, have shown to provide an effective first step in alleviating abject rural poverty (Mack et al., 2004). According to Rural Self-Help Development Association (RSDA) (2011), throughout Africa village poultry are a valuable asset to local populations as they contribute to food security, poverty alleviation and promote gender equality, especially in the disadvantaged groups (HIV and AIDS infected and affected people, women, poor farmers etc.) and less favoured areas of rural Africa where the majority of the poor people reside. The study of Moreki et al. (2010a) in Chobe district of Botswana reported the main reasons for rearing village chickens to be family consumption (75%), source of income (75%), prestige (36%), traditional healing ceremonies (6.82%) and barter (6.82%). These findings clearly show that village poultry have a bearing in the lives of rural populace. Pica-Ciamarra & Otte (2009) in India concluded that backyard poultry farming remains important for rural households, as it ensures a steady flow of high quality food and, through cash income, reduces vulnerability.

2. Advantages of small livestock over larger stock

Unlike larger stock such as cattle, small livestock require less space; they are less capital intensive and are easy to manage as they can be reared within or near homesteads. This makes it much easier for women who are mainly carers of sick people and children to look after both the sick and small livestock simultaneously; hence cutting on labour costs. The rearing of small livestock near or within homesteads ensures regular supply of food to the families in terms of eggs, meat and milk. Lengkeek et al. (2008) argued that PLHWA are less able to perform heavy work, to work for long periods or follow strict work schedules; hence the need to rear smallstock such as a poultry which are easy to keep as they require few inputs. According to Winrock International (1992), livestock contribute directly to the sustainability of the farming systems by providing manure, which is the principal soil amendment and fertilizer available to large numbers of African farmers. A recent study of Simainga et al. (2010) in Zambia reported that the majority of the respondents in Mongu and Kalabo districts used manure from village chickens to fertilize gardens in order to produce vegetables for the households. Figure 1 shows vegetables that were fertilized with chicken manure in Botswana.

According to Sitholimela (2000) in South Africa, the advantages of goats over cattle include: they are easily handled by women and children, e.g., they can be easily milked, dewormed and vaccinated; they require less feed; produce significant quantities of meat and milk for households' consumption; have a short generation interval and produce more progenies. In addition, they are easy to sell to meet immediate households' needs and can be bartered for household commodities such as grain and seeds. To the majority of rural communities in the developing countries, livestock is regarded as "a walking bank" or "a bank in the hoof" because they provide readily available petty cash in times of need.

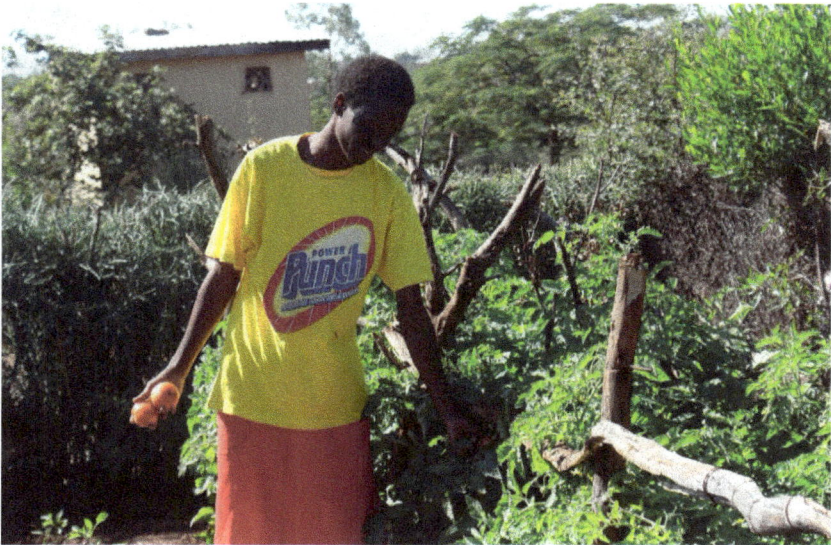

Fig. 1. Tomato plants fertilized with manure

3. The first rung on the livestock ladder

Small livestock, especially village poultry can provide the start of the owner climbing the "livestock ladder", leading to other livestock species such as goats and cattle (Dolberg, 2003). Botswana Network of People Living with HIV/AIDS (BONEPWA) (2010) reported that from October 2005 to October 2010, the beneficiaries of a chicken project supported by Swedish International Development Corporation Agency (SIDA) purchased 250 goats from the proceeds of chickens. Figure 2 shows chickens that were sold to buy goats while the purchased goats are shown in Figures 3 and 4. In a recent field day held in Bobonong in

Botswana, one beneficiary of SIDA supported project reported having bought a cow from the chicken proceeds. This clearly indicates that the rearing of small livestock enables rural families to start owning larger livestock such as cattle, which are considered status symbols in most African countries. BONEPWA (2010) concluded that the rearing of small livestock provides their owners the opportunity to climb the societal ladder by owning larger stock.

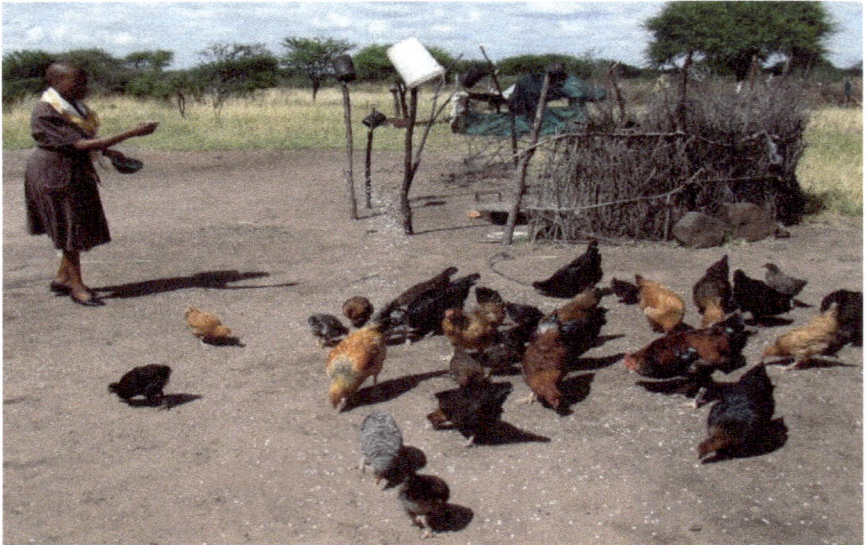

Fig. 2. Part of the chickens that were sold to buy goats

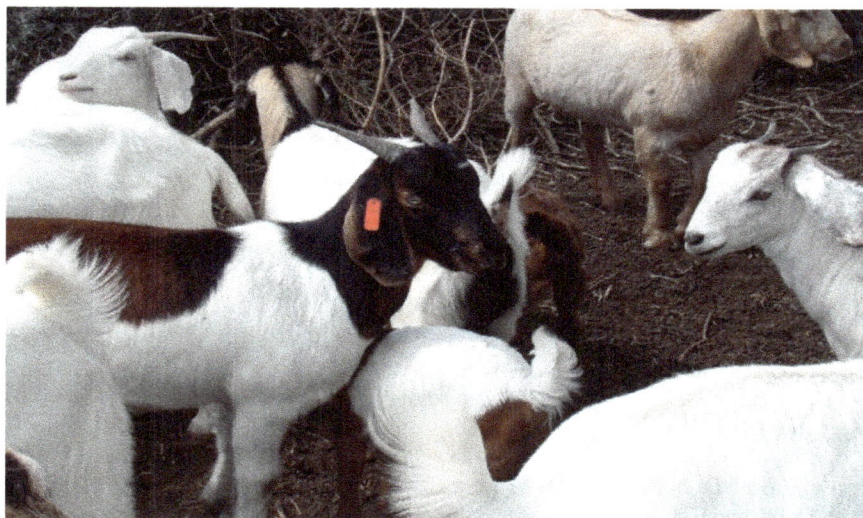

Fig. 3. Some of the goats bought with money from chicken sales

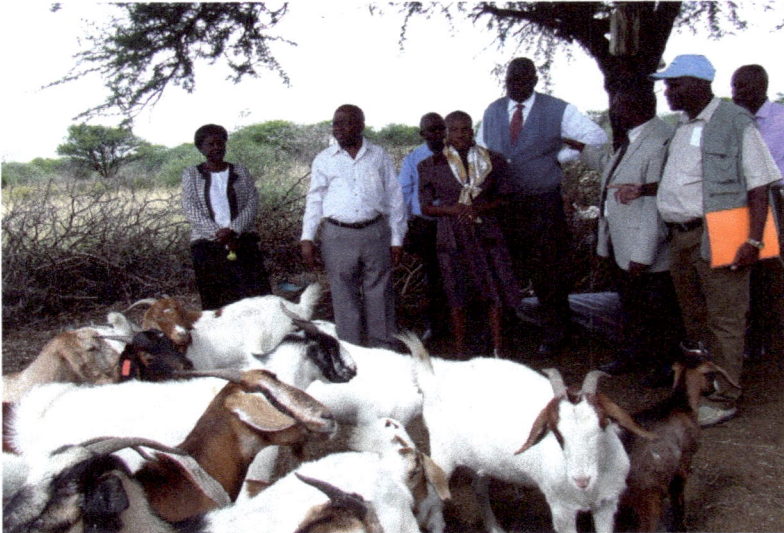

Fig. 4. Goats being appreciated by development workers in Botswana

4. Nutrition and household income generation

The roles played by small livestock in household nutrition and income generation are briefly discussed in the sections below.

4.1 Nutrition

Livestock products such as meat, egg and milk products supply proteins, vitamins and minerals and extra energy, and help to strengthen muscles and the immune system. People with weak health (immune system) are more vulnerable to infections, including diseases transmitted by animals or through contaminated food and water. Even people with access to anti-retrovirals need a balanced diet to fully benefit from such treatment (FAO, 2005).

As shown in Figure 5, goats provide milk which is a balanced diet. Milk is a rich source of nutritionally available minerals (Allen & Miller, 1981) and it contains more of calcium and phosphorus than cow and human milk (Jenness, 1978). From human nutrition's view point, milk and milk products are a source of selenium which plays an important role in the immune system. Goat milk increases the resistance of the body against AIDS. Selenium helps to protect the organism against oxidation stress, participates in the synthesis and metabolism of thyroid hormones, proteosynthesis, it is important for reproduction and its anti-carcinogenic effect plays an important role as well (Schrauzer, 2000). Melse-Boonstra et al. (2007) reported that observational studies on selenium and HIV and AIDS consistently show a positive association between selenium status and delayed disease progression or increased mortality. The study of Barrionuevo et al. (2003) showed that goat-milk has an important and beneficial effect on the bioavailability of copper, zinc and selenium. Belewu and Adewole (2009) concluded that goat milk is affordable, available and nutritious; hence a wide variation of knowledge on the nutrition and hypollergic characteristics of goat milk could promote the direct use of the milk in the nutrition of orphans and vulnerable children.

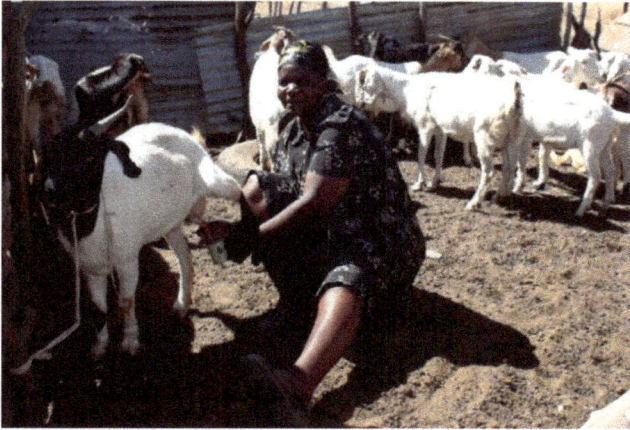

Fig. 5. A woman milking a goat in Bobonong, Botswana

Good nutrition is crucial for PLWHA who need more calories and protein than uninfected individuals. Malnourished HIV-infected people progress more quickly to AIDS and nutrition is critically important to people on retro-viral therapy. The ways of improving the nutrition component of mitigation strategies include promoting block farming, school gardening, community kitchens for orphans and vulnerable children, home-based care nutrition support and nutrition campaigns and training (Economic Commission for Africa, 2006). The rearing of village poultry in Botswana, Lesotho and Zambia has also demonstrated played by village chickens a crucial role in nutrition and food security among PLWHA. RSDA (2011) in Lesotho reported that some people consider village chickens as an option to mitigate HIV and AIDS after realizing that chickens can be the easiest way of obtaining daily nutritional requirements. Moreki et al. (2011) in their study in Botswana reported that all the respondents (46) acknowledged the contribution of chickens in human nutrition. In that study, the respondents said chickens provided relish and hence were the main supplier of good quality protein to the households. Furthermore, the sale of chickens contributed to improved habitable shelter. The proceeds from the sale of chickens contributed to the purchase of building materials for construction of houses. Figure 6 shows the house that was painted following sale of chickens in Nata in Botswana.

Eggs, in particular, offer a great nutritional bargain: they contain approximately 315 kilojoules and are one of the best quality food sources known. Eggs supply an array of vitamins such as A and B12, and they are one of the best food sources of vitamin K, a bone-boosting nutrient. In addition, eggs provide choline, a B vitamin that plays a role in brain development (Alders et al., 2003). Also, eggs are an ideal carrier for enriching human diets with important dietary minerals such as selenium and iodine. Jacques (2006) stated that selenium is involved in the proper functioning of the immune system or inhibiting the progression from HIV to AIDS. The disease is reported to be less prevalent in countries with high selenium soil content than those with low selenium content. Selenium is involved in the conversion of thyroxine (T4) to triodothyronine (T3), indicating its importance in the functioning of the thyroid gland. Seafoods are a rich source of selenium, as are some livestock products, including eggs and chicken meat.

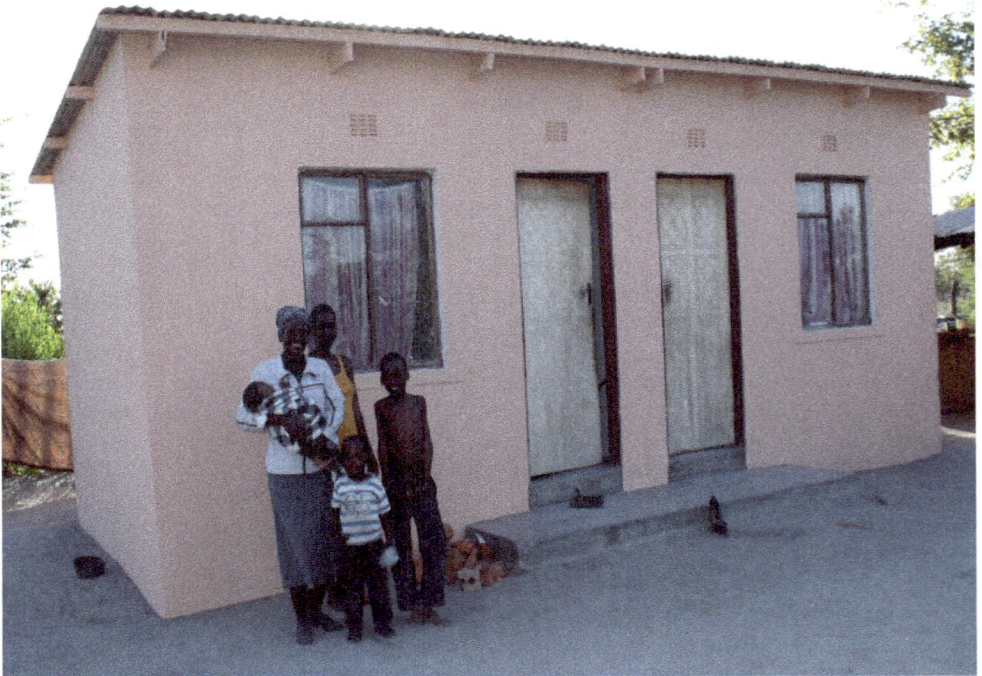

Fig. 6. House painted using money from chicken sales in Botswana

Some of the mitigation strategies mentioned previously attempted to provide some ideas for those working with livestock and communities to mitigate the impact of HIV/AIDS on livestock production and household food security. In addition to these potential interventions, it is important to consider the nutritional needs of the affected individuals and households, review existing support institutions (whether it be extended family, community-based organisations, etc.) and assess, with the community, and particularly those affected, the best way forward to ensure livestock production within, or for, those households. Labour and financial constraints of households must be considered before strategies are discussed or plans developed.

4.2 Income generation

Small livestock can provide income generation for family activities such as education, nutrition, health and clothing. Copland and Alders (2009) stated that village poultry have constantly commanded a price premium over commercial birds and there is a wide market demand for village poultry products. In Zambia, Simainga et al. (2011) reported that income from sale of chickens and eggs was used for groceries, school fees and uniforms, transport to hospitals or medical facilities, medication and talk time (air time).

5. Ownership of small livestock

Generally, small livestock are owned by women. In Botswana, Mrema & Rannobe (1996) reported that women own more goats than their male counterparts who have more resources and can afford to own cattle. Furthermore, village poultry are owned and managed by women and children and are often essential elements of female-headed households (Alders et al., 2003; Guéye, 2004; Bagnol, 2005). The study of Moreki et al. (2010b) showed that 83.2% of women owned chickens compared to 16.8% for men. A recent study (Moreki et al., 2010c) also showed that 73.5% of women own goats. The authors argued that, chickens are generally regarded as livestock that women raise mainly because they are perceived to be of less commercial value than other livestock such as cattle. In the opinion of Moreki et al. (2010b), in Botswana men tend to be responsible for cattle and larger animals and women for smaller animals such as sheep, goats and poultry. These results led Moreki et al. (2010c) to conclude that sheep and goats rearing plays an important role in food security, in addressing issues of gender imbalances, as well as, in poverty eradication in furtherance of the Millennium Development Goals (United Nations, 2010).

6. Marketing

Small livestock and products are sold on a one-on-one basis, which is referred to as direct marketing. Usually, small livestock are sold when there is immediate need for cash. Unlike in commercial livestock, no cold chain is required as stock is sold live and products raw. Recently, Simainga et al. (2011) in Zambia reported that women, especially mothers are involved in chicken sales than men, indicating that women owned chickens and decided on their sales, as well as, how money was used. However, it is likely that women consulted their spouses on how the money was used.

7. HIV and AIDS and small livestock production

Smallstock play a vital role in many rural livelihoods, providing food, income and security. The products of smallstock are rich in protein, minerals and vitamins. They are sources of income and manure for use as compost or fuel, and a store of wealth and insurance. Small livestock may enable women to have more economic independence if they control the income earned from the sale of livestock and their products. Tending to the ongoing every-day requirement of smallstock can normally be integrated into the time and labour constraints facing many HIV/AIDS affected households (Anon, 2006).

According to BONEPWA (2010), the majority of support group members infected and affected by HIV and AIDS in Botswana has attested that through ownership and sale of small livestock (i.e., chickens, guinea fowl and goats), they were able to reduce the number of patients that default from taking anti-retroviral drugs, as they are able to sell chickens to buy medication and food, and also pay for transport to the hospitals for treatment. The effects of HIV and AIDS scourge at household level has reduced since beneficiaries are now able to feed their households resulting in reduced dependency on government hand-outs, family members and relatives. Some of the patients who were bedridden due to AIDS have recovered and are caring for their livestock. This has led to one support group member to say *"we are finding ourselves to be useful members of the community since we are back into our productive lives after spending a long time in sick beds"*. This indicates that small livestock production plays a pivotal role in food and nutrition security, as well as, restoring self-esteem among the affected community members.

8. Conclusion

This review has demonstrated that small livestock have an important role to play in poverty alleviation, improving food and nutrition security, as well as, in economic empowerment of PLWHA and other vulnerable groups. Successful HIV and AIDS mitigation strategies involving goats and chickens in Botswana, Lesotho and Zambia indicate that small livestock play a vital role in the fight against the HIV and AIDS scourge, mainly through provision of nutrition and income generation. Therefore, support from government and non-governmental organizations is crucial if the benefits are to be extended to the rest of the rural communities, the majority of whom are poverty-stricken

9. Acknowledgements

The authors wish to acknowledge assistance they received from BONEPWA+, RSDA and Golden Valley Agricultural Research Trust in Botswana, Lesotho and Zambia, respectively

10. References

Alders, R.; Cambaza, A.B. & Harun, M. (2003). Village chickens, food security and HIV/AIDS mitigation. Retrieved from
   www.kyeemafoundation.org/content/.../HIV-AIDS%20paper%20Nov03.pdf
Alders, R.; Bagnol, B.; dos Anjos, F. & Young, M. (2007a). Promotion of HIV/AIDS mitigation and wildlife conservation through improved village poultry production in Southern Africa, Retrieved from

http://www.fao.org/AG/againfo/home/events/bangkok2007/en/background_4.html

Alders, R.; Bagnol, B.; Harun, M. & Young, M. (2007b). Village poultry, food security and HIV/AIDS mitigation. LEISA Magazine 23.3 September 2007.

Alders, R.; Bagnol, B.; Chicamisse, M.; Serafim, J. & Langa, J. (2009) The role of village chickens in HIV/AIDS mitigation in Manica and Sofala provinces of Mozambique. In, Alders R.G., Spradbrow P.B. and Young M.P. (eds) 2009. Village chickens, poverty alleviation and the sustainable control of Newcastle disease. Proceedings of an international conference held in Dar es Salaam, Tanzania, 5-7 October 2005. ACIAR Proceedings No. 131, 235 pp.

Allen, J.C. & Miller, W.J. (1981). Transfer of selenium from blood to milk goats and non-interference of copper with selenium metabolism. Journal of Dairy Science 64: 814-821.

Anon (2006). HIV/AIDS and small livestock development. Retrieved from http://www.smallstock.info/issues/HIV.htm

Bagnol, B. (2005). Improving village chicken production by employing effective gender-sensitive methodologies. Retrieved from http://aciar.gov.au/files/node/11133/PR131%20part%201.pdf

Barrionuevo, M.; Lopez Aliaga, I.; Alférez, M.J.M.; Mesa, E; Nestáres, T. & Campos, M.S. (2003). Beneficial effect of goat milk on bioavailability of copper, zinc and selenium in rats. Journal of Physiology and Biochemistry 59: 111-118.

Belewu, M.A. & Adewole, A.M. (2009). Goat milk: A feasible dietary Based approach to improve the nutrition of orphan and vulnerable children. Pakistan Journal of Nutrition 8: 1711-1714.

Botswana Network of People Living with HIV and AIDS (2010). Annual Technical Report – October 2009 to September 2010: Village chicken component. Gaborone, Botswana.

Conroy, C. (2005). Participatory Livestock Research: A Guide. ITDG Publishing. The Netherlands. 3-4. ISBN 1-85339-577-3.

Copland, J.W. & Alders, R.G. (2009). The comparative advantages of village poultry or smallholder poultry in rural development. In, Alders R.G., Spradbrow P.B. and Young M.P. (eds) 2009. Village chickens, poverty alleviation and the sustainable control of Newcastle disease. Proceedings of an international conference held in Dar es Salaam, Tanzania, 5-7 October 2005. ACIAR Proceedings No. 131. 207-209.

Dolberg, F. (2003). Review of household poultry production as a tool in poverty reduction with focus on Bangladesh and India. FAO Pro-Poor Livestock Policy Initiative Working Paper No. 6. Food and Agriculture Organizations of the United Nations. Rome.

Economic Commission for Africa (2006). Mitigating the impact of HIV/AIDS on smallholder agriculture, food security and rural livelihoods in Southern Africa: Challenges and action plan., Retrieved from www.uneca.org/sros/sa/publications/HIV-AIDSandAgriculture.pdf

FAO (2003). Measuring impacts of HIV/AIDS on rural livelihoods, Retrieved from http://www.fao.org/sd/2003/PE0102_en.htm

FAO (2005). Ministerial Seminar on *Education for Rural People in Africa: Policy Lessons, Options and Priorities* hosted by the Government of Ethiopia 7-9 September 2005, Addis Ababa, Ethiopia. Retrieved from http://www.fao.org/hivaids/publications/Addis_ERP-AIDS.pdf

Guèye, E.F. (2004). Gender aspects in family poultry management systems in developing countries. http://www.fao.org/ag/AGAinfo/themes/en/infpd/documents/papers/2004/1 2gender318.pdf

Hlanze, Z.; Gama, T. & Mondlane, S. (2005). The Impact of HIV/AIDS and Drought on Local Knowledge Systems for Agrobiodiversity and Food Security. Retrieved from ftp://ftp.fao.org/docrep/fao/009/ag251e/ag251e00.pdf

Jenness, P.E. (1978). The nutritive value of dairy products. Dairy Industries International 43: 7-16.

Lengkeek, A.; Koster, M. & Salm, M. (2008). Mitigating the effects of HIV/AIDS in small-scale farming. Agromisa Foundation, Wageningen. ISBN Agromisa: 978-90-8573-090-3. Retrieved from http://www.anancy.net/documents/file_en/Agrodok-45-Mitigating_the_effects_of_HIV_AIDs_in_small-scale_farming.pdf

Jacques, K.A. (2006). Zoonotic disease: Not just from birds, not just in the flu. In, T.P. Lyons, K.A., Jacques and J.M. Hower (eds.) Nutritional biotechnology in the feed and food industries: Proceedings of Alltech's 22nd Annual Symposium, Lexington, Kentucky, USA. 23-26 April 2006. Nottingham University Press, UK. 149-159.

Mack, S.; Hoffmann, D. & Otte, J. (2004. The contribution of poultry to rural development, Retrieved from http://193.43.36.103/AG/AGAInfo/themes/en/infpd/documents/papers/2004/contribution1618.pdf

Melse-Boonstra, A.; Hogenkamp, P. & Lungu, O.I. (2007). Mitigating HIV/AIDS in Sub-Saharan Africa through selenium in food. Farmer Publication, Lusaka. Golden Valley Agricultural Research Tust (GART). 11.

Mohiddin, A. & Johnston, D. (2006). HIV/AIDS mitigation strategies and the State in sub-Saharan Africa – the missing link? Retrieved from http://www.globalizationandhealth.com/content/2/1/1

Moreki, J.C.; Dikeme, R. & Poroga, B. (2010a). The role of village poultry in food security and HIV/AIDS mitigation in Chobe District of Botswana. Retrieved from http://www.lrrd.org/lrrd22/3/more22055.htm

Moreki, J.C.; Mokokwe, J.; Keboneilwe, D. & Koloka O.A. (2010b). Evaluation of the Livestock Management and Infrastructure Development Support Scheme in seven districts of Botswana, Retrieved from http://www.lrrd.org/lrrd22/5/more22087.htm

Moreki, J.C.; Thutwa, M.; Koloka, O.; Ntesang, K. & Ipatleng, T. (2010c). Utilization of smallstock package of Livestock Management and Infrastructure Development Support Scheme, Botswana, Retrieved from http://www.lrrd.org/lrrd22/12/more22232.htm

Moreki, J.C.; Poroga, B. & Dikeme, R. (2011). Strengthening HIV/AIDS food security mitigation mechanisms through village poultry. Retrieved from http://www.lrrd.org/lrrd23/2/more22055.htm

Mrema, M. & Rannobe, S. (1996). Goat production in Botswana: Factors affecting production and marketing among small-scale farmers. In, Lebbie S H B and Kagwini E (Editors) Proceedings of the Third Biennial Conference of the African Small Ruminant Research Network UICC, Kampala, Uganda. 5-9 December 1994. Retrieved 12 February 2010, Retrieved from http://www.fao.org/wairdocs/ilri/x5473b/x5473b0v.htm

Mutenje, M.J.; Mapiye, C.; Mavunganidze, Z.; Mwale, M.; Muringai, V.; Katsinde, C.S. & Gavumende, I. (2008). Livestock as a buffer against HIV and AIDS income shocks in the rural households of Zimbabwe. Development Southern Africa 25. Abstract, Retrieved from http://www.informaworld.com/smpp/content~db=all~content=a790526994

Pica-Ciamarra, U & Otte, J. (2009). Poultry, food security and poverty alleviation in India: Looking beyond the farm-gate. Pro-poor Livestock Policy Initiative – A Living from Livestock Research Report. Retrieved from www.fao.org/ag/AGAInfo/.../en/pplpi/.../rep-0902_indiapoultry.pdf

Schrauzer, G.N. (2000). Anticarcinogenic effects of selenium. Cell Molecular Life Sciences 57: 1864-1873.

Simainga, S.; Banda, F. & Sakuya, N. & Moreki, J.C. (2010). Health management in village poultry in Kalabo and Mongu Districts in the Western Province of Zambia. Livestock Research for Rural Development 22(9), Retrieved from www.lrrd.org/lrrd22/9/sima22171.htm

Simainga, S.; Moreki, J.C.; Banda, F. & Sakuya, N. (2011). Socio-economic study of family poultry in Mongu and Kalabo Districts of Zambia. Livestock Research for Rural Development 23(02), Retrieved from http://www.lrrd.org/lrrd23/2/sima23031.htm

Rural Self-Help Development Agency. (2011). The study on socio-economic status of village chickens at Ha Molemane (Berea), Phamong (Mohales' Hoek), Tebang, Ha Notsi, and Ribaneng (Mafeteng) of Lesotho. Maseru, Lesotho. pp.111.

Sitholimela, I. (2000). The effect of land tenure system on goat production in Kwazulu-Natal. M. Inst. Agrar. (Animal Production) Thesis. University of Pretoria, Republic of South Africa.

Slater, R. & Wiggins, S. (2005). Responding to HIV/AIDS in agriculture and related activities. Natural Resource perspectives, Number 98, March 2005. www.odi.org.uk/resources/download/1237.pdf

Topouzis, D. (1999). The implications of HIV/AIDS for household food security in Africa. United Nations Commission for Africa, Food Security and Sustainable Development Division, October 1999. Retrieved from www.uneca.org/popia/gateways/Women_Back_doc_4.pdf

United Nations (2010). The Millennium Development Goals Report. The United Nations Department of Economics and Social Affairs (DESA) – June 2010. Retrieved from

http://www.org/milleniumgoals/pdf/MDG%20Report%202010%20En%20r15%2
0-low%20res%2020100615%20-.pdf>

Winrock International (1992). Assessment of Animal Agriculture in Sub-Saharan Africa.
    Morrilton, Arkansas. Winrock International. 12. ISBN 0-933595-76-X. Retrieved
    from HIV/AIDS has severe short- as well as long-term impacts on food security.

Permissions

The contributors of this book come from diverse backgrounds, making this book a truly international effort. This book will bring forth new frontiers with its revolutionizing research information and detailed analysis of the nascent developments around the world.

We would like to thank Nancy Dumais, for lending her expertise to make the book truly unique. She has played a crucial role in the development of this book. Without her invaluable contribution this book wouldn't have been possible. She has made vital efforts to compile up to date information on the varied aspects of this subject to make this book a valuable addition to the collection of many professionals and students.

This book was conceptualized with the vision of imparting up-to-date information and advanced data in this field. To ensure the same, a matchless editorial board was set up. Every individual on the board went through rigorous rounds of assessment to prove their worth. After which they invested a large part of their time researching and compiling the most relevant data for our readers. Conferences and sessions were held from time to time between the editorial board and the contributing authors to present the data in the most comprehensible form. The editorial team has worked tirelessly to provide valuable and valid information to help people across the globe.

Every chapter published in this book has been scrutinized by our experts. Their significance has been extensively debated. The topics covered herein carry significant findings which will fuel the growth of the discipline. They may even be implemented as practical applications or may be referred to as a beginning point for another development. Chapters in this book were first published by InTech; hereby published with permission under the Creative Commons Attribution License or equivalent.

The editorial board has been involved in producing this book since its inception. They have spent rigorous hours researching and exploring the diverse topics which have resulted in the successful publishing of this book. They have passed on their knowledge of decades through this book. To expedite this challenging task, the publisher supported the team at every step. A small team of assistant editors was also appointed to further simplify the editing procedure and attain best results for the readers.

Our editorial team has been hand-picked from every corner of the world. Their multi-ethnicity adds dynamic inputs to the discussions which result in innovative outcomes. These outcomes are then further discussed with the researchers and contributors who give their valuable feedback and opinion regarding the same. The feedback is then collaborated with the researches and they are edited in a comprehensive manner to aid the understanding of the subject.

Apart from the editorial board, the designing team has also invested a significant amount of their time in understanding the subject and creating the most relevant covers. They scrutinized every image to scout for the most suitable representation of the subject and create an appropriate cover for the book.

The publishing team has been involved in this book since its early stages. They were actively engaged in every process, be it collecting the data, connecting with the contributors or procuring relevant information. The team has been an ardent support to the editorial, designing and production team. Their endless efforts to recruit the best for this project, has resulted in the accomplishment of this book. They are a veteran in the field of academics and their pool of knowledge is as vast as their experience in printing. Their expertise and guidance has proved useful at every step. Their uncompromising quality standards have made this book an exceptional effort. Their encouragement from time to time has been an inspiration for everyone.

The publisher and the editorial board hope that this book will prove to be a valuable piece of knowledge for researchers, students, practitioners and scholars across the globe.

List of Contributors

Andrey Bychkov and Shunichi Yamashita
Nagasaki University Graduate School of Biomedical Sciences, Japan

Andrey Bychkov and Alexander Dorosevich
Smolensk Regional Institute of Pathology, Russia

Erik Vakil, Caroline Zabiegaj-Zwick and AB (Sebastian) van As
University of Cape Town, South Africa

Yusuke Okuma, Naoki Yanagisawa, Yukio Hosomi, Atsushi Ajisawa and Masahiko Shibuya
Tokyo Metropolitan Cancer and Infectious diseases Center, Komagome Hospital, Japan

Victor Obiajulu Olisah
Department of Psychiatry, Ahmadu Bello University Teaching Hospital, Zaria, Nigeria

Innocent Ocheyana George
Department of Paediatrics, University of Port Harcourt Teaching Hospital, Port Harcourt, Nigeria

Dasetima Dandison Altraide
Department of Medicine, University of Port Harcourt Teaching Hospital, Port Harcourt, Nigeria

Marco de Tubino Scanavino
Institute of Psychiatry, University of São Paulo, Brazil

Etienne Mahe and Monalisa Sur
McMaster University, Hamilton, Ontario, Canada

Arne N. Gjorgov
Retired Lecturer Epidemiologist, Skopje, Republic of Macedonia

Smit Sibinga, Cees Th and John P. Pitman
ID Consulting for International Development of Transfusion Medicine/University of Groningen, The Netherlands

H. Blake
Division of Nursing, University of Nottingham, B Floor (South Block Link), Queen's Medical Centre, NG7 2HA, Nottingham, United Kingdom

P. Leighton
Division of Primary Care, University of Nottingham, Room 2104, C Floor South 3Block, Queen's Medical Centre, NG7 2UH, Nottingham, United Kingdom

S. Sharma
Department of Psychology, University of Strathclyde, G1 1XQ, Glasgow, Scotland

Antonio Carlos Rosário Vallinoto, Luiz Fernando Almeida Machado, Marluísa de Oliveira Guimarães Ishak and Ricardo Ishak
Federal University of Para, Institute of Biological Sciences, Virus Laboratory, Brazil

Alicja Szulakowska and Halina Milnerowicz
Department of Biomedical and Environmental Analyses, Faculty of Pharmacy, Silesian Piasts University of Medicine in Wroclaw, Poland

Claudia Palladino, María del Palacio Tamarit and Mª Ángeles Muñoz-Fernández
Laboratorio de Inmuno-Biología Molecular, Hospital General Universitario "Gregorio Marañón", Spain

Jose María Bellón
Unidad de Investigación, Fundación de Investigación Biomédica Hospital "Gregorio Marañón", Spain

Francisco J. Climent
Servicio Infecciosas, Hospital "Ramón y Cajal", Spain

Isabel de José
Servicio Infecciosas Infantil, Hospital Universitario "La Paz", Madrid, Spain

John Cassius Moreki
Department of Animal Science and Production, Botswana College of Agriculture, Botswana

Richard Dikeme
Botswana Network of People Living with HIV and AIDS, Botswana